FROM POOR LAW TO COMMUNITY CARE

The development of welfare services for elderly people 1939-1971

Robin Means and Randall Smith

The POLICY PRESS

First published by Croom Helm 1985 ISBN 0 7099 3531 5
Second edition published in Great Britain in 1998 by

The Policy Press
University of Bristol
Rodney Lodge
Grange Road
Bristol BS8 4EA
Tel +44 (0)117 973 8797
Fax +44 (0) 117 973 7308
e-mail: tpp@bristol.ac.uk
Website: http://www.bristol.ac.uk/Publications/TPP/

British Library Cataloguing in Publication Data

A catalogue record for this book is available from the British Library

ISBN 1 86134 085 0

Robin Means is Associate Dean (Primary and Community Care) of the Faculty of Health and Social Care at the University of the West of England, Bristol. **Randall Smith** is Senior Lecturer in the School for Policy Studies, University of Bristol.

Front cover: Photograph supplied by kind permission of John Birdsall Photography, Nottingham.
Cover design: Qube, Bristol.

Printed and bound in Great Britain by Hobbs the Printers Ltd, Southampton.

Contents

Acknowledgements

First edition

The authors of this book owe a considerable debt to a number of organisations which gave us access to their archives, and to a number of individuals who gave us guidance in the use of those archives. Therefore, we would like to thank, first of all, those staff of Age Concern (England), the National Council for Voluntary Organisations, the Centre for Policy on Ageing, the Women's Royal Voluntary Service, the British Red Cross Society, the Public Record Office, the GLC Records Office and the Department of Health and Social Security, who helped in the tracing and collection of material. Roy Parker was especially kind in allowing us to borrow his set of papers submitted to the Seebohm Committee.

Second, we owe a debt to those individuals, listed in the Appendix, who were involved in the events of the period and were willing to give up their time to discuss approaches to social and health provision for elderly people during the period covered by our study. We appreciate that they may not necessarily agree with our analysis of ageing in British Society. We are particularly indebted to William K. Sessions who allowed us to quote from his personal correspondence in the conclusion to Chapter Four.

Third, we have received constructive criticism and support from several academic colleagues. We would especially like to thank Chris Ham, Michael Hill, Chris Phillipson, Phoebe Hall, Moira Martin and Carolyn Taylor. Noelle Whiteside gave us invaluable help in finding our way around the Public Record Office.

Fourth, this book would not have been produced without the administrative support of both the University of Bristol and the School for Advanced Urban Studies. The Publications Committee of the University provided a grant to help with publication costs. Support Staff at SAUS, especially Janet Orme, spent long hours typing the numerous drafts. Sally Strong, the SAUS librarian, was always willing to help in the search for books and journals that were often long out of print.

Finally, the research itself could not have been carried out without funding between October 1981 and September 1983 from the Social Science Research Council (now the Economic and Social Research Council).

Second edition

The production of this second edition would not have been possible without the support and guidance of The Policy Press, and in particular Dawn Pudney.

ONE

Introduction

History lessons

The community care component of the 1990 National Health Service and Community Care Act was meant to have set a clear direction for the provision of welfare services for older people (and for a wide range of other client groups) in the 1990s and beyond. Social services authorities were to be the lead agency with a responsibility to develop user-centred care management, strategic community care planning and a mixed economy of providers based upon a thriving independent sector.

However, the message of many commentators is one of *Care in chaos* (Hadley and Clough, 1996) as local authorities struggle to meet their expanded responsibilities within available resources. A key feature of these critiques is often a comparison of the limitations of the market ideology of the 1990 reforms (efficiency and consumer responsiveness coming from providers competing for 'business') with the more welfare-orientated ideology of the past with its emphasis on a right to free services. Thus, Dominelli and Hoogvelt (1996) complain of the move in social work from needs-led to budget-led provision and from the direct provision of services to the managing of services provided by others.

A rather different line of complaint has been articulated by the 1997 Labour government which has expressed enormous frustration at the continued failure of health and social services to work in partnership to the advantage of those elderly people with both health and social care needs (Means and Smith, 1998, ch 9). This is leading them to explore the potential of some kind of community care authority in which the resources of both agencies would be pooled, an approach which could be linked to the proposal in the NHS White Paper that purchasing in the health service should be driven at the locality level by general practitioners (GPs) and primary care groups (DoH, 1997).

As social scientists with a long-standing interest in the history of welfare services for older people, we remain more convinced than ever that these contemporary debates about future direction and current problems can be very helpfully illuminated by exploring the past. In the context of residential care for both adults and children, Parker (1988) has argued strongly that no informed decisions on how best to move forward can be reached without an understanding of key external factors and "that, in turn, cannot be done satisfactorily without some understanding and appreciation of those forces that have shaped its history" (Parker, 1988, p 3).

The case for drawing on the past has been made eloquently by leading historian Anne Digby:

> **The lesson of history is that it does not repeat itself precisely, yet, on a broader front, certain policy issues, dilemmas, problems and choices do recur in social welfare. To forget the past record of these events is to force each generation to relearn what should already be known, and thus make future developments less satisfactory than they might be. Equally undesirable, however, has been the tendency in some quarters to manufacture mythical virtues which present policy can seek to emulate. Through each of these historical tendencies, current debate on social welfare is made less informed and cogent. (Digby, 1989, p 1)**

It is our view that UK debates about community care have been bedevilled by both these weaknesses. There is a reluctance to learn from a genuine investigation of mistakes and achievements, and there is an even more marked tendency for the 'left' to create a golden age of community care and for the 'right' to deride all that went before.

These thoughts caused us to look afresh at *The development of welfare services for elderly people* (Means and Smith, 1985), our earlier book published by Croom Helm. This had been based upon a two-year grant from the then Social Science Research Council which had allowed us to collect and interpret data from a wide range of sources on the development of welfare services for elderly people. The research covered the period from the outbreak of the Second World War until the reorganisation of the personal social services in April 1971, with welfare services being defined as those services for older people which were to be located within the new unified social services departments. Five main themes were examined:

- the impact of the Second World War on care services for frail and sick elderly people;
- the politics of the 1948 National Assistance Act;
- the development of residential services, 1948-71;

- the development of domiciliary services, 1948-71;
- the restructuring of welfare services for elderly people in the late 1960s and early 1970s.

Our rereading of the book confirmed our view that a genuine engagement with the history of community care had the power to illuminate many contemporary debates. More specifically our book had the capacity to underline among other things:

- the ongoing failure to establish older people as a priority for health and welfare expenditure;
- the periodic anxiety of central government about the public expenditure implications of an ageing population;
- the continued assumption that the lead role in the care of older people should be played by (female) relatives;
- how governments redefine the boundaries between health and welfare over time;
- the long-standing nature of how best to fund what we now call continuing care;
- the long history of argument and debate about which agencies and which professionals should take the lead role in the planning and delivery of welfare services for older people.

Such thoughts led us to work on a second edition of the book in the belief that its relevance to contemporary community care debates justified finding a new and wider audience. The main body of the resultant book is essentially the same as that published in 1985. However, this first chapter and Chapter Eight represent our attempts to return to our core findings and to draw out their relevance to present discussions about how best to shape a community care system for older people which is appropriate for the challenges and possibilities of the 21st century.

The origins of a research project

The fieldwork for the 1985 edition was carried out between October 1981 and September 1983, with the simple objective of exploring the historical development of debates about the respective roles of the family, the state and the voluntary sector in what we called "the care of frail and sick elderly people". This section retraces the origins of our decision to seek funding for a history of community care for older people and how that related to the debates of the late 1970s and early 1980s.

Both authors worked for many years at Bristol University's School for Advanced Urban Studies (SAUS) prior to its incorporation into the School for Policy Studies in 1995. Since the mid-1970s SAUS had organised an extended series of short seminars and workshops for policy makers and practitioners working in the public and independent sectors. In July 1978 Randall Smith was one of the organisers of a seminar on 'Policies for the Elderly' which focused on a discussion document from the Department of Health and Social Security (DHSS) entitled *A happier old age* (DHSS, 1978a). The stated aim of the seminar was to examine "the assumptions behind the current pattern of policies, the objectives of these policies, and the adequacy of the present level and mix of service provision, including the selective contributions of statutory and voluntary sectors in meeting the needs of old people" (Ham and Smith, 1978, p 1). One of the course participants was Robin Means, then nearing the completion of his Certificate of Qualification in Social Work at Warwick University. His presence at the seminar reflected his desire to develop a specialist interest in social work with elderly people. The frustration of that desire within the childcare dominated social services departments of the late 1970s was to be an important factor in his later decision to leave social work practice.

A happier old age represented an important turning point in the debate about the respective roles of the state, the voluntary sector and the family in the care of elderly people. It was the point at which growing concern about 'the fiscal crisis of the state' seemed to meet growing concern about future demographic trends. The document began by stressing that the number of people aged 65 and over had increased by 20% between 1966 and 1976. This increase was especially large among the old old and "by 1986 there will be approximately 24 per cent more people aged 75 and over than there are now" (DHSS, 1978a, p 7). This had created a situation in which "just over £100,000 million, or a third of the total expenditure on the main social programme is attributable to elderly people" (p 10).

The discussion document made it clear that the incremental growth of residential and domiciliary services for elderly people could no longer be guaranteed. It was stressed, for example, that the "development of the domiciliary services has so far largely relied on professional judgement and been influenced by demands pressed against a background of growth in the national economy and rising expectations" (DHSS, 1978a, p 32). The discussion document saw a better use of volunteers and informal caring networks as a major way forward.

> **... it is vital to make the best use of all available resources, to deploy these in a way which gives elderly people – and their relatives – the kind of help they need, and to ensure that those in greatest need are given priority. This means improving co-ordination between the statutory services, and between those services and the whole range of voluntary and informal help available (including family and community support). It also means exploring the scope for innovation especially in providing practical help to meet personal needs; it is here that volunteers and other informal effort can play a major part. (DHSS, 1978a, p 33)**

Issues of priorities and value-for-money were being addressed. In retrospect, *A happier old age* can be seen as a clear statement of the desire of the DHSS to reduce pressure on residential and domiciliary services through an extension of family and community support.

Most of the participants at the seminar were reluctant to accept this message; they had not yet been 'trained' to accept the inevitability of the economic imperative and were content to list those areas where services needed to be expanded and developed. There was a strong emphasis upon the rights of elderly people to services, and it was felt that these rights might well be actively pursued "because the elderly in the future may not be so constrained by their personal histories of deference" (Ham and Smith, 1978, p 49).

The concept of a right to public services was not central to the subsequent March 1981 White Paper, *Growing older* (DHSS, 1981) which was meant to have evolved out of the discussions and submissions encouraged by *A happier old age*. Instead, the primary argument was that:

> **Whatever level of public expenditure proves practicable and however it is distributed, the primary sources of support and care for elderly people are informal and voluntary. These spring from the personal ties of kinship, friendship and neighbourhood. They are irreplaceable. It is the role of public authorities to sustain and, where necessary, develop – but never displace – such support and care. Care in the community must increasingly mean by the community. (DHSS, 1981, p 3)**

By this time, both authors were working at SAUS and were keen to develop their shared interest in elderly people and the personal social services.

Even before the publication of *Growing older*, they were becoming increasingly aware of the speed at which policy assumptions were changing. A political and academic consensus seemed to be developing that residential care was 'bad' for elderly people. The need to focus domiciliary services on priority cases was being stressed. The potential of informal caring networks and the voluntary sector was being put forward as a cheap and humane alternative to public services. A major shift in policy direction for elderly people in the field of personal social services seemed about to take place. The expectations of elderly people and their families about the availability of public services were being lowered.

This raised the issue of whether such a shift represented a form of incrementalism because of the tendency for any new situation to be responded to as "like something already known, or some element of it" (Heclo, 1974, p 315). Or did it represent a more radical shift from previous policy paradigms? Certainly, policy was often being discussed in the late 1970s and early 1980s with very little if any reference to what had happened before. Was there a taken-for-granted assumption that welfare services for elderly people had been a low priority in the past, and so earlier developments were not relevant to a debate about how to cope with the present growth in the elderly population combined with major restrictions on state expenditure?

At the same time, arguments being developed by other researchers on how to respond to this growth were based on assumptions about the nature of medical and social need in old age, about the 'correct' caring role of the family, and about the potential of the voluntary sector (see, for example, Challis and Davies, 1980). Examination of the literature on old age and the personal social services from the 1950s and 1960s led us to realise that these same issues had always been central to arguments about service development in this area.

A second justification for the research was that the development of welfare services for elderly people was a neglected area of study. No previous work had attempted a descriptive mapping of policy change in welfare services for elderly people. Authors such as Heywood (1959) and Packman (1975) have provided a far greater volume of information about the development of childcare services than was available about comparable services for elderly people in the period after the Second World War. Some interesting work on the development of welfare services for elderly people during this period has certainly been carried out. Muriel Brown, in her unpublished 1972 doctoral thesis, looked at the legislative intention behind Part III of the 1948 National Assistance Act, and the different ways in which this was interpreted by a number of local authorities. Julia Parker in *Local health and welfare services* (1965) provided some interesting material on the role of local authority associations and the Ministry of Health in the early evolution of welfare authorities. Kathleen Slack (1961; 1970) had written two excellent accounts of the changing relationship between voluntary agencies and local government over the provision of services for elderly people in London. Greta Sumner and Randall Smith (1969) carried out detailed research on how local authorities responded to the need to provide the Ministry with 10-year development plans on their health and welfare services. Peter Townsend in *The last refuge* (1962) made his penetrating attack on the inadequacies of residential care under the 1948 Act. Other examples could be cited. There was not only a clear case for drawing all this material together but also a case for carrying out original research on how and why these policies evolved in the form they did when they did.

The third justification related to the relevance of the proposed research to key issues facing the social work profession. After the death of Maria Colwell in January 1973, social workers had been heavily criticised by the popular press, the police and the courts. (This criticism is reviewed and then supported by Brewer and Lait, 1980.) As a result, it had become common to talk about the identity crisis in social work. This 'crisis' was recognised by the Secretary of State for Social Services in October 1980 when he requested the National Institute for Social Work to establish a working party to review the tasks of social workers in local authority social services departments (Barclay Report, 1982). This review occurred at a time when government reports were suggesting an increased role for social workers in the support of sick and frail elderly people (DHSS, 1978a; 1981).

We suspected this suggestion would receive little encouragement from social work courses because of their failure to explain to students anything of the past history of welfare services for elderly people, and why they were eventually located within social services departments. A knowledge of this history could be invaluable not just from the point of view of general feelings of identity but also as a means of increasing understanding of practice problems. DHSS funded research (DHSS, 1978b, pp 365-93; Black et al, 1983) had shown that social workers have less commitment to casework with elderly people than other client groups; other authors have noted the tendency for elderly clients to be allocated to unqualified social work staff (Goldberg and Connelly, 1982, pp 92-5). One task of the proposed research was to place these problems within an historical perspective and provide at least a partial explanation of their origins. It was, therefore, hoped that the research would help those responsible for social work courses to address the problems of providing appropriate support for dependent elderly people in a more informed way than had previously been the case.

Theoretical perspectives

Underpinning these justifications for the research was a desire to operate in the political economy of ageing perspective being developed in the late 1970s and early 1980s through the work of authors such as Phillipson (1982), Townsend (1981) and Walker (1981). Such a perspective emphasised the structured dependency of older people as having been created through their removal from the workforce as a response to high unemployment especially in the 1930s. This removal had been made possible through the introduction of state pensions which offered a very poor standard of living to most older people.

Such a perspective stressed it was always unlikely that older people could emerge as a high priority for state expenditure since:

> **... the elderly are an ongoing problem in a society where institutions are geared primarily around issues of production and reproduction, where the facilities in the communities which most people retire into are concerned mostly with the serving of the existing labour force and the reproduction of a new one. (Phillipson, 1977, p 43)**

Political economists such as Gough (1979) were arguing in the late 1970s that such "social expenses" would always be more vulnerable to cutbacks in capitalist societies during periods of fiscal crisis than that which directly supported the accumulation of capital and its reproduction (p 138). Under these circumstances it was perhaps not surprising that Macintyre (1977, pp 39-64), in her brief review of the shifts in central government policy towards the provision of health and welfare services for old age, should find that humanitarian rhetoric about 'community care' often masked a desire to reduce the costs of residential and hospital care.

This low priority for health and welfare expenditure on older people was seen as being justified by reference to the inevitability of illness and enfeeblement in later life. Haber, for example, found that in the late 19th and early 20th century:

> **Most European clinicians seemed to imply that illness and old age are inseparably intertwined, if not quite synonymous. At best the division between the two was extremely subjective. A large proportion of the diseases of old age are attributed to natural, intractable changes in the organism. (Haber, 1983, p 62)**

The term 'chronic sick' summed up this attitude of mind within the medical profession; illness in old age was chronic, inevitable and barely treatable since "the organic difficulties that increased with age made the hope of corrective treatment illusory" (Haber, 1983, p 72).

The whole thrust of the proposed study was to investigate whether similar negative assumptions had underpinned the slow development of welfare services for elderly people in England. If they had, what were the consequences in terms of the details of policy (non) development? This was to be achieved through the combined use of government files from the Public Record Office for the period up to 1952, published government documents, the records of key voluntary agencies and the local authority associations, through a scanning of the secondary literature including professional journals and through the interviewing of key figures from the period (see Appendix).

Changing discourses

Drafting of the research proposal along the lines outlined above was occurring in 1980 in the early period of 18 years of Conservative governments. We had little perception of just how radical a restructuring of the welfare state was to be attempted through the introduction of quasi-market reforms across education, health, housing and the personal social services (Le Grand and Bartlett, 1993). Only 11 years after *A happier old age* (DHSS, 1978a), the 1989 White Paper on community care reflected a move from a tentative concern with rationing to a bold plan to usher in markets, purchaser–provider splits and care management (DoH, 1989). Nor has the pace of change been slowed by the arrival of a Labour government since it seems determined to push through an even more radical review of the principles of the welfare state, which is bound to have a massive impact upon the provision of community care services for older people in future years.

However, the last 18 years have also seen a number of other important changes in how we conceptualise and refer to the central themes of this book. The 1985 edition used welfare services to cover both residential care and the provision of services in the home, with the latter being seen as 'community care'. The 1989 White Paper used the term 'community care' to cover the full spectrum of potential support available to older people from nursing home care to informal care. The first edition also decided to use the expression "frail and sick elderly people" to define the client group focus of the research rather than alternatives such as elderly people with health and social care needs, elderly people with high support needs, disabled elderly people or elderly people with impairments. Although none of the alternatives fully convince, neither do the words 'sick' or 'frail' which no longer feel appropriate for the late 1990s. This is because such words seem to draw upon a medical model of old age and to stress the powerlessness of older people. Nevertheless, it was decided to retain the initial terminology in the middle chapters of the second edition on the grounds that this would be the only way to retain the integrity of what had originally been written.

The initial introductory chapter had been self-critical in reflecting that the dependence of the research on documents generated from the centre had resulted in the giving of:

> **... little credence to the possibility that elderly people themselves have the capacity to influence the content of the services provided; throughout much of this book elderly people and their families appear as passive objects and this is a major simplification of a complex reality. (Means and Smith, 1985, p 9)**

This now seems starker than ever given the immense influence of the disability movement on how most social researchers understand the impact of community care provision upon service users. If starting out today, the research would have had to engage with the social model of disability with its distinction between:

- *impairment:* lacking part or all of a limb, or having a defective limb, organism or mechanism of the body;
- *disability:* the disadvantage or restriction of activity caused by a contemporary social organisation which takes no or little account of people who have physical impairments and thus excludes them from the mainstream of social activities (Oliver, 1990, p 11).

Put even more simply, people have impairments but it is society which disables them. Thus, disability is a political issue requiring disabled people to struggle for their rights as citizens to be full members of the society in which they live (Campbell and Oliver, 1996). How older people with impairments fit into this picture would have been a central concern of the research (Means, 1997, pp 12-25).

It is unrealistic to expect the majority of older people with major impairments to be at the forefront of the disability movement and many require the support of either advocates or professionals who appreciate the importance of 'right conduct' towards vulnerable elderly service users (Goodin and Gibson, 1997). This does not imply the acceptance of a crude political economy perspective which stresses the passiveness of older people. Older people struggle on a day-to-day basis with health and welfare professionals to negotiate their needs and how these might be responded to. However, our position does stress the central importance to them of how the community care system is organised, the values that underpin it and the resources allocated to ensure its implementation.

Outline of the book

Our political economy assumptions about old age as a social problem in a capitalist society suggested older people might be extremely vulnerable during a national crisis. **Chapters Two** and **Three** explore the treatment of 'frail and sick elderly people' during the Second World War, first in respect of evacuation arrangements and then in respect of the 'reform' of domiciliary and residential services. **Chapter Four** discusses the extent to which the 'reform' process was consolidated by the 1948 National Assistance Act. All three chapters are concerned with the conditions under which elderly people do or do not become a priority for service provision by the state.

The second half of the book outlines welfare services developments for elderly people in the period 1948-71. **Chapter Five** looks at the failure of residential provision for elderly people to meet the optimistic hopes of politicians who supported the 1948 Act, and it considers the growth of criticism during the 1960s of all forms of institutional care. **Chapter Six** describes the failure of such criticism to encourage a major expansion of domiciliary services for elderly people and attempts to show how this can be understood only in relation to assumptions about 'family care'. **Chapter Seven** looks at the arguments about which professional groups have the expertise to control the delivery of welfare services to elderly people and how these related to the broad debate about the restructuring of the personal social services in the late 1960s. In **Chapter Eight**, linkages and insights to be gained from past debates and policy developments are drawn together as a contribution to the ongoing discussions about the future of community care provision for elderly people.

TWO

Evacuation and elderly people in the Second World War

Introduction

This chapter discusses the availability of services for frail and sick elderly people in the Second World War, and suggests that the quality of this provision was often influenced strongly by arguments about whether or not these elderly people were war victims. It was often claimed that war victims had a right to special care from the state which avoided any possible stigma through association with Poor Law provision. The social needs of groups not defined as war victims were seen as a low priority in conditions of war.

The chapter therefore begins by providing a brief outline of state provision for elderly people in 1939 followed by a more detailed outline of the limitations of public assistance institutions (PAIs) for the frail and sick. Next the disruption caused first by the establishment of the Emergency Medical Service (EMS) and then by the bombing raids from Autumn 1940 onwards is examined. This will be followed by a consideration of the responses made by central and local government to this situation in terms of billeting and evacuation arrangements. A central theme throughout the chapter is that little attempt was made to direct help to those elderly people most 'at risk' through illness and frailty; rather attention was focused upon those elderly people who might have the capacity to disrupt civilian morale either through their behaviour (for example, in air raid shelters) or through their complaints (for example, to the press).

Before attempting these tasks, the limitation of what has been achieved needs to be stressed. An attempt has been made to unravel policies towards certain groups of elderly people that were being implemented at a time of major civil disruption. To fully examine the bombing raids, the EMS and the evacuation arrangements would require more extensive research than it was possible to carry out. Not only this but the main subjects of the study – frail and sick elderly people – were far from being the central concern of senior civil servants and key politicians. Instead, the disrupted lives of elderly people and the implications of this disruption for Poor Law and evacuation policy tended to be dealt with by relatively junior officials on a case-by-case basis. As Titmuss explains, "the interminable corresponding, interpreting, minuting and accounting on this or that issue went on steadily among the lower and middle ranks of officialdom" (Titmuss, 1976, p 235). An attempt has been made to gain at least a partial understanding of the main types of case raised in this way and, also, an appreciation of what principles or dominant attitudes tended to be applied by officialdom. In so doing, the authors have been enormously helped by Richard Titmuss' outstanding contribution to the Official History of the Second World War (1976).

Finally, it is important to stress that this chapter is not about the experience of elderly people in general during the war but only those who suffered directly as a result of the civil disruption. Actual death rates for middle-aged and elderly men and women declined in the latter half of the war (Titmuss, 1976, p 524). For many elderly people, the war meant a far more active and involved time than they might have experienced if a period of peace had been maintained. There were enormous opportunities and considerable pressure to help on the home front, either as paid workers or volunteers. Many of those organisations which played a leading role in helping elderly people during this period, such as the Women's Voluntary Service (WVS), the British Red Cross Society (BRCS) and the Old People's Welfare Committee (OPWC), probably used volunteers who were themselves over 65.

State provision for elderly people in 1939

The 1931 Census (Marsh, 1965, pp 22-31) indicated that England and Wales had a population of 39,952,000 and that 7.4% of these, or 2,962,000 people, were aged 65 or over. Of this 65 plus population, 1,690,000 were female and 1,272,000 were male. A minority only of these elderly people lived in households that had accrued enough wealth to live off savings during retirement and to meet medical expenses during illness. The majority were not so fortunate and had by 1939 a complex web of potential services available to them.

In 1939, for example, both contributory and non-contributory pensions existed for different groups within the elderly population. These had developed piecemeal since the first pension legislation in 1908. By 1939 the relationship of the two types of pension had become quite complex although Robson made a brave attempt to explain this:

> **The ... legislation bifurcates into two main streams. One stream flows from the original Old Age Pensions Act and is based on the principle of non-contributory pensions payable from the age of 70 onwards, subject to certain tests as to means, nationality, and residence. The other stream flows from the so-called 'insurance' principle, first introduced in regard to other contingencies in 1911, but not applied to old age until 1925, when contributory pensions were created for widows, orphans, and old persons between the ages of 65 and 70 who satisfied certain 'insurance' conditions. The Contributory Old Age pensions scheme was grafted on to the National Health Insurance Scheme for the purposes both of contributions and central administration. At the age of 70 the two streams are joined, for the contributory pensions are then merged in the non-contributory pensions. (Robson, 1948, p 18)**

Non-contributory pensions were means-tested for some groups but not others and administered by the Customs and Excise in conjunction with the local pension committees of local authorities: 1,140,832 such pensions were issued in March 1939 (Board of Trade, 1940, p 86). On the other hand, there was no means test for the contributory pensions, which were administered by the Ministry of Health. An estimated 755,340 of these pensions were being drawn in 1939 (Board of Trade, 1940, p 89). It is hard to disagree with Robson that it was "all incredibly and senselessly complicated" (Robson, 1948, p 18).

Some groups of elderly people, however, were still not covered by this legislation; for example, those 65- to 70-year-olds who failed to meet the contribution conditions. Others received a pension that was just not sufficient to meet all their food, clothing, heating and other expenses. Such elderly people had the option of applying to the public assistance committee of their local authority for outdoor relief under the provisions of the 1930 Poor Law Act. This required them to undergo a household means test and the whole process was very unpopular because of the stigmatising history of the Poor Law.

This mechanism for 'topping up' pensions was reformed through the 1940 Old Age and Widows Pension Act. Local authority responsibility was replaced by a system of supplementary pensions to be administered nationally by the Unemployment Assistance Board, which was renamed the Assistance Board. Section 10 of the Act stated "the administration of supplementary pensions shall be conducted in such a manner as may best promote the welfare of pensioners". The Minister of Health claimed the new Act reflected the view of local authorities that "the responsibility for pensions was primarily that of the state and that this task should not have to be assumed by them" (*Hansard*, House of Commons, vol 357, 20 February 1940, col 1199). The response to the new scheme was enormous. It was expected that about 400,000 would apply, 125,000 more than had been receiving poor relief, but:

> **Pensioners began to apply to the board on 10th June 1940. Over 125,000 claims were received in the first four days. The daily figure reached a peak of 60,000 on 18th June and it did not fall below 30,000 until 4th July. A total of 1,275,000 applications had been lodged by the time the first payments were made on 3rd August. (Deacon, 1981, pp 519-20)**

Many pensioners had refused to apply for Poor Law help despite financial hardship and Deacon has shown that the unexpected claims were concentrated in the more prosperous regions where the stigma of relief had been greatest (Deacon, 1981).

The medical needs of elderly people were met in an equally complex way. A pensioner who had contributed to a health insurance scheme remained entitled to primary healthcare from a health insurance panel doctor but this was not true of his wife unless insured in her own right. As a result, many elderly people had to pay privately for such help although there was one alternative. This was to seek help from the public assistance committee of the local authority under the Poor Law regulations. Different local authorities organised access to general practitioners under this legislation in different ways, but the general principle was that persons in receipt of outdoor relief and others who were without the means of providing themselves with medical attention were entitled to use the district medical service of the public assistance committee (Marshall, 1948).

Finally, there were various forms of institutional provision for elderly people in 1939. Three types of hospital existed. The voluntary hospitals were run on a charitable basis and concentrated on the 'acute sick'. Public health hospitals were those that had been removed from the Poor Law system by the 1929 Local Government Act, and they also tended to focus on the 'acute sick'. The 'chronic sick', which was seen as including most sick elderly people, tended to be catered for in those hospitals that were still administered by public assistance committees; these mixed institutions provided 56,000 hospital beds in 1938 out of a total of 176,000 beds in all three types of hospital (Abel-Smith, 1964, p 382). Other elderly people were defined as not requiring medical treatment but still needing institutional care. They were accommodated in the non-hospital parts of PAIs. In 1939, such institutions housed nearly 150,000 people (Board of Trade, 1940, p 94) and the bulk of them would have been aged 65 years or more. These elderly 'inmates' were disqualified from receiving a pension unless they were admitted specifically for medical treatment and even then pension rights were lost after three months.

Public assistance institutions and the 1929 Local Government Act

According to Engels, the 1834 Poor Law Amendment Act was "the most open declaration of war of the bourgeoisie upon the proletariat" (Engels, 1969, p 308) with its policy of offering relief only to the 'able-bodied' in the workhouse. More recent commentators have stressed the boredom (Crowther, 1981) rather than the brutality of workhouse life together with the extent of local variation in practice (Digby, 1978). It was not until the 1929 Local Government Act that major organisational change was attempted within the Poor Law system. This Act provided that the powers, duties and assets of the 625 Poor Law unions should be transferred to counties and county boroughs, each of which would be required to form a public assistance committee. The workhouse was to become the PAI. But as Gilbert has pointed out:

> **In effect the measure transferred the administration of the Poor Law to the major authorities but left any reform of the Poor Law, beyond certain useful but minor administrative changes, such as county-wide supervision of institutions, to the initiative of the local authority itself. Poor Law relief remained Poor Law relief and pauperism remained pauperism except for a few small modifications. (Gilbert, 1970, p 229)**

Indeed, the law governing the granting of relief was merely consolidated in Section 14 of the 1930 Poor Law Act, which restated Elizabethan principles of family responsibility, namely:

> **It should be the duty of the father, grandfather, mother, grandmother, husband or child, of a poor, old, blind, lame or impotent person, or other poor person, not able to work, if possessed of sufficient means, to relieve and maintain that person.**

The principle of family responsibility was still to be upheld and destitute groups, whether elderly people or not, could only be offered relief after a test of their means; sons and daughters still had to make a financial contribution to the upkeep of any old person received into institutional care. Regulations about aspects of the institutional regime such as clothing, other personal possessions, leaving the institutions and visiting rights were not liberalised, but merely recodified.

Arguments about the impact of the 1929 Act upon institutional provision for elderly people must be tentative because the main period investigated for this book begins in 1939. However, it can be argued that there is little evidence of reforming zeal from either central or local government. Some local authorities built separate units for elderly people, especially in the period just before the Second World War and this development was encouraged by the Ministry of Health. Roberts (1970, pp 23-5) indicates that such reforms were discussed at some length during the 1937 Public Assistance Conference of the local authority associations. Birmingham, for example, had opened three such units although elderly people were carefully selected for these homes. One home was reserved for "women of the more gentler type" (*Birmingham Post*, 27 June 1940) while another was for men of "the merit class" (City of Birmingham, 1940, p 15). However, such reforms seem to have affected only a relatively small number of authorities.

Some pressure for a more general change in the internal running of the large PAIs did exist. Olive Matthews, who was later to be very active in the OPWC, called for a general attempt to bring more colour into the lives of old people in institutions "through contact with visitors from the outside world, by providing occupations as well as entertainments, and by introducing more variety into their food, clothing and surroundings" (Matthews, no date). In *Housing the infirm*, she made detailed proposals in all these areas on how the routine of PAIs should be changed. Some liberalisation in these areas may well have occurred in many institutions although this is something to be denied or confirmed by other research.

One of Matthews' proposals was for 'pocket money' to be paid to elderly inmates on the grounds that:

> **Pocket money gives an added spice to life. It is one thing to be given weekly rations of sweets or tobacco – it is quite another thing to be able to choose and buy for yourself. Many of us remember the pleasure of receiving a small weekly sum when we were children.... It is very much the same for old people in Institutions. (Matthews, no date, p 13)**

A considerable campaign built up around this issue[1]. It included MPs, trades councils and some individual local authorities placing pressure upon the Ministry of Health for a change in the regulations. The 1938 Poor Law Amendment Act enabled local authorities to pay up to two shillings 'pocket money' per elderly person per week from their rates, although the Association of Municipal Corporations (AMC) opposed the Act on the grounds that it would be preferable to withdraw the pension disqualification for those in PAIs[2]. In other words, the AMC did not wish to finance the scheme from the rates. The 1938 Act gave local authorities a permissive power rather than a statutory duty to pay pocket money and as late as 1944 Samson (1944, p 15) claimed that many local authorities were not using these powers.

So far it has been suggested that the period 1929-39 saw some improvements in the treatment of elderly people in PAIs, but that these were often fairly marginal. However, one result of the 1929 Local Government Act may well have worsened the position of many elderly people in Poor Law care. Councils were authorised but not required under the 1929 Act to transfer Poor Law infirmaries from public assistance committees to public health committees. The object of this innovation was to enable the standard of the work carried out in these hospitals to be improved and brought up to that which existed in the best of the voluntary hospitals. Amulree claimed such progress was soon attained by these appropriated hospitals but only at the cost of further extending their reluctance to offer treatment for the 'chronic sick'. The end result was that "the Relieving Officers had not the power to order the admission of such a patient into a Public Health hospital, and so the statutory right of admission of the destitute, which was one of the most valuable features of the Poor Law, began to be lost" (Lord Amulree, 1951a, p 13).

The result of such policies was almost certainly a shortage of beds for elderly people who were ill. The remaining Poor Law infirmaries tended to concentrate upon them as a group but lacked sufficient beds and skilled medical personnel to cope with the overall demand or complex needs. One solution to this problem was to allow the 'chronic sick' to take up non-hospital beds. McEwan and Laverty provide an excellent description of how this system worked in Bradford in the period just before the establishment of the National Health Service (NHS):

> **In the Public Assistance Hospitals [The Park and Thornton View] ... patients are discharged or returned from the chronic sick wards to the ambulant or 'house' section.... In The Park, where the chronic sick wards were overcrowded, the most fit [but often frail] patients had to be sent to the ambulant wards to make room for admissions to the hospital section. There was, in consequence, a proportion of sick or disabled people in the ambulant section, where they had to remain, often confined to bed, there being no room for them in the hospital. (McEwan and Laverty, 1949, p 7)**

McEwan and Laverty were quite clear that this pressure on beds for elderly patients had been increased by the redesignation of several municipal hospitals in Bradford after 1929. As they explain, "many of the new and aspiring municipal hospitals got rid of their undesirable chronic sick ..., sending them to Public Assistance Institutions to upgrade their own medical services" (McEwan and Laverty, 1949, p 8).

In brief, institutional care for frail and sick elderly people prior to 1939 had many limitations. The growth of pension legislation had eased the situation of some elderly people outside the institution and the bulk of elderly people remained in the community with or without such financial help. For a minority of those over 65 years of age who were in PAIs, small residential units were available, although access was often restricted to those considered to be socially above the average inmate. There was considerable confusion about the boundaries between sickness and frailty. Above all, as Roberts pointed out, most elderly inmates continued to sleep "in large dormitories, sat on hard chairs, looked out on cabbage patches diversified by concrete, were separated according to sex and, except on one day a week, could not pass the gates without permission" (Roberts, 1970, p 26). What would be the impact of the Second World War upon this state provision and could such facilities be considered appropriate for war victims?

The creation of the Emergency Medical Service and the hospital treatment of elderly people

Both Titmuss (1976, pp 54-86) and Abel-Smith (1964, pp 424-9) provide detailed accounts of the planning for the Emergency Medical Service (EMS) before the outbreak of the Second World War. This was dominated by a fear of the huge casualties that could be expected from air attack. Estimates of civilian casualties proved far greater than ever materialised. A target of 300,000 beds for an EMS was agreed upon by the Ministry of Health and this required the discharge of 100,000 patients from existing hospitals on the outbreak of war. When war was declared these instructions were vigorously carried out and 140,000 patients were discharged from hospitals in just two days (Titmuss, 1976, p 193). The age composition of the patients is not known but many of them would have been those classified as the elderly chronic sick. In an article written at the time, Morris (1940) stated that these events created enormous suffering and led to many unnecessary deaths. She claimed that:

> **... the people who fared worst of all were the chronically sick, the bedridden, the paralysed, the aged, people suffering from advanced cancer or from tuberculosis who were discharged in their hundreds from public institutions to their own homes, where they could get little, if any, care, where in all too many cases they were regarded as an intolerable burden on their relatives, and even to houses from which all their relatives had been evacuated to the country. (Morris, 1940, p 189)**

For the first 12 months of the war, no bombing raids materialised. The beds reserved for the EMS remained empty, awaiting civilian casualties. The civilian sick, on the other hand, had to compete for places in the remaining hospitals and PAIs that were not part of the EMS scheme. These hospitals became badly overcrowded because they were under a statutory obligation to accept patients in need of hospital care. The Nuffield Foundation survey of old people (see Chapter Three) spoke of a breakdown of provision for the 'sick and infirm aged' and how "cases have come to the notice of members of the Committee of aged persons dying in circumstances of great squalor and loneliness because local authorities, although asked, have been unable to fulfil their legal obligations to receive them into an Institution" (Rowntree, 1980, p 63).

Attempts were made in the period September 1939 to September 1940 to ease this situation by making use of the EMS staff and beds for the civilian sick. For example, in February 1940 a regional officer for the Ministry of Health claimed that:

> **At the present time many of the PAIs which still have chronic inmates are staffed for emergency hospital purposes with the very best London specialists. These gentlemen apparently find that time is hanging on their hands and it might be of considerable advantage to both sides if they could be asked to see and treat some of the aged chronic cases[3].**

This suggestion was seen by Ministry officials in London as "bristling with complications"[4], especially over payment problems although it was finally agreed there was no objection so long as it could be done by informal arrangements within the institution itself. The extent to which this practice was adopted within the EMS is not known.

Many of the EMS beds were in the voluntary hospitals and these were paid for by the Ministry of Health irrespective of whether they were in use. As Abel-Smith points out, the Ministry of Health made numerous attempts to persuade voluntary hospitals to be flexible in their use of these beds for the civilian sick but such approaches received a less than sympathetic response since:

> **The hospitals were receiving about £100,000 a week for keeping their beds empty. Any reduction in casualty beds meant a reduction in subsidy. In October 1939, the Ministry hastened to point out that urgent civilian cases should be admitted to hospital, but hesitated to take any further action because of the 'storm of criticism' it feared from the voluntary hospitals. But in December 1939, the number of beds reserved for casualties was reduced to 20 per cent, and hospitals were allowed to use 'frozen beds' for civilians up to a maximum of 66 per cent total occupancy for all purposes. (Abel-Smith, 1964, p 429)**

Abel-Smith indicates there was little response to this proposal, and this was borne out by Ministry of Health files[5].

Mass bombing raids: the initial response

The first year of the war had, therefore, brought considerable hardship to many frail and sick elderly people. The situation was to be made far worse with the impact of bombing raids from 23 August 1940 onwards. Minns has graphically described the scale of these raids for London alone:

> **Not counting the thousands of small incendiary bombs that women and householders often swept off roofs and doormats, over 50,000 high explosive bombs fell on London between September 1940 and May 1941. The September 1940 raids alone caused the temporary or permanent loss of homes of 40,000 to 50,000 people a week. By December 1940 the death toll from bombing in London was 12,696 with 20,000 seriously wounded. By May 1941 over 1,400,000 people in London had been made homeless and 1,150,000 houses damaged. (Minns, 1980, p 65)**

Numerous authors have described the disruption caused and the extent to which air raid precaution arrangements struggled to cope with the social problems generated (see, for example, Titmuss, 1976, pp 239-51; Minns, 1980, pp 3-16; Harrison, 1976; Calder and Sheridan, 1984, pp 73-111). In such an emergency situation, it seems reasonable to ask whether sick and frail elderly people should expect to receive a high level of consideration from the government. This chapter and the next suggest that such consideration was offered only when their plight was seen as a threat to the morale of the rest of the civilian population.

A good example of this concern with civilian morale in general rather than with the specific needs of elderly people can be seen from the response to the large numbers of frail elderly people who began to gather in the public air raid shelters in the Autumn of 1940. *The Lancet* indicated how:

> **The shelter became a dormitory instead of a temporary refuge. To the most popular, people came from long distances, bringing their bedding, and friends found places for old people, the bedridden and infirm while the queues waited outside. Gross overcrowding has resulted, and the lack of sanitation and sanitary supervision, of heating and ventilation, coupled with lack of sleep, nervous stress and improvised meals, has brought the danger of typhoid and dysentery, and, more menacing still,**

> **respiratory diseases. (*The Lancet*, 1940, 'Infection in the shelter', 12 October, p 455; for a more general discussion of attitudes to shelter inhabitants, see Harrison, 1976, pp 110-26)**

A committee under Lord Horder was set up to investigate conditions and recommended after only four days that certain groups such as "the aged, the infirm and the bedridden" should be evacuated because their inclusion in shelters "added to the difficulty of supervision, increased the risk to health and lowered morale", while they were perceived as "a serious encumbrance in the presence of an incident" (Ministry of Health and Ministry of Home Security, 1940, p 3). (For a more general account of shelter conditions and how this led to the setting up of the committee, see Lord Horder, 1941.)

The detailed mechanisms of the first evacuation scheme for elderly people have not been uncovered. It seems that the medical officers of health from metropolitan borough councils[6] took responsibility to visit the shelters and they decided who needed nursing care. These people were then removed by train to EMS hospitals throughout the country. Four thousand elderly people were transferred from London to emergency hospital beds in the next 22 months until the suspension of the scheme in December 1940. Titmuss stressed the unsatisfactory nature of this evacuation process:

> **Many did not want to be separated from their normal surroundings; married couples wanted to remain together; in some instances, the fear of being treated as a pauper was much more real than the fear of bombs. It became clear that the problem went far beyond the scope and resources of the emergency medical service. Not all the aged and infirm who were unable to stand the strain of shelter life were necessarily in need of hospital care. Many were still active enough to lead useful lives in more normal conditions. To confine them all indiscriminately to bed involved not only a waste of hospital resources but the risk of making them permanently bedridden. (Titmuss, 1976, p 451)**

What is not known is how these elderly people were processed on arrival at EMS hospitals throughout the country. Did many lose contact with relatives? Were some placed in non-medical beds in PAIs and so lost the right to a pension? How many moves did some of these people suffer?

What happened to their belongings and homes in London? However, more is known about the attitude of central and local government towards the scheme. One London County Council (LCC) report referred to it as "the scheme for clearing aged persons from air raid shelters" (GLC Records Office, 1940). Another LCC document referred to how "the 'shelter' patients ... were so dealt with not merely because they were in need of immediate medical care and attention but also because they are regarded as persons permanently unsuitable for retention in an evacuation area"[7]. The reason that action was taken over the issue appears to have been the development of concern about possible epidemics being caused by certain sick, old and perhaps often rather poor shelter inhabitants. Many of these may have been people with no fixed abode as some Ministry of Health reports referred to them as shelter derelicts[8]. The fears of the general civilian population were seen by state officials as needing to be allayed. Whether this operated in the interests of elderly shelter inhabitants is another matter.

In the early weeks and months of the bombing raids, therefore, the EMS was receiving large numbers of 'chronic sick' cases from public air raid shelters. A further group of elderly patients for this service were coming from the rest centres. These had been established in evacuation areas and were designed to meet the immediate needs of those whose homes had suffered war damage. During the planning stage, it was assumed people would either return to their own homes or find a billet after a very short stay. As the chief assistant of the LCC's social welfare department explained:

> **... elaboration of the service has been avoided in order that the people shall not regard the centres as hostels in which they can stay indefinitely but shall be encouraged to make their own arrangements, with such assistance as may be necessary, to resume a normal family life.[9]**

When the raids arrived, it became clear that planning arrangements had overestimated the level of civilian casualties and underestimated the level of homelessness and property damage (Titmuss, 1976, pp 3-53). The rest centres became blocked with homeless people, and major alterations in the scheme had to be effected. One group that was seen as especially creating difficulties was the so-called 'unbilletables'. As the Chief Officer, Rest Centre Services in London, outlined:

> **... reports came in from all sides of the admission of invalids**

> **and aged persons who were unsuitable either to be fitted in households or to look after themselves in furnished accommodation. (GLC Records Office, 1940)**

This was seen as a 'disposal' problem and the Ministry of Health were asked to evacuate these notified cases to beds in London hospitals from where they could be taken to accommodation outside London. The size of this operation was quite large. No figures were found for the period up to 9 October 1940. After that date and up to 31 October, 561 people were transferred from rest centres to EMS beds.

At first glance, this scheme seems to raise fewer issues than the air raid shelter scheme, especially when it is appreciated that hostels were being established by the Ministry of Health for some of those who did not need medical care (see later). However, the Chief Officer of the Rest Centre Service was expressing the view to LCC councillors in November 1940 that the scheme was "still far from satisfactory". He listed numerous problems, most of which revolved around the confusion of the elderly people themselves about what was happening to them and the illogicality of placing people in hospitals because they were unbilletable rather than because they needed medical treatment. The criterion of admission for this group was not medical need, although many may have needed medical treatment. The examples provided by the Chief Officer suggest some of these elderly people may have suffered terrifying ordeals. He claimed:

> **Many old persons object to going to hospital. Whatever explanation is given to them they are afraid that they are going to receive treatment; the married couples are afraid of being separated. The hospitals which have suffered heavily from bombing appear to them to be less safe than the Rest Centres. In one case a man was put in a surgical ward and ran away the following morning. In another a woman left because she had to sleep on the fourth floor.**

He went on to describe how:

> **Complaints have been received from those who have been evacuated under this scheme that they have been placed in accommodation in danger areas on the outskirts of London. In another case a respectable married pair complained that they had been put in a workhouse where they were only allowed**

to meet for a short time in the afternoon. (GLC Records Office, 1940)

Were such problems inevitable given the general conditions prevailing in Autumn 1940? Later in this chapter it will be seen how a more clearly defined policy towards elderly people did emerge, even if it was restrictive in its definition of state responsibility to elderly people in wartime.

From these two schemes (evacuation from air raid shelters and evacuation from rest centres), hospitals and PAIs in rural areas (both inside and outside the EMS) received large numbers of elderly people. There was also a general transfer of 'chronic sick' cases from LCC hospitals to country hospitals. Titmuss estimated this number as 3,500 (1976, p 451). Such evacuation arrangements were not restricted to London. Evacuation plans in June 1940 for 19 coastal towns included a programme of removal of invalids from institutions and private homes to institutions in reception areas[10]. However, such mass evacuation of 'chronic sick' cases to safer areas ended in December 1940. The extension of bombing raids to other urban areas in December 1940 placed increased pressure on emergency hospital accommodation in reception areas and the 'chronic sick' were seen as blocking bed reserves.

The shift in policy can be seen from the extension of evacuation arrangements to a further 12 coastal towns in April 1941. The bedfast were excluded from the scheme on the grounds that previous bedfast evacuees had permanently blocked EMS beds so that "there is now hardly any accommodation of the same kind available for any similar movement in the future[11]. It was agreed that "as a general policy a 'stay put' doctrine must be adopted for invalids in the 31 coastal towns". The evacuation plan concluded that the new arrangements seemed "to accord with the military objective which is that the population of the towns should be reduced in advance so that there is less danger of them flocking out on to the roads in the event of invasion". The sick and frail, many of whom were elderly, could not 'flock out' so were expendable in terms of the military objective.

'Chronic sick' patients already in EMS hospitals were often seen as blocking bed reserves. There were complaints from the beginning that members of the Civil Nursing Reserve and Red Cross "joined these organisations to nurse soldiers and air raid casualties, and protest loudly at being called to nurse the chronic sick" (*British Medical Journal*, 1941, letter from Leonard Parsons, Birmingham, 11 June, pp 100-1). Elderly patients were moved out of EMS beds and Titmuss argues that:

> **... some of the chronic sick were consequently shifted from one place to another, amid much confusion [and] hardship and many complaints resulted from these attempts to move patients from good hospitals to which they had been transferred in the first instance. (Titmuss, 1976, pp 451-2)**

There was considerable sensitivity from the government to any suggestion that war victims were being treated as "paupers"[12]. This charge was made by the newly formed Old People's Welfare Committee[13] (see Chapter Three); this organisation suspected many elderly evacuees in such hospitals were treated more as Poor Law inmates rather than as patients. Their survey of EMS beds in hospitals and PAIs revealed a less than satisfactory situation. Many patients were not allowed up even when fit to be so; others received inadequate treatment and some were placed in the same wards as "mental, senile and poor law cases"[14].

The boundaries between EMS beds and beds in PAIs were not always clear, especially since the EMS often took over only part of a hospital or institution. One solution to pressure from the 'chronic sick' on EMS beds was to remove some of them to the non-medical beds of PAIs. This raised the issue of pension rights. The Ministry of Health took the following position in relation to this issue:

> **In order to continue to be eligible to receive a non-contributory old age pension, a pensioner who is evacuated from an air-raid shelter or rest centre to an EMS hospital under the scheme for the aged and infirm must continue to satisfy the statutory conditions.... If the Emergency Hospital was a Public Assistance Institution the question might arise whether he was an inmate of a workhouse or other Poor Law institution ... if so, and the pensioner was not admitted for the purpose of obtaining medical or surgical treatment he would be disqualified from receiving a non-contributory old age pension.**[15]

This would suggest that those officials who decided whether medical or surgical treatment was still needed were in a powerful position over the elderly infirm residents of EMS hospitals and PAIs. However, this situation was subsequently eased by the development of hostel accommodation for homeless and evacuated elderly people (see next section).

At least hospitals and PAIs which were outside the main conurbations and coastal towns were fairly free of direct danger from bombing raids.

This was not true of such institutions in the evacuation areas. Beds in all types of institution in London became blocked as top floors were left empty for safety reasons[16]. One Ministry of Health report stated that "the top floor wards of hospitals in London cannot be regarded as suitable accommodation for chronic sick because of danger to nursing and other staff"[17]. No mention was made of the danger to the patients. Numerous institutions suffered damage as a result of the bombing raids although statistics on this do not seem to have been collected nationally. Attempts were made to raise this as an issue. The former medical officer of health for the LCC wrote to the *British Medical Journal* that:

> **I am informed from absolutely reliable sources that there are still hundreds, if not indeed thousands, of 'chronic sick' patients being maintained in institutions in those of our large towns which have been repeatedly bombed during the last few months. I am also informed that, despite the fact that many 'chronic sick' patients have been killed and others seriously injured and that in some instances the buildings in which they are housed have been seriously damaged with consequent great discomfort to both patients and staff, the Ministry of Health obstinately declines to remove these unfortunate bedridden patients to places of comparative safety and comfort outside our large towns. (*British Medical Journal*, 1941, Letter from Frederick Menzies, former Medical Officer of Health for the LCC, 7 June, p 868)**

In June 1941 the matter was raised in the House of Commons. The Minister of Health (E. Brown) replied that the desirability of such removal was accepted. However, it was difficult to achieve this objective because of "the urgent demands on existing accommodation for the acute sick, for casualties and service sick, for transferred industrial workers and civil defence personnel, and for others who had an at least equal claim to priority, and the need for keeping a large number of beds immediately available for emergency purposes" (*British Medical Journal*, 1941, 'Medical notes in Parliament', 21 June, p 950). He pointed out that 8,000 such cases had been removed from the London area – 4,000 from PAIs and 4,000 from those found in the public air raid shelters and temporarily accommodated in London institutions.

The air raids had created massive disruption for most sections of the civilian population. This was especially true for the sick and frail elderly people. Social and medical care for these groups was in danger of breaking down. EMS hospitals were reluctant to take such cases. PAI beds had been reduced. Rest centres were struggling to cope with the volume of demand from the 'aged and infirm'. This was despite the setting aside of certain of these centres as reception units for this group. However, the Chief Officer of the Rest Centre Service in London warned that "there is a tendency for aged persons to find these centres so comfortable that they do not desire to move" (GLC Records Office, 1940). Nevertheless, such centres still had to perform their other functions, and so they could not be allowed to become permanent hostels. It is interesting to speculate on why so many of the elderly residents of these rest centres were reluctant to move on. Was it a reluctance to move into PAIs, whether or not part of the EMS? Whatever the reason, this difficulty, and the others reviewed in this section, led to attempts by civil servants to formulate a more clear-cut policy in relation to elderly people.

Towards a policy? The laws of settlement and removal

The main elements of this 'policy' are examined in the next three sections, but it is useful to begin by listing each of these as a basis for considering what options were excluded from the package. Elderly people were encouraged to find their own billets outside evacuation areas. Hostels were established for those elderly people made homeless by enemy action. Hostels were found for some 'able bodied' elderly evacuees from the London area.

The crucial feature of both types of hostel (homeless hostels and evacuation hostels) was that people were seen as residents not inmates; they were not covered by any of the Poor Law legislation and they did not have to give up their pensions. An Evacuation of the Aged Committee was established by the Ministry of Health to aid the development of these schemes; this made considerable use of the main voluntary organisations. One feature of these schemes was that they encouraged the evacuation of large numbers of elderly people from urban areas (the home authority) to safer areas (the reception authority). This was especially true of those elderly people who found billets with relations, friends or strangers in areas considered safe from bombing raids.

Did all this represent a coherent response from the state to the medical and social needs of elderly people in wartime? Titmuss was in no doubt that it did not. Above all there was the problem of who paid for evacuated elderly people. The financial arrangements involved a complex division of responsibility between the home authority, the reception authority and central government.

Despite the payment of billeting allowances by central government, there was still a clash between "the philosophy and practice of localism, by which every neighbourhood was held responsible for the support of its own poor and sick people" and "how this principle collided with the need for social help on a national scale during the Second World War" (Titmuss, 1976, p 234). Titmuss stated:

> **In a great many ways, this collision resolved itself into not one but a whole series of administrative and organisational problems. That is one reason why it was never seen and faced by the government as a simple problem. Even in the Ministry of Health, the struggle to find a way through a medley of scattered principles and precedents rarely reached the higher administrative levels. (Titmuss, 1976, p 235)**

Examination of the relevant Ministry of Health files suggests that there is considerable truth in Titmuss' comment, but certain reservations do need to be made. A mass of correspondence on individual cases does exist. This tackles such issues as pension rights[18], the maintenance of furniture and homes of those evacuated[19] and how to interpret the laws of settlement and removal under the Poor Law acts[20]. The last issue proved particularly complex and time-consuming. It was a frequent occurrence for billeted elderly people to ask for institutional care because of increased frailty. However, this raised the issue of who was financially responsible for them – the reception authority or the home authority. There was general agreement that the law placed the responsibility on the home authority but the mechanism for enforcing this was cumbersome, to say the least. A removal order had to be obtained by the reception authority from two justices of the peace. The removal order then had to be suspended if the evacuated person was not to be forced to return to the home authority with the attendant danger from bombing raids. The suspension could be granted on the grounds that "any person named therein is unable to travel by reason of sickness or other infirmity, or that it would be dangerous for him to do so" (Exley, 1932, pp 97-8). The expenses of relief were only recoverable under a suspended removal order if a copy of it was served on the relevant council within 10 days. In these circumstances:

> **... the removing council may at the end of every quarter send**

> **to the council against whom the order is made an account of the costs incurred in the relief of any person named in the order, and may recover the amounts reasonably expended by them (or so much thereof as may remain unpaid) in any county court the district whereof is wholly or partly comprised in their county or county borough. (Exley, 1932, p 98)**

As the war progressed, tension increased between reception and home authorities. Evacuees needed to live in their reception authority for only three years to obtain a right of settlement in the reception authority. This suggested that financial responsibility for Poor Law care might fall on the reception authority even after the evacuees had returned to their home authorities. In other words, if the elderly evacuees returned to London and the other major cities after the war and subsequently went into PAIs the home authorities could themselves use the removal procedure to obtain the costs of relief from the old reception authority.

Such administrative issues were complex and took up a great deal of civil service time at the Ministry of Health as local authorities continuously clamoured for an opinion on specific cases. However, it is not the case, as Titmuss argued, that such issues always remained the province of junior officials and that no attempt at policy formation was made. As early as October 1939 the County Councils Association (CCA) had complained to the Ministry of Health about the need for "agreements on procedures between Public Assistance Authorities in evacuating areas and reception areas"[21]. In January 1940 the Permanent Secretary at the Ministry of Health called a conference of the CCA, the AMC and the LCC on *Public assistance in wartime*[22]. The LCC proposed that it should have to reimburse a reception authority only if the inmate was in receipt of relief at the time of evacuation; this would, of course, greatly reduce the financial obligations of the LCC under the existing law of settlement and abode. This proposal was rejected by the other two associations and it was finally agreed that:

- if a person who changes his place of residence during the war was in receipt of relief immediately before removal, any relief granted after removal, should be paid or reimbursed by the same council as that other relief;
- in respect of all other cases of relief the existing law of settlement and removal and the existing machinery should continue to operate.

Ministerial acceptance of this approach was confirmed by *Circular 2000*, 'Public assistance', issued on 19 April 1940 (Ministry of Health, 1940b)[23], which called for the above arrangements to operate where local authorities could not agree a mutual suspension of removal orders. The above arrangements involved the suspension of Article 5 of the 1930 Relief Regulation Order and local authorities were asked to "reduce to a minimum the amount of investigation undertaken".

After the publication of the Beveridge Report (1942) (see Chapter Three), the Ministry of Health came to accept that the old system of poor relief would be swept away in postwar reforms. This could be seen from their response to the request of the CCA for "such legislation as is necessary to ensure that the period during which evacuated persons are resident in reception areas shall not be reckoned either for the purposes of the law relating to settlement and irremovability or as residence within the meaning of any statutory enactment on the subject"[24]. The official ministerial reply was that it was not convenient to introduce legislation at the present time. Handwritten comments, however, make the point that "the whole business is artificial having regard to the probable demise of the Poor Law after the war"[25].

Towards a policy? The dispersal of elderly people from London

This discussion of policy has so far, however, focused only on the activities of one division of the Ministry of Health, the Public Assistance Division. Titmuss' emphasis upon localism and lack of policy does carry weight in relation to the activities of this division with its concern to maintain the existing Poor Law system. The Evacuation Division of the Ministry of Health was also concerned with the social care of some elderly people, even if its primary focus was on young children and their mothers. This division did engage in a policy debate with local authorities, other central government departments and voluntary organisations about the boundaries of its responsibilities to elderly people.

The core of this debate was whether the responsibilities of the Evacuation Division should be to the elderly 'infirm' as a class or only to those physically disrupted or made homeless by the war. Pressure did exist from several quarters for a wide definition of responsibilities. As indicated in the first half of this chapter, arrangements were developed from Autumn 1940 onwards to evacuate elderly people from public air raid shelters and rest centres. The Chief Officer of the Rest Centre Service of the LCC was in no doubt that this created enormous anomalies:

> **The anomalies are so obvious and striking that officials administering this scheme are at a loss to explain them. The aged person who is taken to a shelter is removed. The aged person who goes into a rest centre is removed. But the aged person who is bedridden and cannot get to an air raid shelter ... cannot be dealt with.... While the difficulty of securing satisfactory hostel accommodation outside London is appreciated, it is still felt that this problem has not been faced sufficiently boldly or with sufficient realism. (GLC Records Office, 1940)**

Such views received support from Sir Henry Willinck who had been appointed in September 1940 as Special Commissioner to coordinate services for London's homeless. After the war he remarked how "in the earlier years, in particular, the break up of families caused both by evacuation and by the destruction of homes by bombing left many thousands of old people in tragic isolation" (Sir Willinck, 1961, p vii). More specifically in Autumn 1940 this led him to ask the Ministry of Health to support more hostel provision for the elderly 'infirm', provision that he felt should be supplied as part of the evacuation arrangements rather than as public assistance provision[26]. The Assistance Board[27] and the newly formed Old People's Welfare Committee[28] (see Chapter Three) were also concerned not only at the lack of provision, but also with the stigma associated with what did exist. An early meeting of the OPWC complained of the failure to make a "distinction ... between people who were mentally deficient or suffering from some incurable disease or sexual perversion and the ordinary decent old people"[29].

The argument, then, was that the war had disrupted the lives of sick and frail elderly people. As a result, many were having to seek admission to PAIs even though they were often not the kind of old person normally associated with such provision. Others were bedridden in their own homes and in terrible danger from the bombing raids. No evacuation arrangements existed for these groups unless they were picked up in public air raid shelters or had moved to rest centres, having been made homeless. Overall, frail and infirm elderly people were 'victims' of the war but they were often being treated as local authority public assistance department cases rather than as evacuation cases.

The Evacuation Division of the Ministry of Health was quite clear-cut in its policy towards elderly people. One priority was the establishment of schemes to ensure the reduction of the elderly population of London.

Their second priority was the establishment of mechanisms for ensuring the elderly homeless were treated as 'war victims'. The elderly 'infirm' as such were not a high priority in either policy.

The programme of voluntary dispersal of elderly people from London seems to have been strengthened by the blockages experienced in the public air raid shelters and rest centres in November 1940. It was a humane alternative to forced removal. However, as early as June 1940, a scheme existed to encourage elderly people to leave towns in evacuation areas by finding their own private billets. *Circular 2060* on 'Evacuation of civil population – Special scheme' stated that "in order to facilitate such arrangements the Local Authorities in these towns have been authorised to assist persons in need by the payment of travelling expenses and it has been decided that billeting allowances may be made available if necessary to the householders who provide them with accommodation" (Ministry of Health, 1940a)[30]. The size of this scheme was considerable. By March 1941, 17,000 'aged and infirm' people had been issued with free travel warrants from the London region alone[31]. However, it was questioned whether this scheme was adequate, especially for the large numbers of frail elderly people who found it difficult to make such private arrangements. Were they to be left to the mercy of either the bombs or PAIs?

With the onset of the main bombing raids, the Ministry of Health decided to take further steps to ensure the evacuation from London of those elderly people who were unable to make private billeting arrangements. In November 1940, the Evacuation of the Aged Committee was formed as "a small executive body including representatives of the London County Council and the principal voluntary organisations interested in the matter"[32]. The Ministry of Health saw the task of the committee "to supplement the arrangements for the evacuation of old people from London" in which "the purpose was to mobilise voluntary effort, to discover premises that might be suitable for hostels and to assist the local authorities to start such hostels"[33]. Although the Ministry of Health did finance hostels "for a very small number of old people from certain of the other heavily attacked evacuation areas"[34], the bulk of evacuation hostels were for elderly people from the London region and the Evacuation of the Aged Committee seemed to be exclusively concerned with London. It focused on stimulating both hostel development and the offer of billets to elderly people. The processing of the applicants at the London end was the responsibility of the Education Department of the LCC. In June 1941 it was dealing with a backlog of 1,200 people[34].

Why was this scheme established? The main reason was concern with civilian morale during the bombing raids. Elderly people were blocking rest centres and public air raid shelters. They were also fleeing London by train without arranging billets at the other end. This combination of circumstances led the Quaker Relief Organisations to establish a series of hostels at their Meeting Houses in reception areas in the Autumn of 1940 (Staley, 1943). The Evacuation of the Aged Committee can be seen as an attempt to extend and coordinate such voluntary effort. The Ministry of Health asked the main voluntary organisations (National Council of Social Service [NCSS], the WVS and the BRCS) to carry out a search for private billets on the grounds that "the Minister attaches the greatest importance to the removal of as many old people as possible from London at the present time, both from the point of view of their health and safety and to lighten the task of civil defence"[35]. The NCSS circular to its branches about the scheme stressed that "many of these old people spend a large part of their time in emergency rest centres and shelters where they are not only unhappy and uncomfortable themselves but where they are also a source of anxiety and difficulty to others"[36]. However, although these billets and hostels were designed to help the difficult-to-place who were blocking emergency arrangements in London, they were still only suitable for the relatively 'able bodied'; those in need of regular nursing and social care were excluded.

It is interesting that the NCSS circular was marked confidential and stressed that nothing should appear in the press about the scheme. The desire for secrecy was probably two-fold. The primary task was seen as removing those who were creating problems rather than assessing overall demand for evacuation. Second, there may have been sensitivity about the bias of provision towards London rather than other areas in danger from bombing. Despite this a press notice was released by the LCC in December 1940 – with or without Ministry of Health approval – entitled 'Homes wanted for aged Londoners'[37] and this was picked up by most national newspapers (for example, *Daily Herald*, 'Can you give them shelter?', 17 December, 1940). However, when the *Picture Post* approached the LCC in March 1941 they were discouraged from providing a story on the evacuation scheme on the grounds "that the wide circulation of *Picture Post* might give rise to false ideas of the scope of this business and that it would be wiser to take no action"[38].

As already indicated, the London processing of applicants was carried out by the Education Department of the LCC. The number of private billets found was very limited. By November 1941, only 285 had been placed in private billets, whereas 1,158 had been placed in evacuation hostels[39]. Officers of the Education Department assessed each applicant for evacuation. Such criteria as 'personal cleanliness' and 'class of person (well educated, working class etc)'[40] were used and it may be that the 'well educated' and 'clean' middle-class applicant was more likely to be perceived as suitable for a private billet. The rest were offered hostel places so long as they were able to look after themselves. A brief summary of the scheme in November 1941 described the hostels in the following way:

> **Those so far opened accommodate numbers varying from eight to ninety old people. Cook-housekeeper in charge: she does the cooking. Old people look after themselves, make their beds, prepare vegetables, keep rooms tidy. Heavy scrubbing and cleaning done by domestics.**[41]

The evacuation hostel scheme constantly faced two main problems. First, many of the applicants were too frail for such hostels; they could no longer manage in the community but they wished to avoid going into PAIs. Second, elderly people often deteriorated in health after arriving at hostels and this created a problem of where they should be sent.

There were constant complaints from local authorities that those sent to hostels were too frail. For example, the Public Assistance Officer, Monmouth, wrote to the LCC's Education Department:

> **I have to refer you to my letter of the 14th instant herein and to state that Mr D was found to be suffering from incontinence of urine and mentally queer. It therefore became necessary to remove him from Cwmbran House, Pontnewydd to Regent House Public Assistance Institution, Chepstow – please inform his sister.**[42]

In November 1941, the Cambridge region were complaining that "the criteria of able-bodiedness has been stretched too far"[43]. The response of officers from the Education Department to these pressures was to argue for special provision for the 'elderly infirm'. The Evacuation Division of the Ministry of Health refused to consider this option. They suggested that the 'infirm' should be placed in LCC hospitals outside London. The public health officer for the LCC responded by claiming that "there are already more chronic sick in our acute and chronic hospitals than I like and I am unwilling to add to their number"[44]. He did not specify what the 'chronic sick' outside existing hospital provision were meant to do.

The next response of the Education Department was to approach the Rest Centre Service. It pointed out that:

> **Ever since the present scheme came into operation, we have found that in spite of all our efforts to weed out unsuitable applications some old people of the wrong categories have slipped through in the parties for the hostels. The kind of people who have created difficulties for the staff of the hostels are those who, on arrival, have been found to be suffering from some chronic sickness; those who are too infirm to look after their personal needs; those who are dirty (and in a few cases verminous); and those who are abusive or unmanageable.[45]**

The request was for the use of a rest home (see next section) as a clearing house; six beds could be reserved for elderly evacuation applicants and a three- or four-day assessment carried out. The matron could produce a report and "if any of the old people did not pass muster, they would be returned whence they came, ie to home address or hospital". This request was refused on the grounds that rest homes were only for those rendered homeless by bombing "and that the old people who came to you for evacuation may not meet these requirements"[46].

Demand for evacuation places varied considerably according to the extent of bombing raids. Demand was high in Autumn 1940. The same occurred on 16 and 19 April 1941 when the raids brought 'a flood' of evacuation requests, totalling 354 for the week ending 26 April[47]. The spring raids encouraged the Ministry of Health to ask local authorities to extend their evacuation hostel provision[48] and a further attempt was also made to find private billets[49]. However, by December 1941 a situation had been reached in which the supply of evacuation places was exceeding the demand[50] and by July 1942 the Education Department was asking the Ministry of Health to suspend the scheme[51]. It was agreed that the 'able-bodied elderly' had decided to remain in London and await developments, that is, to see if the raids restarted. The trickle of evacuation requests came mainly from relatives trying to get rid of "difficult old people" who had "reached their second childhood, and have become 'problem children'"[51]. The Ministry of Health agreed to suspend the scheme[52], and the Evacuation of the Aged Committee ceased to function. Therefore the only means of evacuation for elderly people not made homeless by the war became the private billeting arrangements under *Circular 2170*.

Towards a policy? The establishment of hostels for the homeless

The previous section dealt with the development of policy towards evacuation hostels for elderly people from London. This section considers what arrangements were made for elderly people made homeless by the war. The eventual extent of provision for both types of hostel can be seen from Table 1, which lists those funded by central government and run by local authorities. Hostels were also provided by certain voluntary organisations. Total figures for these are not known, although the largest provision was made by Quaker Relief Organisations which had 27 hostels offering 305 places in July 1942.

Table 1: Hostels for the aged (local authority places)

	London region	
	Number of hostels	*Accommodation*
Hostels for evacuees	–	–
Hostels for homeless	43	1,730
Hostels for bedridden	3	125
Total	**46**	**1,855**
	12 regions of England and Wales	
	Number of hostels	*Accommodation*
Hostels for evacuees	80	1,863
Hostels for homeless	80	2,572
Hostels for bedridden	15	510
Total	**175**	**4,945**

Source: PRO HLG7/322, *Evacuation of aged and infirm.* These figures have been taken from *Regional Organisation Administration* 377, 'Hostels for old people', 21 July 1942

It has been argued that central government pursued two important 'policies' in relation to elderly people and evacuation during the period of the mass bombing raids. Elderly people were encouraged to leave London. There was a concern to treat all homeless civilians, including elderly people, as war victims and not potential PAI cases. What is less clear is the extent to which these two policy concerns were reflected in a neat division into the two types of hostel listed in Table 1. It is not known how many of the people dealt with by the Evacuation of the Aged Committee were in fact homeless and the same information is also lacking for the residents of Evacuation Hostels. The Ministry of Health summary report for 1941-42 mentioned how:

> **In many parts of the country hostels have been established, under the management of local authorities, for aged homeless who cannot be billeted or make their own arrangements with relatives and friends.... A number of aged but able-bodied homeless from the evacuation areas have also been taken into the 200 hostels set up under the Evacuation Scheme in reception or neutral areas. (Ministry of Health, 1942a)**

This would suggest that the distinction between the two types of hostel became blurred as the war progressed. Despite this difficulty, this section focuses on the development of policy towards hostels for the homeless.

As already indicated, the first hostels for victims of the bombing raids were established without government support by the Quaker Relief Organisations as a response to those elderly people who had fled London in panic. They were homeless because of the war but in an indirect way. Later residents were selected by Quaker relief workers in London on the basis of their homelessness or general isolation. According to Staley, they often dealt with cases "too delicate for the Authorities" such as old people "whose lives had been shamefully hard because of poverty, poor education and squalid homes, and particularly loneliness" (Staley, 1943, p 20).

The exact influence of these Quaker hostels upon Ministry of Health thinking is not known. However, it is clear that after the initial panic measures reviewed earlier in this chapter, central government accepted the need for hostels for elderly people made homeless by the war. This would stop rest centres being blocked by homeless people who lacked relatives to live with or who were unsuitable for billeting. It avoided the charge that war victims were being treated as 'paupers'.

By January 1941, local authorities were running 25 hostels for 'LCC homeless aged cases'[53] of which 10 were run by Surrey, six in Wales and a further three in the South West. These hostels were for 'the aged homeless who were able bodied'[54] but who were not able to find a billet with friends or relatives. The same criterion was used for hostels established by the Quaker Relief Organisations (Staley, 1943, pp 18-20). Such provision had two main deficiencies.

First, such accommodation did not meet the needs of the homeless elderly 'infirm' and, as already indicated, this led to a blocking of EMS beds. Where these beds were in former PAIs there was also the taint of pauperisation, especially when medical treatment was completed. Willinck (Special Commissioner for London) continued to press the Ministry of Health for the establishment of 200-300 bed hostel infirmaries although it was stressed that the only question under discussion was provision for the 'aged and infirm' made homeless by enemy action[55]. The outcome of these negotiations was an instruction in September 1941 to senior regional officers of the Ministry of Health that:

> **The most satisfactory solution for both the able-bodied and the infirm is the establishment of special hostels, preferably on the periphery of target towns.... The net cost should be charged to the local authorities' homeless persons account.**[56]

The figures already provided on hostel development show that this was a stimulus to growth although provision for the 'infirm/bedridden' remained quite limited, probably because of the shortage of nursing staff. Slightly more problematic was the lack of use made of the beds created for the 'infirm'. In July 1942 only 55 beds out of 510 for the 'bedridden' were occupied in hostels outside the London region[57]. The reasons for this are not known. Was it lack of staffing? The lull in the bombing raid? A desire to save the accommodation for an emergency?

Second, nearly all provision was outside London and the main conurbations. Some of the homeless were very keen to leave the main urban areas, but others were reluctant to leave their homes. Many seemed to prefer a rest centre in London to the thought of a hostel, for example in Lancashire[58]. Not all elderly people wished to leave London, especially after the initial adjustment to the bombing raids. This is confirmed by Nixon in *Raiders overhead*. The author was a civil defence warden during the war and she felt elderly people were a 'liability' during bombing raids. However, many refused to be evacuated out of London, even after being made homeless: "the blind, the crippled, and the very old would say, 'Yes, Miss; thank you, Miss; I'll go, Miss' but they never went" (Nixon, 1980, p 62). The first attempt to tackle this issue was in the Ministry of Health *Circular 2251* on 'Hostels' in December 1940 which announced the setting up of the London Hostels Association Ltd to make "provision in the London

Civil Defence Region of residential hostels for persons, who, through circumstances arising out of the war, are in need of accommodation in such hostels". The scope of the association would be:

> **... the provision of accommodation for persons made homeless by direct enemy action ... they intend also to deal with elderly persons who are not in need of medical or nursing care but who have lost their homes or are not capable of looking after themselves under war conditions.**[59]

This non-profit making organisation was financed by the Exchequer, and the Ministry of Health hoped this would reduce the pressure for the establishment of local authority hostels for the homeless in the London Region.

The eventual provision of hostels in the London region by a number of different organisations was considerable: 46 hostels for the aged homeless provided 1,856 beds, of which 1,188 were occupied in July 1942[60]. Facilities for the elderly infirm proved much more modest. Three hostels existed with 126 beds but only 15 patients[60]. Once again it is difficult to interpret the reasons for this and it may be these hostels were not properly staffed.

The last two sections have attempted to specify central government policy towards evacuation hostels and hostels for the elderly homeless. It has been argued that this policy centred on the desire both to reduce the elderly population in London and also to establish arrangements by which the elderly homeless were treated as war victims rather than potential inmates of PAIs. There was consistent resistance from the Evacuation Division of the Ministry of Health to any attempt to define their responsibility as extending to "the elderly infirm as a class" because of the disruption caused by the war. However, such conclusions are tentative for a number of reasons. Many of the relevant negotiations about evacuation hostels, homeless hostels and rest homes have not been uncovered. The sources of uncovered information were biased heavily towards London. It is impossible to estimate the rigidity of the distinction between an evacuation hostel and a homeless hostel.

Evacuation and the flying bomb raids

After the main bombing raids ceased, hostel provision was reduced and the occupancy rates in the remaining hostels were often low, especially outside London (Staley, 1943, p 30)[61]. At first, the Ministry of Health refused to consider the possibility of these empty beds being used for elderly people trying to avoid entry to PAIs. The OPWC were told in July 1943 that "pressure on hostel accommodation is severe and it is not easy to arrive at an agreement in view of the many conflicting claims"[62]. Such a statement was surprising given the hostel vacancy figures (see Table 2). By the beginning of 1944 the Evacuation Division was showing signs of relenting and they offered OPWC a 'trickle arrangement' by which they could nominate 26 'able-bodied' cases and 12 'infirm' cases for hostel places[63].

Table 2: Accommodation for aged evacuees and homeless persons

Hostels	*Total accommodation*	*Number of Inmates*	*Vacancies*	*% of accommodation vacant*
Local authority	2,325	1,301	1,024	44
Voluntary	742	616	126	17
Total	**3,067**	**1,917**	**1,150**	**37**

Source: PRO HLG7/322, *Evacuation of aged and infirm.* These figures have been taken from *Regional Organisation Administration 377*, 'Hostels for old people', 21 July 1942

Such negotiations were ended by the flying bomb raids which began in June 1944. The Evacuation Division defined three groups of elderly people placed at risk by this development:

1) homeless elderly people in rest centres and rest homes;
2) elderly people in public air raid shelters;
3) elderly people living in their own homes who are unable, by reasons of infirmity, to go to shelters.

It was argued that "our first duty is clearly to the homeless aged" and no commitment should be made "for the removal of persons in classes (2) and (3) above"[64]. The shortage of accommodation for elderly homeless people in London was to be eased by the removal of some of them to hostels in other regions. By 19 July 1944, over 500 such transfers had taken place. In addition to this, 6,224 elderly people had found private billets under *Circular 2170* between 12 June and 14 July 1944[65].

However, the various pressure groups complained at the lack of provision for elderly people who were not homeless, that is, they campaigned for a scheme similar to the one run by the LCC Education Department from November 1940 to July 1942. The Charity Organisation Society, for example, wrote that "great hardship is being experienced by old people who have been bombed out in these raids or in previous raids and who are therefore very nervous and unsuited for shelter life and by invalids who lack mobility which also makes them additionally nervous"[66]. The Evacuation Division backed down on its original policy on the grounds that "a demand is being voiced for the evacuation of aged and infirm persons who cannot make private arrangements to go to relatives or friends"[67]. A total of 740 hostel places were found for 'able-bodied' evacuees and the voluntary organisations were asked to renew their search for private billets and voluntary homes.

The hostel places were not allocated by the LCC Education Department as in 1940-42. The reason for this is not known. Instead, the Evacuation Division of the Ministry of Health established a selection panel. It was chaired by a senior officer from the LCC and other members were from the Charity Organisation Society, the OPWC, the WVS and a medical officer from the Ministry of Health. It is not known whether panel members were perceived by the Evacuation Division as appropriate individuals or representatives of their organisations. The panel employed the following eligibility criteria for applicants:

1) Applicants must be in normal health and able to attend to themselves, to make their beds and keep their quarters clean.
2) Applications can be considered from the following persons only:
   a) elderly able-bodied persons who are in the care of a mother with young children or an expectant mother, who will leave for a safe area if the applicant is evacuated;
   b) elderly able-bodied people who have been shocked or blasted by enemy action;
   c) elderly able-bodied people (including married couples) who are living alone[68].

The emphasis was again on the needs of 'able-bodied' elderly people before the frail and sick. It is likely that these criteria were supplied to the selection panel by the Ministry of Health. A total of 400 people were evacuated in the first four weeks[69]. By 14 September 1944, 852 elderly people had been evacuated by the panel although over 500 applicants were refused such help because of 'infirmity'[70].

This evacuation scheme does not mean that elderly people were given a higher priority for evacuation in the second half of the war. When the Public Assistance Division was asked by the Evacuation Division about the possible removal of elderly people from London institutions, it was agreed this might be possible "in isolated cases ... but this arrangement is not to be publicised in any way". It was stressed that:

> **The guiding principle should clearly be to make the best use in the national interest of the limited amount of accommodation in large houses, camps, hostels, etc which is available in the reception areas; as that accommodation is limited, its use must be determined by a system of priorities; babies and expectant mothers clearly have first claim and the infirm or aged equally clearly last claim.[71]**

The end result of such assumptions was that the bulk of 'infirm' elderly people remained in London during the period of the flying bomb raids.

As the danger from these raids receded, the Ministry of Health agreed with the LCC in October 1944 that the selection panel should be wound up on 12 December 1944[72]. The WVS were not happy about this and at first refused to accept the closure of the panel because of the need to help those elderly people whose homes had been bomb damaged. As late as March 1945[73], the WVS was still trying to obtain permission to use hostel places outside London for those with bomb damaged homes. The Evacuation Division felt this was not the main problem: "we are likely to be faced shortly by a clamour from the old people evacuated so great a distance to be allowed to return to the vicinity of London"[73].

The termination of evacuation arrangements

In February 1945 the Ministry of Health estimated that there were 50,000 evacuated old people in reception areas of which 3,000 were in local authority and voluntary hostels[74]. By early 1945 there was general agreement among civil servants about the need to wind up the various evacuation arrangements. With regard to elderly people, one major difficulty had been identified:

> **How long will the 'homeless' label remain attached to these people? In other words how long will the homeless aged continue to receive preferential treatment over other aged who are without accommodation or who are living in unsatisfactory conditions?[75]**

It was recognised that any attempt to place hostel residents in PAIs could cause a public outcry; this would not be seen as the way to treat war victims. At the same time, there was a desire to end central government financial responsibility for such cases. The preferred solution was seen as persuading voluntary organisations to take over such hostels[76].

The regional inspectorate of the Ministry of Health were told in March 1945 how to deal with 'the residual problem'[77] of old people. For elderly evacuees living with relatives in reception areas, the billeting allowance was to be withdrawn but the elderly person would be allowed to claim an increased supplementary pension from the Assistance Board. Those in private billets would be visited by Assistance Board officers to see if the billeting allowance could be withdrawn without the elderly evacuee being in danger of losing his or her accommodation. Voluntary hostels would also no longer receive billeting money, but the residents would again be able to claim maintenance costs from the Assistance Board. Local authority hostels would continue with financial support from central government but voluntary organisations would be encouraged to take them over. Privately, however, it was accepted that this was unlikely to occur in the London region where several of the hostels were located. A briefing to the Minister of Health for a deputation from the NOPWC noted how "the arrangement is likely to be less welcome to County Authorities in the London Region such as the LCC, Surrey County Council, and East and West Ham County Boroughs, who administer a number of hostels for the aged with marked success"[78].

At the same time, it was appreciated that a major problem would be the number of elderly evacuees wishing to return to the London region, many of them lacking homes or an ability to care for themselves. As a result, the LCC was given permission to establish additional rest home accommodation sufficient for 250 elderly people[79]. The BRCS was asked to bolster this provision further by establishing their sick bays in Middlesex as permanent hostels for the 'infirm'. These bays were privately owned but had been staffed by the BRCS for the duration of the war. The BRCS showed little interest in negotiating possible rental charges and nothing came of this proposal[80]. The NOPWC complained to the Ministry of Health about lack of sufficient funds to take over evacuation hostels or to establish new residential homes[81]. The Friends Relief Service was also finding it difficult to establish arrangements by which voluntary organisations could take over its hostels (personal correspondence with Professor Roger Wilson and William K. Sessions).

The reasons for these problems have not been clarified by the research. Were the voluntary organisations blocked by the local authorities? Were they short of funds? Did they prefer to establish new hostels for the 'able-bodied' elderly rather than take over ones where many of the residents were already very 'infirm'? Was the main problem just the length of time such negotiations inevitably take? The picture is confusing. Although voluntary organisations did manage to open new hostels for elderly people in the period 1945-48 (see below), little movement occurred over the actual evacuation hostels. This failure tended to encourage a hardening of attitudes in the Ministry of Health towards elderly evacuees. In August 1945, an assistant secretary claimed:

> **... the majority of these chronic cases are of the type who would in the normal course of events have become a poor law responsibility had they not been evacuated and it seems there is no alternative but to try to arrange for their admission either to a PAI in the reception area; or to return them to an institution in the area of the authority to which they would have been chargeable but for evacuation.**[82]

This official made the point that many of the evacuees had been in reception areas for over three years so that their home authorities could use the law of settlement to make them chargeable to the reception authorities.

The issue of 'how to deal with aged evacuees' was discussed at an internal meeting of Ministry officials in August 1945. Two options were considered, namely that either elderly evacuees should become a Poor Law responsibility or that an interim scheme should be established on the lines of that proposed for child evacuees. Attitudes at the meeting were mixed. Some pointed out that there could be little justification in giving preferential treatment to evacuees and so they should be looked after under the Poor Law system. Others pointed out "as a practical consideration, that whilst school children did not write to their MPs the aged certainly would do so if they are forced into the position that – as they would see it – solely by virtue of the loss of their home by enemy action and their subsequent evacuation, they must become poor law cases and lose all their old age pensions"[83]. It was finally decided that hostel residents who remained in the reception areas should be retained under the government evacuation scheme.

This policy was outlined in *Circular 195/46* (Ministry of Health, 1946a)[84] which dealt with "aged persons who are without suitable accommodation to which to return". The Circular described a complex set of arrangements for evacuation and homeless hostels. Voluntary organisations were again encouraged to take them over while those run by district councils were to be transferred to county councils. Every attempt would be made to empty these hostels of the 'displaced aged' so that central government funding could be ended. However, so long as a particular hostel had to be kept open for elderly evacuees, the Minister would be prepared to allow the filling of vacant places by the admission of 'specially selected public assistance cases' provided that no suitable accommodation was available for such cases in existing PAIs and that payment was made for them by the council. It was hoped that this arrangement would allow the gradual takeover of such property by the local authority:

> **The war-time financial arrangements by which the responsible authority was reimbursed any net deficiency on the running of a hostel will continue so long as the hostel is mainly used by 'displaced aged' but should the position arise when a hostel contains a preponderance of public assistance cases, the Public Assistance Authority will be requested to consider taking over the hostel ... for Poor Law purposes in which case 'displaced aged' who could not be transferred to another hostel would remain in the hostel with the status of evacuees. (Ministry of Health, 1946a)[84]**

Central government would continue to reimburse public assistance authorities any net additional expenditure occurred in respect of the 'displaced aged' admitted to PAIs for lack of other suitable accommodation. Central government financial support would also be offered to local authorities with regard to those returning to their original home areas. A number of these elderly people had by reason of evacuation acquired settlement in the reception area and would, if admitted to a PAI, therefore, be legally chargeable to the public assistance authority for the reception area. The Circular concluded by stressing that 'displaced aged' persons admitted to PAIs should not incur disqualification for the receipt of a pension even though they may not be in the institution for the purposes of receiving medical treatment.

These arrangements continued until 5 July 1948 when the National Assistance Act was implemented. During this period, the Ministry of Health encouraged local authorities to take over financial responsibility for evacuation and homeless hostels so that they could be used as residential accommodation under the new legislation. The LCC was especially keen to acquire several of the rest homes on a permanent basis, although this was often complicated by the fact that much of this property had been requisitioned for war purposes[85]. The other main problem in this period was the level of 'infirmity' of many of the hostel residents. As the regional inspectorate were informed:

> **The majority of 'displaced' aged persons have been accommodated in hostels for a number of years, and many of them have deteriorated in health and physical capacity to the extent that they now require constant medical and nursing care. Had it not been for the acute shortage of beds most of the aged in this condition would have been transferred to hospital. In addition, hostels for the infirm (ie evacuees and homeless persons requiring hospital treatment) were established some years ago, and many of the residents have by now reached the condition where they may be regarded as in need of hospital treatment.[86]**

This was seen as problematic since "after the appointed day, local authorities will have no power to provide accommodation for the sick". The inspectorate were, therefore, encouraged to visit all the hostels and arrange for the transfer to hospital of all those in need of medical care.

The final closing down of the government evacuation scheme occurred on 5 July 1948 and the detailed implications of this were announced a month earlier in *Circular 85/48* (Ministry of Health, 1948a)[87]. This confirmed the ending of billeting arrangements, the closure of remaining evacuation hostels and the ending of all forms of central government subsidy to local authorities under evacuation arrangements. The Circular stressed that those in need of medical treatment needed to be transferred to hospital so that "on 5th July 1948, no sick persons remain in hostels for the 'displaced aged' or 'infirm'". Finally, future financial responsibility for hostel residents in need of care and attention was to be defined by their ordinary residence as laid down in Sections 24 and 32 of the National Assistance Act.

Concluding comments

It is possible to predict some of the main arguments that will be made against the thrust of the analysis in this chapter. Suffering is inevitable in war. It is appropriate that personnel involved in 'war work' should be given highest priority for medical care. Children and young mothers should be given a higher priority in evacuation arrangements than elderly people who have already lived most of their lives. The chapter fails to appreciate the full gravity of the situation facing Britain in the period June 1940 to July 1942.

These views have been put with great precision by William K. Sessions, who worked with Quaker Relief Organisations during the war. In personal correspondence, he has made the following set of points:

> **In this context I think your phrase 'the low priority given by government to elderly people in a war situation', although technically and academically correct, is unfair, except in the sense that not all the eventualities were foreseen and/or planned for before they happened. I see it as a question of priorities for the statutory authorities. The government was concentrating its brain power on (i) whether and when Hitler would make a combined operation landing against Britain – virtually defenceless since the Dunkirk near-annihilation of June 1940; (ii) how to counter the air raids and bring down the enemy bombers; (iii) how to support and reinforce the fire services to prevent London and other big cities being completely engulfed in flames etc. etc. Good pre-planning had been done for the evacuation of the priority classes of children and mothers with very young children. Meantime the adult population of all ages did not, I believe, expect also to receive priority treatment. Certainly I recall no anti-government, no anti-authority resentment amongst voluntary bodies and here I am speaking right through to the end of the war.**

The authors do not disagree with much of this argument; they also suspect 'the adult population of all ages' did not expect priority evacuation treatment.

At the same time, this approach neither confronts nor explains certain aspects of evacuation 'policy' towards elderly people. The eventual evacuation arrangements that were made for this group were not directed always to those most 'in need'.

In his November 1940 report, the Chief Officer of the LCC's Rest Centre Service expressed dissatisfaction at how evacuation arrangements offered 'help' to those elderly people able to reach rest centres and air raid shelters but not to "the aged person who is bedridden". A small number of evacuation hostels were eventually established for the 'infirm' but the general thrust of provision was towards the evacuation of the 'able bodied' (GLC Records Office, 1940); this was true in the initial bombing raids and remained true in the flying bomb raids. The main response of government reflected concern about the impact of elderly people upon the morale of others. Priority was given to those whose suffering was visible to the general population and whose behaviour disrupted other arrangements. All elderly people made homeless by bombing raids were seen as war victims and had to be protected from PAIs. 'Able-bodied' elderly people in the London region were also treated as war victims. 'Able-bodied' elderly people in the rest of the country and 'elderly infirm' people in general were not treated in this way; their requests for institutional care could only be met through the Poor Law system.

An important defence of these arrangements was that, in the words of an assistant secretary in the Evacuation Division, "we have not available the resources that would enable us to undertake to provide for the aged infirm as a class"[88]. Nursing and care staff may not have been available to run a more extensive system of hostel provision. However, this does not excuse the indifference accorded to sick and frail elderly people. It may not have been possible to meet their demands in a war crisis but this does not justify references to them as if they lacked value as human beings. They were described as 'the unbilletables' or 'shelter derelicts'. They were a 'disposal problem' or they 'blocked beds'. They were not 'potential effectives'. The top floors of PAIs were closed to save the lives of staff rather than inmates. It may be that these attitudes were strongest towards the poor working class elderly people who were seen as already drifting towards PAIs before the war. The Second World War may have ushered in a general concern for civilian morale but this does not mean hostile attitudes towards the 'undeserving poor' were completely swept away by the onset of war. However, the next chapter shows how such attitudes were modified as the war progressed.

The above analysis does not mean to infer that elderly people were passive victims of the war who were incapable of having their own influence upon events. The arrival of many elderly people in 'safe areas' but without billets in Autumn 1940 encouraged the opening of the first hostels. The later reluctance of the homeless elderly to leave the London region encouraged the expansion of LCC rest homes. Complaints from elderly people and their relatives about PAI conditions encouraged the establishment of evacuation and homeless hostels, and ensured their continuation until July 1948 when the National Assistance Act came into force; civil servants and politicians appreciated that elderly people write letters and have the capacity to define themselves as deserving war casualties in need of special provision. Their complaints were to become part of the argument for a general reform of the Poor Law system itself – the implications of this for PAIs during the 1940s is one of the themes of the next chapter.

This chapter ends with a quotation from Richard Titmuss which encapsulates many of the nuances about the evacuation arrangements for elderly people that have been outlined:

> **The problem of the aged and the chronic sick had been serious enough in peacetime; in war it threatened to become unmanageable. Thousands who had formerly been nursed at home were clamouring for admission to hospitals when families were split up, when homes were damaged or destroyed, and when the nightly trek to the shelters became a part of normal life for Londoners. Yet everything, except humanitarian considerations - which often take second place in war – spoke against these poorest and most helpless members of the community. Because they occupied beds for indefinite periods it was wasteful to admit them to specifically equipped and staffed emergency scheme beds. To nurse them was not only uninteresting but often unpleasant; the work soon dampened the enthusiasm of newly enrolled VADs who had expected to nurse soldiers and not incontinent and senile old people. It was moreover agreed in the jargon of the day that the emergency hospital service must give priority to 'potential effectives'. (Titmuss, 1976, p 448)**

During the first years of the Second World War, elderly people were not seen as 'potential effectives'. As the war progressed, however, such attitudes did begin to shift; the humane treatment of dependent groups became an important symbol of 'post-Beveridge' Britain.

Notes

[Much of the material referred to in this and the following chapters has been collected from the departmental files of the Ministry of Health. There are two main sources for this material. Much of the pre-1952 material is located in the Public Records Office. These will be referred to in the notes as PRO files and their PRO index number will follow. However, much of the relevant material at the time of the fieldwork was still located at the DHSS and these files were being processed prior to handover to the PRO. These files will be referred to in the notes as DHSS files and their original departmental index number will follow; these files will be given a new number on transfer to the PRO.]

[1] DHSS 94003/7/2A, *Public assistance institutions: Reception and welfare.*

[2] DHSS 94003/7/5, *Poor Law Amendment Act 1938: Representations by associations of local authorities.*

[3] DHSS 94003/5/24, *Public assistance institutions: Inmates: Specialised treatment for aged chronic cases by emergency medical staff.* See letter from Mr Rowdell, SE Regional Office, Ministry of Health, 26 February 1940.

[4] Ibid; see various handwritten responses from Ministry officials to Rowdell letter.

[5] See, for example, PRO MH 76/138, *Hospitals general: Release of beds from London hospitals.*

[6] GLC Records Office: LCC, Education Officer's Department. File EO/WAR/2/40 *Aged and infirm.* See also undated joint report to the Civil Defence and General Purpose Committee by the Education Officer and the Chief Officer of the Rest Centre Service. A short discussion of the evacuation of elderly people from air raid shelters is also provided in the Report by the Chief Officer, Rest Centre Service, dated 26 November 1940 (GLC Records Office, 1940).

[7] GLC Records Office: LCC, Education Officer's Department. File EO/WAR/2/40. Letter from Education Department Officer to G.White, Ministry of Health, Emergency Hospital Service, Section 9, Surrey, 25 February 1941.

[8] DHSS 99063/11/1A, *Social welfare: National Council of Social Service: General correspondence and Executive Committee 1940-46.* Memorandum from Miss Puxley (Assistant Secretary) to Mr Turner (Principal Secretary), 21 October 1941.

[9] GLC Records Office (1940). 'Public Assistance Department: Memorandum on the Emergency Rest Centre Service for persons rendered homeless through enemy action' from E. King (Chief Assistant), 4 September 1940.

[10] PRO HLG7/84, *Evacuation: Special scheme.* See Ministry of Health (1940).

[11] PRO HLG7/84, *Evacuation: Special scheme.* See 'Special scheme: Lines of suggested revision in light of changed situation', April 1941.

[12] See for example, PRO MH 76/368 for copy of ROA 482 on 'The aged and infirm homeless', 4 September 1941.

[13] Age Concern Archives: Box One: *Historical and early activities.* Minutes of OPWC meeting, 27 February 1941.

[14] Ibid; correspondence from 4 July 1941 to 5 May 1942 about survey of aged evacuees in EMS hospitals.

[15] DHSS 94003/1/47, *Public assistance institutions – General,* Paper on 'Removal of old age pensioners to EMS hospitals' by Mr Deans (Superintending Clerk, Old Age Pensions Branch), 31 October 1940.

[16] GLC Records Office. See various reports in *LCC Social Welfare Committee: Minutes of Proceedings No 6, 1939-44.*

[17] PRO CAB 102/716. *Miscellaneous Papers 1938-43 used in the completion of 'Problems of social policy': Emergency Medical Service,* Minutes of Conference between LCC and Ministry of Health on 'Chronic sick', 8 October 1940.

[18] DHSS 94003/1/47, *Public assistance institutions – General.*

[19] DHSS 94014/1/97, *Relief: Payment of rents of evacuated persons.*

[20] DHSS 94014/1/108, *Relief: General: Effect of evacuation on public assistance authorities in receiving areas.* DHSS 94014/1/124, *Relief: Circular 2000: Effects of war on administration of Poor Law.* DHSS 94014/1/125, *Relief: General: Correspondence arising out of Circular 2000: Effect of war on administration of poor relief.*

[21] DHSS 94014/1/108, Letter from CCA, 7 October 1939.

[22] Ibid; minutes of meeting, 25 January 1940.

[23] A copy of this can be found in DHSS 94014/1/124.

[24] DHSS 94014/1/125, Letter from CCA, 22 April 1942. See also *CCA Gazette Supplement*, February 1942, pp 32-3: 'Public assistance – Evacuation: Settlement and removal', and May 1942, p 100: 'Public assistance – Evacuation (settlement and removal)'.

[25] DHSS 94014/1/125, handwritten note, 17 July 1942.

[26] PRO HLG 7/395, *Care of the homeless: Accommodation of aged and infirm.* See various memoranda from Sir Henry Willinck.

[27] PRO AST 7/557, *Welfare: Homes and hostels.* For example, Ibberson (Principal) complained to Reid (Secretary, Assistance Board) that "the need for hostels for the aged (other than those bombed out) has been acutely aggravated by the disturbance of their normal life caused by the war and the position has been aggravated locally by the commandeering of PA Institutions", Memorandum 9 August 1941.

[28] A general account of the setting up of the OPWC and the influence of the Assistance Board is provided in Roberts (1970, pp 41-51). The creation of the OPWC and the link between this development and concern about elderly people in wartime will be further explored in Chapter Three.

[29] Age Concern Archives: Box Files 1-4, *Early and historical activities.*

[30] A copy of this can be found in DHSS 94003/1/47.

[31] GLC Records Office: LCC, Education Officer's Department. File EO/WAR/2/41 *Aged and infirm.* Report for Evacuation of the Aged Committee, March 1941.

[32] GLC Records Office: LCC, Education Officer's Department, File EO/WAR/2/40, Memorandum from Russell Smith to Savage, 7 November 1940.

[33] PRO HLG 7/395, Memorandum from Barter to Rucker, 5 May 1941.

[34] PRO HLG 7/534, *Evacuation of the aged and homeless.* See copy of ROA 422 on 'Evacuation of old people', 27 June 1941.

[35] PRO MH 76/363, *Regional Organisation Administration Nos 201-250.* A copy of *Circular 2213* is attached to ROA 241 on 'Government evacuation scheme – Evacuation of the aged', 21 November 1940.

[36] Ibid. NCSS letter on 'Evacuation of the aged' attached to ROA 241. A copy of the NCSS letter and related correspondence can be found in Age Concern Archives: Box One, *Historical and early activities.*

[37] GLC Records Office: LCC Education Officer's Department, EO/WAR/2/40. See Press Notice, 13 December 1940.

[38] GLC Records Office: EO/WAR/2/41, minute from Williams, 4 March 1941.

[39] GLC Records Office: EO/WAR/2/43, report on the 'Evacuation of the aged and infirm', 12 November 1941.

[40] GLC Records Office: EO/WAR/2/40, letter from Education Department, London Council of Social Service, 22 November 1940.

[41] GLC Records Office: EO/WAR/2/4, 'Evacuation of aged and infirm: Summary of scheme', 3 November 1941.

[42] GLC Records Office: EO/WAR/2/41, letter, 18 March 1941.

[43] GLC Records Office: EO/WAR/2/43, letter, 14 November 1941.

[44] GLC Records Office: EO/WAR/2/41, letter from LCC Public Health Department, 15 April 1941.

[45] GLC Records Office: EO/WAR/2/43, memorandum from Middlemiss to Ruck, 13 October 1941.

[46] Ibid. Undated respone from T.Clark to Middlemiss.

[47] GLC Records Office: EO/WAR/2/41, memorandum from Leadbetter to Middlemiss, 25 February 1941.

[48] PRO HLG 7/534; see copy of ROA 422 on 'Evacuation of old people', 27 June 1941.

[49] Ibid; "It is proposed now to see if a solution to this problem can be found by utilising the assistance of various agencies which are willing to try to find groups of suitable voluntary billets for these old people in certain selected neutral and reception areas".

[50] GLC Records Office: EO/WAR/2/43, memorandum from Leadbetter to Middlemiss, 2 December 1941.

[51] Ibid, Middlemiss to Leadbetter, 16 July 1942.

[52] Ibid, Leadbetter to Middlemiss, 24 July 1942.

[53] PRO HLG 7/322, *Evacuation of aged and infirm,* memorandum from Howell James (Ministry of Health) to Ure (Assistance Board), 23 January 1941.

[54] PRO HLG 7/395, *Care of the homeless: Accommodation of aged and infirm.* See ROA 482 on 'The aged and infirm', 4 September 1941.

[55] PRO HLG 7/395, memorandum from Sir Henry Willinck, 24 January 1941.

[56] Ibid; see copy of ROA 482 on 'The aged and infirm', 4 September 1941.

[57] PRO HLG 7/322; see copy of ROA 337 on 'Hostels for old people', 21 July 1942.

[57] PRO MH 76/365, *Regional Organisation Administration, Nos 301-350*; see ROA 339 on 'Evacuation of old people from London', 9 April 1941 which states that "London County Council have found old people reluctant to go to Lancashire".

[59] GLC Records Office: LCC, Education Officer's Department, File EO/WAR/ 2/40. Contains a copy of Ministry of Health (1940c).

[60] PRO HLG 7/322; see copy of ROA 337 on 'Hostels for old people', 21 July 1942.

[61] See also PRO HLG 7/332, *Evacuation of aged and infirm,* Memorandum from MacKinnon to Duke, 27 March, 1943.

[62] PRO HLG 7/332, memorandum from MacKinnon to Samson, 30 July 1943.

[63] Ibid. See correspondence between Strong and Samson, 11 March 1944 and MacKinnon and Green, 15 March 1944.

[64] PRO HLG 7/333, *Evacuation (1944) aged and infirm persons policy*; paper by Rowland on 'Evacuation of aged persons from London', 6 July 1944.

[65] Ibid. These figures are abstracted from a memorandum by Rowland, 19 July 1944.

[66] Ibid; letter from the Charity Organisation Society, 13 July 1944.

[67] Ibid; memorandum from Rowland, 19 July 1944.

[68] Ibid; undated publicity handout on 'Government evacuation scheme'.

[69] Ibid; Evacuation Panel Report, 8 August 1944.

[70] Ibid; Evacuation Panel Report, 15 September 1944.

[71] Ibid; memorandum from Wilkinson to Rowland, 24 August 1944.

[72] Ibid; memorandum from Willinck, 6 October 1944.

[73] Ibid; memorandum from MacKinnon to Wilkinson, 20 March 1945.

[74] PRO HLG 7/535, *Homeless: Evacuation of aged and infirm: Provision for their return.* Figures abstracted from minutes of meeting on the 'Winding up of the government evacuation scheme for old people', 1 February 1945.

[75] Ibid; memorandum from Andrew to Wilkinson, 12 January 1945.

[76] Ibid; minutes of meeting on the 'Winding up of the government evacuation scheme for old people', 1 February 1945.

[77] Ibid; ROA1183, *Government evacuation scheme: Residual problem – Old people.*

[78] Ibid; notes prepared for the Minister of Health for deputation from NOPWC and London OPWC on 'The return of elderly evacuees to London', 10 April 1945.

[79] Ibid; memorandum from Carruthers, 10 May 1945.

[80] Ibid; minutes of meeting between Ministry of Health officials and BRCS, 21 June 1945.

[81] Ibid; minutes of meeting between Ministry of Health officials and NOPWC, 20 June 1945. Similar complaints had been made at an earlier deputation on 26 April 1945. Age Concern Archives: Box Files 1-4.

[82] PRO HLG 7/535; memorandum from MacKinnon to Lindsay, 9 August 1945.

[83] Ibid; minutes of meeting on 'How to deal with aged evacuees', 30 August 1945.

[84] A copy of this can be found in PRO HLG 7/535.

[85] PRO HLG 7/118, *Termination of government evacuation scheme*; letter from Thigh to O'Gara, 3 November 1947 and memorandum from O'Gara to Carruthers, 10 November 1947.

[86] Ibid; draft letter to Regional Inspectors, November 1947.

[87] A copy of this can be found in PRO HLG 7/118.

[88] PRO HLG 7/395; memorandum from Barter to Sir Arthur Rucker, 5 May 1941.

THREE

Civilian morale and elderly people: the emergence of 'reforms' in residential and domiciliary welfare services

Introduction

Chapter Two outlined the complexity of evacuation arrangements during the Second World War and suggested this had a deleterious impact upon some sick and frail elderly people. Evacuation policy was seen as driven by a concern for the morale of the civilian population rather than as an attempt to meet the needs of dependent groups.

This chapter continues the theme of the importance of civilian morale and charts its relevance to the emergence of social policy reforms for elderly people in the period 1942-48. As the war progressed the care of elderly people 'at risk' became seen as important by the government because of the desire to be perceived as sympathetic to the needs of deserving groups. Subsequent to the publication of the Beveridge Report (1942), sensitivity to issues of social justice combined with the improved war situation opened the way for voluntary groups to argue for reforms in both residential and domiciliary services for older people. The extent and form in which the government responded to these pressures is a central feature of this chapter.

The Beveridge Report

The Inter-Departmental Committee on Social Insurance and the Allied Services was appointed in June 1941 by the Minister without Portfolio with terms of reference "to undertake, with special reference to the interrelation of schemes, a survey of existing national schemes of social insurance and the allied services including workmen's compensation, and to make recommendations". The committee was chaired by Sir William Beveridge and he soon came to dominate the review. His biographer, Jose Harris, claims this was because "the official members were all heavily engaged on other aspects of wartime administration, most of them had been evacuated out of London, and none of them had the time to prepare detailed alternatives to Beveridge's proposals" (Harris, 1977, p 385). As a result, it was decided that the final report should be signed by Beveridge alone and it became widely known as the Beveridge Report.

The report proposed a comprehensive system of insurance to meet the financial needs of those in sickness, unemployment and old age. It also envisaged the creation of some form of national health service and the replacement of the remaining poor law legislation. The report reflected a continuation of previous trends in state intervention rather than any really dramatic change in form and content. For this reason, George has described the report as "a middle-of-the-road document and like all such documents it represented no real threat to the position of the ruling class" (George, 1973, p 24).

The report, when published on 1 December 1942, received an enthusiastic response from the Labour movement and trade unions – an enthusiasm shared by the media, much of the business community and many backbench Conservative MPs. Harris (1981) suggests some civil servants and ministers (including Churchill) were less receptive because of concern about costs and a possible deflection of public attention away from war aims. Overall, however, a consensus seemed to be emerging "in favour of state planning and centralised bureaucratic control" (Harris, 1981, p 259) as envisaged by Beveridge. Disagreements tended to be over the timing and not the content of the proposals, although old age pensions were a notable exception (see Chapter Four). The White Paper on social insurance was presented to Parliament by the coalition government in 1944 although the 1946 National Insurance Act was steered through Parliament by the following Labour administration (Ministry of Reconstruction, 1944).

A crucial point about the report was that it coincided with the improved fortunes of Britain in the Second World War. It was published three weeks after El Alamein. The immediate threat from bombing and invasion was receding. As Addison explains:

> **From the time of the Beveridge Report, reconstruction became a priority for the government and a major focus of political**

> **debate. The report's implications reverberated throughout the remaining years of the war. (Addison, 1975, p 17)**

Titmuss has argued that the reason for this reverberating influence was the centrality of "the elusive concept of civilian morale" as "an imperative for war strategy" (Titmuss, 1963, p 82). The Second World War, unlike previous wars, depended on the efforts of the whole population rather than mainly on the armed forces so that it was not until three years of war that the enemy could claim to have killed as many British soldiers as women and children. As a result, "the war could not be won unless millions of ordinary people, in Britain and overseas, were convinced that we had something better to offer than our enemies – not only during but after the war" (Titmuss, 1963, p 82).

This chapter confirms the centrality of concern about civilian morale in government debates about social policy developments in the period during and just after the Second World War. In relation to welfare services for elderly people, this concern was expressed in discussions about the inadequacies of PAIs, and the early development of domiciliary services. It will be further shown how voluntary organisations were both a source of pressure for new services and also an avenue through which new services could be established. These organisations also wished to engage in the reconstruction debate[1] and so clarify their own role in relation to the proposed restructuring of state services.

Voluntary organisations and elderly people in the Second World War

Numerous voluntary organisations were involved in debates about services for elderly people in the Second World War and this section concentrates upon those that appeared to be most influential, namely, the British Red Cross Society, the Women's Voluntary Service and the National Old People's Welfare Committee. All three organisations not only pointed to service deficiencies but claimed a capacity to provide services themselves. They not only engaged in a debate about the need for reforms, but also actively attempted to influence conceptions of the division between the responsibilities of the state and those of voluntary organisations.

The above list excludes the National Federation of Old Age Pensions Associations (NFOAPA), which was formed in March 1939 and campaigned vigorously for pension reform (for a brief history, see Dunn, no date). In many ways its style resembled the abrasive approach of 1960s pressure groups such as Shelter rather than the more staid 'non-political' approach of the organisations examined in this book. For example, the Association's evidence (Beveridge Report, 1942b) to the Beveridge Committee was very different in form and presentation from that provided by most other organisations. It called for a pension of thirty shillings a week for every man and woman on reaching sixty "to be given as a right and just reward for services rendered in producing the wealth of the country" (Beveridge Report, 1942b, p 238). It attacked the rules and regulations of the Assistance Board which led to a failure to deal with "the total social welfare of the aged" (p 242). It criticised voluntary organisations for attempting to run hostels and homes for old people since:

> **... they cannot touch even the fringe of what is required, are administering palliatives, mitigating the evil, which by a National effort needs totally eradicating. It is a National responsibility which should and must primarily be that of the Government, and not that of a voluntary organisation. (Beveridge Report, 1942b, p 242)**

At the same time, it did not see institutional provision as meeting the main needs of sick and frail elderly people. Such people preferred to live in their own homes, perhaps with regular visits from the district nurse. Adequate pensions would reduce the numbers who felt it necessary to apply for institutional care. The minority who did require such care needed a homely atmosphere. There was a danger that "authorities who are now scrapping their barrack-like workhouses will replace them by modern palaces of hygiene" (Beveridge Report, 1942b, p 241).

The above analysis may have led the NFOAPA to concentrate its efforts on campaigning about pensions and to ignore issues of social and medical provision for frail and sick elderly people. There was no evidence that the NFOAPA was included in any of the Ministry of Health discussions about such issues, discussions that are reviewed in the rest of this chapter. At the same time, the Association's analysis and frame of reference clashed very clearly with the perceptions of most officials from the Ministry of Health. Its campaigning style was unlikely to have been appreciated. A positive decision may have been taken to exclude the Association from the relevant discussions although no evidence was traced of any NFOAPA attempt to establish such a dialogue. (The process of exclusion for voluntary groups who use a frame of reference not acceptable to the state is discussed in the context of local government by Dearlove, 1973.)

The British Red Cross Society (BRCS) is a very different type of voluntary organisation (for a general history, see Oliver, 1966). The basis of their work is still the Geneva Convention of 1864 which encouraged the formation of voluntary societies to help the wounded in time of war. Although Britain signed the 1864 convention, it was not until 1870 that 'the National Society for aid to the Sick and Wounded in War' was formed. This soon became known as the British Red Cross Society. In the First World War, it was involved in the provision of nursing facilities, forming 1,920 Voluntary Aid Detachments. During the Second World War, the BRCS played a major role in the staffing of the EMS and so the organisation was constantly involved in questions of who should nurse or look after the 'chronic sick and infirm' (for a detailed history of the BRCS activities during the Second World War see Cambray and Briggs, 1949). However, not all the work of the BRCS was of a nursing nature. A more general welfare function was also developing:

> **Welfare as a distinct branch of Red Cross work started during the 1939-45 War, a good deal of social help being given in air-raid shelters, and to civilian air-raid casualties, combined with First Aid treatment. It was also found that many needs of Service patients in hospital could be met by Red Cross members who were not nurses, but who could serve the patients by writing letters, giving entertainments, and in many ways providing the diversion and occupation so necessary to recovery. (Gilmour, 1951)**

The development of this welfare function led the Ministry of Health to include the BRCS in early discussions about meals on wheels and home help services. It also led the BRCS to develop its own residential homes for elderly people.

The Women's Voluntary Service (WVS) was formed in 1938 as "a new women's organisation sufficiently flexible to cope with unimagined difficulties likely to arise in Civil Defence" (Beauman, 1977, p 6). The initiative came from the Home Office and seems to have represented a desire both to mobilise volunteers to perform specific functions and also to establish an organisation that could reduce the danger of civilian panic during bombing raids. This was reflected in the principles agreed between the Home Secretary and the WVS founder, the Dowager Marchioness of Reading:

The aims of the organisation should be:

- to stimulate the enrolment of women in the Air Raid Precaution Services so as to bring the number of women in those services up to mobilisation strength as soon as possible;
- to bring home to all women, especially women in the household, what air raids mean and what they can do for their families and for themselves. (Graves, 1948, p 2)

The new organisation consisted of an advisory council representative of all the main women's organisations in the country, and a small executive committee of selected persons. The WVS would offer their services only when invited by local authorities, and all their costs would be paid by the Home Office.

Was the WVS a voluntary organisation? Rooff, in her classic 1957 study of *Voluntary societies and social policy*, defined such organisations as providing "some form of social service, which control their own policy, and which depend in part at least upon financial support from voluntary sources" (Rooff, 1957, p xiii). The WVS does use volunteers but has always been very heavily dependent on central government funds. Lady Reading described it as "a national voluntary service ... existing primarily to serve central and local government in the carrying out of legislation helpful to the life of the nation" (Lady Reading, 1948). It is perhaps more appropriate to perceive it as starting out as an arm of state security which is also available in civil emergencies and to support people in difficulty.

The WVS does present itself very clearly as a voluntary organisation and in the 1940s was treated in negotiations with Ministry of Health officials over welfare services as such an organisation. For this reason, it is treated here, as elsewhere, as if it were part of the voluntary sector but with the reservation that it does have a security function that places it in a very different relationship to central government than other voluntary organisations. It was directly responsible to the Ministry of Home Security during the operation of the Second World War and had a senior civil servant seconded as its General Secretary from 1938-40 (this was Dame Mary Smieton; see Graves, 1948, pp 5-8).

During the early stages of the war there was considerable debate about the boundaries of the Women's Voluntary Service work[2] . How narrowly should civil defence work be defined? For example, in April 1940 the Ministry of Home Security asked the General Secretary of the WVS to make sure they were consulted before new work was undertaken "so that we shall be in a position to satisfy ourselves (or outside critics) that there is no more suitable body available to undertake the work, and that it is not so far removed from a reasonable interpretation of 'civil defence' that, however, beneficial the work, it is clearly outside the scope of our powers to subsidise it from Home Office or Home Security Funds"[3]. In July 1940, the Ministry of Home Security expressed its concern to the Ministry of Health about "the increasing absorption of the Women's Voluntary Service organisation in activities which go far beyond the sphere of civil defence"[4].

Despite these doubts the WVS became heavily involved in service provision for the civilian population. This was true in relation to evacuation arrangements, rest centre services and communal feeding facilities. For example, the 1942 Annual Report indicated they had 1,145 mobile canteens intended primarily to help civilians in the aftermath of bombing raids but which, while standing by, served outlying units of the forces, and dockers and industrial workers on a temporary basis[5]. Mechanisms were eventually established by which the WVS could be financed by government departments other than the Ministry of Home Security and the Home Office[6].

With regard to services for elderly people, the WVS played a major role in the period 1942-48. It was given major responsibility for the evacuation of elderly people during the flying bomb scare of 1944 (see Chapter Two) and it initiated developments in residential care, the home help and meals on wheels services.

The National Old People's Welfare Council (NOPWC) is the last voluntary organisation to be considered in this section. It was established at the time of the mass bombing raids but its genesis preceded that period. As the NOPWC has undergone several changes of name it is perhaps important to begin by outlining what these were:

- Autumn 1940-January 1941: Committee for the Welfare of the Aged
- January 1941-May 1944: Old People's Welfare Committee
- May 1944-July 1955: National Old People's Welfare Committee
- July 1955-December 1970: National Old People's Welfare Council
- January 1971 onwards: Age Concern.

George Haynes, the Secretary of the National Council of Social Services (NCSS) explained the establishment of the original Committee in a letter to the BBC in the following words:

> **When the Assistance Board was charged with the administration of supplementary pensions for old people, its officers realised something of the loneliness suffered by the old age pensioners**

> **under their care and it was mainly for this reason that the Board suggested to this Council the desirability of setting up a representative Committee to co-ordinate and extend work for the welfare of old people. This Committee was formed in the autumn of 1940 and meets under the Chairmanship of Miss Eleanor Rathbone, MP.[7]**

As early as May 1940, a principal officer from the Assistance Board was expressing concern to the Ministry of Health about the inability of visiting officers from the Board to perform all the functions of the old relieving officer[8]. This officer also raised the issue with Dorothy Keeling who had been seconded to the NCSS from the Liverpool Personal Service Society to establish a national system of Citizens Advice Bureaux (Keeling, 1961, p 137). She obtained permission from NCSS to hold an exploratory meeting to consider the establishment of "a national committee for the care and general welfare of the aged". At this stage, the focus was on the general isolation and loneliness of old age rather than the disruption caused by the war. This had changed by the time of the exploratory meeting on 13 September and the subsequent conference on 7 October 1940. Delegates from the 12 organisations attending heard how elderly people had lost the support of relatives who had been called up in the armed forces or evacuated out of London. Domestic help could no longer be bought because of labour shortages. Those needing residential care were being offered places in large PAIs. There were too few voluntary homes, no general register and no system of inspection of those homes that did exist. Such problems led to a decision to form the 'Committee for the Welfare of the Aged' to coordinate the work already being done for the old and to extend its scope; the new committee would be convened by the NCSS (Roberts, 1970, pp 30-40)[9].

In her commissioned study of the NOPWC, Roberts mentions certain organisations, including the Ministry of Health, which failed to respond to invitations to the conference. She claims "the fact that they did not reply was as likely to have meant that their headquarters had moved or been bombed out of London as that they were uninterested or felt unable to help" (Roberts, 1970, p 32). However, in the case of the Ministry of Health, sections of it were hostile to the new organisation and remained so for some considerable time[10]. The Public Assistance Division of the Ministry of Health refused to send representatives to the meetings on 13 September and 7 October 1940 not only because they were too busy but also because they felt certain

Assistance Board officials were manipulating the situation to increase pressure on the Ministry of Health to establish 'reforms' in service provision for elderly people[11].

Individual cases raised by the new committee with this division tended to be about those removed from rest centres and public air raid shelters (Roberts, 1970, pp 34-5). Where had they been sent and how were they being treated? Were they being treated as war victims or as inmates of PAIs? Such enquiries upset the Public Assistance Division which complained that "although they cheerfully assume that the Public Assistance Department is concerned, it is clear that most of the cases they are troubled about, although maintained in PAIs are not Poor Law cases at all but various sorts of lodgers, shelter derelicts, rest centre EMS cases, evacuees"[12]. In other words, they were the responsibility of the Evacuation Division of the Ministry of Health.

The new committee appears to have quickly learnt the importance of this distinction and to have established simultaneous negotiations with both divisions over service provision for elderly people. No attempt will be made to outline all the activities of the OPWC/NOPWC during the War. Below are some of the key areas in which it became involved.

- *Support for evacuated elderly people:* as already indicated OPWC felt considerable concern about the future of those evacuated from rest centres and public air raid shelters at the height of the mass bombing raids. They established visiting schemes (see Chapter Two) and frequently complained about the regimes within these supposedly EMS establishments.
- *Campaign for increased provision for the 'elderly infirm':* OPWC pointed out the lack of hostel provision for the 'elderly infirm' and called for a major expansion of provision in this area. As seen in Chapter Two, the Ministry of Health always opposed this as impractical in wartime although they did increase hostel provision for 'infirm' people who had actually been made homeless from the bombing raids.
- *Voluntary hostels:* OPWC argued the need for a general expansion of voluntary hostel provision. Many elderly people needed some form of institutional care because of the disruption caused by the war. However, many groups failed to qualify for existing hostels for evacuees and the homeless or felt this provision to be inappropriate. Unless voluntary hostel provision could be increased, such people would be forced to seek admission to public assistance institutions.
- *Old people's homes advisory service:* OPWC attempted to collate information about private billets, private homes and voluntary homes.

It accepted referrals from elderly people seeking such accommodation and attempted to place them. This service generated a considerable volume of work: from 17 October to 21 November 1942, 124 applications were received and 54 people were placed[13]. The work proved time-consuming and expensive. The casework specialists at the NCSS felt that the organisers of the advisory service lacked the expertise to assess each applicant[14], and the service was handed over to the Charity Organisation Society on a trial basis in July 1944[15].

- *The development of local committees:* these developed slowly in the period 1940-46 and then speeded up after the publication of a model constitution in February 1946. Roberts claims this stressed that "the primary function of a local committee was less to take action itself than to co-ordinate action already being taken by existing bodies and to make action possible by inducing co-operation between different agencies" (Roberts, 1970, p 74). Samson (1944, p 42) claims that 70 such committees existed in 1944 while the 1952 Progress Report of the NOPWC referred to 12 regional, 49 county and 831 local OPWCs (NOPWC, 1952, p 3).
- *Reform of PAIs:* OPWC was very critical of the larger PAIs and campaigned for major reforms. Samson, when secretary of the OPWC, explained the situation in the following way:

> **These buildings are not easy to improve or adapt and are often such as to defy all efforts to produce anything akin to a homelike atmosphere.... The residents – termed 'inmates' – are generally accommodated in very large wards, and the homogeneaity of the equipment, the precision of its arrangement and the scrupulous tidiness which is everywhere apparent, inevitably conduce to an institutional atmosphere. (Samson, 1944, p 46)**

The next section looks at how pressure for reform of residential provision for elderly people built up in the 1940s, and the influence upon this pressure of wartime experience of smaller hostels and voluntary homes.

The campaign for reform of public assistance institutions

This section examines developments in residential care for elderly people from 1941 to 1948. The 1948 National Assistance Act abolished the term 'public assistance institution' and placed on local authorities the duty to provide accommodation to all who needed care and attention, regardless of their financial circumstances. The central message of Aneurin Bevan (Minister of Health) when introducing the Bill to Parliament was that "the workhouse is to go" and was to be replaced for elderly people by 'special homes' for up to 30 residents (*Hansard*, House of Commons, vol 443, 24 November 1947, col 1609). The detailed politics of the 1948 Act are explored in Chapter Four. This section looks at the build-up of pressure on the Ministry of Health to 'reform' PAIs. This pressure was often organised by voluntary organisations and effectively used the general public interest in postwar reconstruction.

Chapter Two explained how evacuation hostels and rest homes for elderly people were seen as being for war victims and so the restrictions associated with PAIs were seen as inappropriate. For example, residents kept their pension. A pamphlet on rest homes in London stated that residents:

> **... must contribute to their maintenance if able to do so. Full cost is 30s. Those unable to pay this amount will be expected to contribute their income less 3s.6d. a week to be retained for pocket money (6s. for married couples).**[16]

The resident was also offered far more freedom than that available to most inmates of PAIs. They could be "visited by their friends at all reasonable times". They could also go out whenever they wished and could take up to 14 days leave without being considered to have left the home.

As already seen, attempts by OPWC to persuade the Ministry of Health to extend such provision to all 'elderly infirm' people received a blunt refusal on the grounds that they were a low priority in wartime. The OPWC, therefore, decided to exploit its special relationship with the Assistance Board. As early as August 1941, one of its leading members (Margaret Hill) was putting the case to a senior official of the Board about "the great need for accommodation in residential homes for old people who have not suffered directly from bombing but who owing to various difficulties cannot manage for themselves at the present time"[17]. The OPWC argued for Assistance Board support in setting up voluntary hostels for this group on the grounds that Section 10(4) of the 1940 Old Age and Widows Pension Act placed on the Board a duty to promote the welfare of elderly people. OPWC were asking for a special high rate of supplementary pension for voluntary hostel residents so that the running costs of hostels could be met. Both the Public Assistance and Evacuation

Divisions of the Ministry of Health opposed this plan[18]. Nevertheless, the Assistance Board decided to go ahead[18] as explained by the chairman of the Board in December 1941:

> **The Board have had under consideration the position of pensioners who are not in need of continuous medical or nursing services but are nevertheless so shaky that it would clearly be in their interests that they should have special care and attention which may not be available in their homes. We have, therefore, arranged to facilitate the setting up of hostels for old people who cannot otherwise receive the attention which they need. We have agreed to increase the supplementary pension normally given to a sum which should be sufficient to provide the person with an income of 30s. per week. This, we understand, would enable many voluntary organisations to establish and maintain such hostels. (Speech on 'The welfare of the aged' by Lord Soulbury to NCSS)**

This last statement proved too optimistic. By December 1945, the Assistance Board was funding residents in only 26 such hostels (Assistance Board, 1946). Despite this, they created a considerable stir both within the Ministry of Health and from the local authorities.

The Evacuation Division of the Ministry of Health argued that the new hostels were outside their province since the hostels were not catering for evacuated or homeless people. At first, the Public Assistance Division seemed sympathetic to the case for voluntary hostels. It stated that the public assistance powers of local authorities might be used to help voluntary organisations set up hostel schemes so that "the immediate problem, therefore, is to see how far Public Assistance powers can be used to help the old people ... by co-operation with the interested voluntary organisations and without stressing the powers under which the local authorities give their help"[19] (that is, Poor Law legislation). This position, however, hardened after a meeting between civil servants from this division and representatives from the public assistance departments of the London County Council, Surrey, Kent[20] and Middlesex. The local authority side made four main points:

- Public Assistance Authorities in the Home Counties can, even in existing circumstances, provide for all old people requiring hostel treatment;

- the suggestion that provision by local authorities is more expensive than by voluntary agencies is based on a fallacy;
- local authority homes are superior to anything that a voluntary agency would provide;
- the Poor Law stigma is overemphasised[21].

The OPWC was informed by an Assistant Secretary at the Ministry of the flavour of these discussions and he warned that "we could not properly give any general promise of help in the establishment of new voluntary homes by certifying that materials or equipment wanted for the purpose were required urgently and necessarily in the national interest"[22].

Leading members of OPWC attempted to overcome this resistance by a direct approach to the Minister of Health (Ernest Brown). They complained about the lack of cooperation they were receiving from ministry officials. They stressed that one result of a growth of voluntary hostels would be a release of chronic sick hospital beds occupied by patients who were able to get up daily and needed only limited care[23]. After these meetings, senior officials from the Public Assistance Division tended to be less hostile to voluntary hostels in direct negotiations with OPWC. A willingness to help with finding buildings and equipment was expressed so long as no attempt was made to create "a privileged class of necessitous aged persons"[24]. Internal correspondence suggests that such officials remained unconvinced of the need for such voluntary provision. A Principal Secretary referred to a ministry view "that the provision of homes for the aged is properly a function of local authorities to be undertaken as a charge on local rates, and that the establishment on a voluntary basis of a further organisation for the purpose subsidised from exchequer funds will be indefensible"[25].

This last comment could also be taken to represent a fear that OPWC proposals would lead to a system of voluntary provision for the middle class and PAI provision for the working class. Before the war, the Ministry of Health had seemed actively to encourage a dual system of local authority provision – large institutions for the 'undeserving' and special small homes for the 'deserving' (see Chapter Two). Such a policy became more problematic in wartime. Voluntary hostels might help to deflect attention away from the inadequacy of PAI provision by 'creaming off' the more middle-class applicant. At the same time, government support for such a dual system could easily lead to criticism of unfair social provision at a time when the war effort demanded civilian unity. However, at the beginning of 1943 there was still no sign of a general acceptance from central and local government that PAIs needed major reform.

It is dangerous to point to newspaper correspondence in one national paper as triggering off a more defensive attitude to PAIs especially when it has not proved possible to establish a direct link between this correspondence and departmental thinking. The letters began to appear in March 1943 in the *Manchester Guardian* and covered numerous aspects of conditions in such institutions. Extracts from these letters were presented by Samson in *Old age in the new world.* She claimed the initial letter called 'A workhouse visit' "aroused extraordinary interest in various part of the country"(Samson, 1944, p 47). It is not known if the OPWC initiated this correspondence through one of its members, but they certainly contributed to the later correspondence.

The initial writer spoke of a workhouse visit to "a frail, sensitive, refined old woman" of 84 who was forced to live in the following regime:

> **But down each side of the ward were ten beds, facing one another. Between each bed and its neighbour was a small locker and a straight-backed, wooden uncushioned chair. On each chair sat an old woman in workhouse dress, upright, unoccupied. No library books or wireless. Central heating, but no open fire. No easy chairs. No pictures on the walls.... There were three exceptions to the upright old women. None was allowed to lie on her bed at any time throughout the day, although breakfast is at 7 am, but these three, unable any longer to endure their physical and mental weariness, had crashed forward, face downwards, on to their immaculate bedspreads and were asleep. (Samson, 1944, p 47)**

The response to the letter was sufficiently intense and voluminous to encourage an official from the Public Assistance Division of the Ministry of Health to provide an interview (Samson, 1944, pp 48-9) on the criticisms to a *Manchester Guardian* reporter. The official asked that all examples of bad conditions should be sent to the Ministry although he admitted that the desired standard was sometimes difficult to achieve in wartime. He stressed that staff shortages during the war had led to an emphasis on care rather than the provision of activities but that OPWCs "had been excellent in helping with amenities". Old people could wear their own clothes in PAIs as long as they were suitable. Where this was not the case, the clothes provided were not uniforms and they "shall not be recognisable as 'workhouse' clothes". Overall he emphasised that "the war has interrupted the early stages of substantial improvements in the care of old people ...

but experiments in requisitioned country houses and evacuation hostels have brought valuable lessons for the future". He thought these had shown that older people were better suited in smaller units than had been envisaged before the war. The shift in policy appears considerable compared to the earlier hostility to the OPWC and complacency about conditions in PAIs.

The extent to which residential provision for elderly people had become more of an important public issue was confirmed by the decision of the Ministry of Health to provide an advisory member to the Nuffield Foundation survey committee on the problems of ageing and the care of old people. The third objective of the Nuffield Foundation is, in the words of the Trust Deed, "the care and comfort of the aged person". The Secretary of the Foundation in his foreword to the eventual report claimed the survey committee was established to provide the Foundation with a proper basis on which to decide future action in pursuit of this objective (L. Farrer-Brown, 1980).

Age Concern Archives suggest the genesis of the committee may have been more complex. The Chairman of the Trustees of the Nuffield Foundation had shown interest in the Old People's Home Advisory Service in May 1943 and expressed concern that its closure was being considered because of the size of the problem and the lack of casework expertise among OPWC staff. A subsequent meeting was held between OPWC and the Secretary and Chairman of the Nuffield Foundation in June 1943. OPWC expressed a hope that Nuffield might fund the advisory service after some kind of more general investigation[26].

This triggered off the idea of a survey committee and by Autumn 1943 the Ministry of Health was being asked to offer support. This was given and the Chief General Inspector for PAIs was appointed as observer with discretion "to make available to the inquiry body any relevant facts and figures in the possession of the Ministry"[27]. Seebohm Rowntree was appointed chairman in January 1944 and the report was published in 1947. By this time, negotiations over the 1948 National Assistance Act (see Chapter Four) were well advanced and there was already agreement on the need to abolish the remaining Poor Law legislation, including that covering residential institutions.

The first half of the Nuffield Foundation report deals with the incomes of elderly people, and the second half with housing, homes and institutions. The report makes the case for sweeping away PAIs and replacing them with smaller homes (personal correspondence with Professor Roger Wilson, 10 May 1983). The report pointed out that many PAIs were built in the early decades of the 19th century, were structurally inadequate, and:

> **Day-rooms in such institutions are usually large and cheerless with wooden windsor armchairs placed around the walls. Floors are mainly bare boards, with brick floors in lavatories, bathrooms, kitchens and corridors. In large urban areas such institutions may accommodate as many as 1,500 residents of various types, including more than a thousand aged persons. (Rowntree, 1980, p 64)**

In some of these institutions "rules are harsh or harshly administered while residents often showed acute apathy". This was not to say that some institutions were not of more modern design and more flexible over rules but these were apt to be something of 'showpieces' because local authorities carefully selected residents on the basis of "character, background, and alertness" (Rowntree, 1980, p 65). However, bad conditions were not limited to the public sector. For example, in some homes run for profit but not registered as nursing homes "the staff ratio ... is lower than it should be, sometimes as low as 1 to 15" (p 69) and the committee came across some shocking cases of cruel exploitation or neglect of old people. The report called for a system of statutory inspection for all voluntary and private homes.

The survey report recommended the provision of four main types of local authority home. The first of these was 'small homes' since "all normal old people who are no longer able to live an independent life shall be accommodated in small homes rather than in large institutions" (Rowntree, 1980, p 75) and these would cater for between 30 and 35 residents. Second, as an interim measure, medium sized institutions for up to 200 residents should be established. They should be home-like in their atmosphere and there should be a large degree of personal liberty. Third, there should be some 'general purpose institutions' because "a small proportion of old people may be permanently unsuited, by nature or temperament, to either of the foregoing types of institutions" (Rowntree, 1980, p 76). Finally, there should be separate institutions for 'senile dements'. The report received considerable press coverage. An editorial in *The Times* on 15 January 1947 spoke of the 'Claim of the aged'. *The Daily Herald* ran a feature on 'Old people exploited in homes'; the *Daily Express* referred to 'Scandal of old folks homes' and the *Daily Mail* claimed 'Old folks live in shadows'[28].

The Nuffield Foundation survey committee was not the only source of pressure upon the Ministry of Health to reassess the role of PAIs. A limited number of articles and booklets also appeared which extolled the virtues of the small voluntary hostel, in which pension rights were retained and such homes were compared favourably to the large impersonal PAI. In January 1944, 'An old people's hostel' by Marjorie Rackstraw appeared in *Social Work (London)*. She painted a picture of a voluntary home in Hampstead where "crotchetiness and cantankerousness seem to dissolve in this calm" (Rackshaw, 1944, p 3); she concluded that "if all the Poor Law Institutions could be turned into factories and these small Hostels or Homes peppered all over England, Scotland and Wales, what a much happier country it would be, not only for the old people themselves, but for their relatives and friends, and also for those not yet old who begin to look forward to the future with apprehension and dread" (Rackshaw, 1944, p 4).

In Autumn 1943, the Friends Relief Service (FRS) produced a 45-minute 16mm silent film, entitled *Those who are old* (Staley, 1948, p 32) which focused on what had been learnt about the needs of elderly people in residential care from the evacuation hostels. In July 1945 a 30-page pamphlet on *Hostels for old people* (FRS, 1945) was published by the same organisation so that "as much as possible of the benefit of the experience of FRS and its predecessor bodies should be available to others working in the same field" (Staley, 1948, p 33). The central theme of the pamphlet was that:

> **It is beginning to be recognised – as much by Local Authorities who run them as by those who criticise them from the outside – that the large Institution is no adequate answer to the needs of the aged and that the dread of ending one's days there is very natural. Smaller, homelier places are needed whether they be provided by a Local Authority or by a voluntary hostel. (FRS, 1945, p 4)**

By this time, such views had become firmly accepted within the Public Assistance Division of the Ministry of Health. In September 1945, the Chief General Inspector not only stressed the need for change to his regional inspectorate but also the key role that the voluntary sector might be able to play in this process. He stressed that "voluntary agencies can help local authorities substantially by trying out various forms of institutional assistance for the 'new poor'"[29]. He also argued that residents in PAIs should be kept active and interested through good diets, plenty of books, and suitable games while "the term 'resident' in place of 'inmate' has advantages". Such elderly residents

> **... would probably be best housed in small Homes and the experience of wartime emergency services and experiments such as Mrs Hill's [a leading member of OPWC] voluntary hostels in Middlesex and East Ham Homes for bombed-out people suggest that small homes can be not only more satisfactory to the residents but at least as economical in cost if a suitable unit is chosen. (Hill, 1961, pp 23-39)**

However, the memorandum does admit that the two major obstacles to the development of hostels along these lines were lack of staff and lack of premises.

Over the next 15 months, before the publication of the Nuffield Report, the Ministry of Health received a growing pile of complaints from pressure groups, local authority associations and professional associations about inadequate hospital and residential provision for elderly people. Not all agreed on the need to base provision on small homes but nearly all agreed on the need to reform PAIs. Much of this correspondence was an attempt to influence the proposed 'reform' of the public assistance system that will be considered in detail in the next chapter. However, this pressure also influenced Ministry of Health officials in the Public Assistance Division who had to maintain a system that was soon to be ended. The National Association of Administrators of Local Government Establishments, for example, stated that they were seriously concerned at the prospect of uncoordinated policy over hostels for elderly people[30]. In April 1946, the AMC informed the Ministry of Health of the following resolution passed by its Social Welfare Committee:

> **That when the forthcoming legislation relating to the amendment of the Poor Law is under consideration provision should be made to enable local authorities to provide hostels or similar accommodation for aged persons who may not be capable of being entirely on their own.**[31]

In October 1946 the National Association of Local Government Social Welfare Officers attacked "the present deplorable conditions whereby the aged and chronic sick are deprived of the necessary care and attention to alleviate their pain and discomfort"[32]. The publication of the Nuffield Survey followed in January 1947 and this encouraged an even greater volume of complaints from MPs, individuals and organisations[33].

The NOPWC also continued to criticise the quality of provision for both those in chronic sick hospitals and PAIs. Fred Messer MP (Chairman of NOPWC and a member of the Nuffield Survey Committee) wrote to Bevan in October 1946[34] about these issues and this led to a major deputation to the Ministry of Health in November 1946[35]. At that meeting, Olive Matthews from the NOPWC called for an extension of freedom within PAIs along the lines she had suggested before the war in *Housing the infirm* (Matthews, no date). The response of the Ministry of Health to such criticism was *Circular 49/47* (Ministry of Health, 1947a)[36] on 'The care of the aged in public assistance homes and institutions', which one civil servant saw as the direct result of the above deputation[37].

This Circular drew the attention of local authorities to the Nuffield Survey (Rowntree, 1980) and mentioned forthcoming legislation (the 1948 National Assistance Act) but stated that in the meantime, public assistance authorities should consider what action could be taken immediately to improve arrangements for existing elderly residents. The Circular called for the resumption of the building of small homes and made it clear that the Minister would be prepared to consider schemes for the acquisition and adaptation of suitable premises for this purpose. The daily routine of the larger homes should also be improved to provide more freedom, especially in the following areas:

- visiting hours every day of the week;
- freedom to wear your own clothes;
- each resident should have their own wardrobe, chest of drawers or locker;
- clocking in and out regulations should be ignored.

The Circular also called for a general smartening up of the inside and outside of all PAIs through better chairs, pictures and handrails.

Issuing the Circular does not appear to have greatly reduced the worries of ministry officials about the ways in which the management of many of the larger PAIs could be open to scandal. On 9 October 1947, officials from the Public Assistance Division met under the chairmanship of their Assistant Secretary who explained that:

> **... the purpose of the meeting was to consider methods of securing a more effective 'follow up' to the reports made by the Inspectorate of their visits to Homes and Institutions for old people. The care of the aged was arousing considerable public attention, and the Department must not lay itself open**

> **to charges of inactivity such as were implied in the Curtis Report in regard to the supervision of Children's Homes[38].**

The officers agreed on the need for a careful filing of complaints from inspectors of homes and a follow-up system to make sure that the response of the local authority was known. The meeting ended with the compilation of "a list of authorities considered likely to require stimulus, in order that the relevant administrative files might receive special and early attention".

The attitude of central government to PAIs was very different in 1948 compared with 1942. They had become an embarrassment and were seen as out of keeping with other social reforms of postwar reconstruction. The extent of this embarrassment can perhaps be best judged when it is appreciated that *Circular 49/47* was mainly a restatement of previous circulars from over 50 years previously. Macintyre points out how:

> **Circulars issued by the Local Government Board in 1895 and 1896 laid down principles of workhouse administration for the elderly in complete contrast to those set out ... two decades earlier. The elderly were to be given a better diet, tobacco, more privacy in their sleeping arrangements, better physical facilities and allowed to receive visitors and pay visits themselves. (Macintyre, 1977, p 47)**

These circulars had never been implemented by local authorities. The issue of institutional regime had faded from public view as debate became focused on such issues as pensions and mass unemployment. Townsend has claimed there was "a conspiracy of silence" (1964, p 17) although it was shown in Chapter Two how this was beginning to ease in the period just before the Second World War. The re-emergence of this reform movement was blocked by the war. It was not until the end of the main bombing raids and the publication of the Beveridge Report that such letters as 'A workhouse visit' and the pressure group tactics of the OPWC brought any major response from the Public Assistance Division of the Ministry of Health. What is less clear is the extent to which a sympathy towards reform was speeded up by the return of a Labour government in 1945 and the development of detailed plans to reform the public assistance system (see Chapter Four). Local authority associations and local authority officials probably began to feel a need to distance themselves from the old system of institutional care, which they seemed reluctant to attempt when the OPWC 30 shilling hostels were first established with Assistance Board support.

The development of domiciliary welfare services for elderly people

The opening section of this chapter stressed the importance of considerations of civilian morale in the genesis of social policy development in the period 1942-48. This general point is now illustrated by outlining the early growth of home help and meals on wheels services for elderly people.

The home help service

The first statutory power to permit the appointment of home helps was contained in the 1918 Maternity and Child Welfare Act, and these powers continued under the 1936 Public Health Act (for a brief review of this early history, see Burr, 1949, p 3). Local authorities were empowered to provide home help assistance during a mother's lying-in period, whether the confinement took place at home or elsewhere. The duties of home helps were seen as being the ordinary domestic duties usually undertaken by the mother including cleaning, cooking, washing and the general care of children. Burr (1949), Nepean-Gubbins (1972) and Richey (1951) all describe how this service was extended to households containing sick and frail elderly people in December 1944 through Ministry of Health *Circular 179/44*. Burr claims:

> **The Minister of Health was distressed at the position of sick or infirm persons who were unable to obtain either hospital accommodation – which was much limited in the number of beds – or help in the homes of which they were particularly in need. Moreover, it was apparent that many of these sick or infirm people, many of whom were aged, were quite unable to pay for the service they required. (Burr, 1949, p 3)**

Richey paints a similar picture stressing that "during the war the plight of many households where the mother or housewife was laid aside or absent by acute illness or other family emergency, induced the Government to authorise measures of emergency help" (Richey, 1951, p 1).

This would suggest that the main drive behind this policy was the wish to prevent sick and frail elderly people from having to enter residential or hospital care. As the Chief General Inspector at the Ministry of Health explained in 1945,

> **... the general tendency of the various proposals being discussed and in some cases being carried into effect is to keep as many old people as possible in their own homes, or houses specially built for them, for as long as they can look after themselves, or can do so with some daily or weekly assistance with some of their household duties[39].**

Was this how and why the home help service was extended to elderly people during the Second World War? Or was it a concern with civilian morale in general rather than the needs of elderly people in particular that was the main reason for the reform? This second view was stated quite bluntly in a Ministry of Health letter to the Metropolitan Boroughs' Standing Joint Committee in June 1944:

> **... as you know, the Minister of Labour and our own Minister are concerned about the hardship which is arising owing to lack of domestic help in private households where there is sickness or where there are aged or infirm persons and the deleterious effects which this may have on service and civilian morale.[40]**

Concern about the lack of domestic help available for private householders surfaced quite early in the war. According to the Census of 1931 (Markham/Hancock Report; Ministry of Labour and National Service, 1945, p 4) 70,409 males and 1,332,224 females were classified as domestic servants. Of these 35,693 males and 1,142,655 females were in private service. In 1931, nearly half a million private families or 4.8% of all private families employed resident domestics; rather more than three quarters of this total (that is, 375,000 or 3.7% of private families) had a single servant apiece. Such numbers were dramatically reduced after the outbreak of the Second World War. Male servants were called up into the armed services. Many female servants moved into the aircraft and munitions industries. Others merely took advantage of increased job opportunities in the early part of the war to move into other forms of work.

This was raised as a problem by certain MPs for a variety of reasons.

Middle-class families were struggling to cope with sickness among their children and elderly relatives (*Hansard*, House of Commons, vol 383, 22 October 1942, col 2072; speech by Eleanor Rathbone). Sick elderly people were failing to gain admittance to hospital and so needed domestic servants to look after them (*Hansard*, House of Commons, vol 385, 26 November 1942, col 840; speech by Sir Leonard Lyle). People with large homes were reluctant to offer billets for the homeless and other groups, if they could not obtain servants to carry out the domestic chores (*Hansard*, House of Commons, vol 374, 7 October 1941, col 1091; speech by Sir Henry Morris Jones). A report produced by the Ministry of Labour and National Service summed up the situation in the following way:

> **The overriding claims of aircraft and munitions have swept the vast majority of maids, trained and untrained alike, into essential national war work. But total war has brought great sufferings and hardships to countless households; especially to families which include the aged, the sick, and young children. Family life among the middle and upper classes in this country has for generations rested largely on the assumption of domestic help of some kind being available.... The single-handed care of an old-fashioned house with stone passages, coal fires and an antiquated range has proved a heavy task during the war for a mistress bereft of her maids. There is much evidence of strain and consequent ill health. (Markham/Hancock Report, 1945, p 4)**

This quotation underlined the extent of concern to maintain the availability of working-class women as domestic workers for middle-class professional families. It was felt that "the demand of the girl who has had a modern education, for personal liberty and self expression is much too strong for any acceptance of an existence wholly circumscribed by home work" (Markham/Hancock Report, 1945, p 8). The report called for a raising of the status of domestic work by establishing it as a form of day work, rather than residential work, in which servants would receive training from a new organisation called the National Institute of Houseworkers (Markham/Hancock Report, 1945, p 11).

However, by the time of this report, local authority home help services had already been extended to households with sick and infirm elderly people. Some pressure for such a change had existed prior to the war. In

August 1939, one MP had called for "an extension of power to local authorities to enable them to provide a service of home helps generally, in cases of non-infectious illness and also to assist aged persons, similar to the existing service of home helps for expectant and nursing mothers and children under five years of age" (*Hansard*, House of Commons, vol 350, 3 August 1939, col 2650; speech by Mrs Adamson). The then Minister of Health (Colonel Elliott) refused to introduce new legislation (*Hansard*, House of Commons, vol 350, 3 August 1939, col 2651). As already indicated, the availability of domestic help continued to be raised in the period 1939-44 although the government response tended to be that it would show sympathy by allowing domestic servants to find frail elderly employers who needed help with household chores. In May 1944, the Joint Parliamentary Secretary to the Ministry of Labour explained this policy in the following way:

> **In these cases we will do our best to supply help. We give these jobs high priority, and if necessary, if there are no mobile older people available, we will allow young mobile people of ages at which they would normally be sent to the factories, to go to those houses; and in cases where there is doubt whether hardship exists and whether a young person who would otherwise be employed in the highest military production should be allowed to go to the household, we ask our women's panels to advise us. (*Hansard*, House of Commons, vol 399, 4 may 1944, col 1572)**

However, he also indicated that negotiations were taking place with the Ministry of Health and local authorities to see if existing home help arrangements could be extended to include other groups such as sick or frail elderly people.

By 1944 there had already been some extension of existing home help arrangements under the 1936 Public Health Act through central government encouragement of local authority and voluntary organisation activity[41]. In November 1942, the Minister of Health issued to all local authorities in England Circular 2729, informing them that the Minister of Labour and National Service had agreed to regard home helps employed under their maternity and child welfare scheme as doing "work of national importance". This Circular recommended that women over 40 should be encouraged to take up this work where it was needed, and that the need should be made known both to the Labour Exchange and to the local offices of the WVS. This seems to have encouraged the WVS to become more involved in this issue; they were already offering volunteers to carry out domestic chores in "the larger old-fashioned type of house" where "the householder is willing to give board and lodging to four or more workers"[42].

The pressure for some form of extension of the home help service was building up. A WVS report explains the pressures in the following way:

> **By the autumn of 1943 it was clear that prompt and vigorous action must be taken if the nation's health, and its war effort, were not to be gravely affected. Much compassionate leave had to be granted to service men and women, and there was considerable absenteeism among women munition workers. Later that year a serious widespread influenza epidemic led to an appeal by the Ministry of Health to the St John Ambulance Brigade, the British Red Cross Society and WVS. The three organisations mutually agreed to give what help they could, and to circulate the appeal to their members.[43]**

The Ministry of Health wrote to borough and district councils (*Circular 2897*) suggesting that they should use their powers as widely as possible to provide home helps, and stating that the Ministry's Chief Medical Officer had informed medical officers of health of the voluntary help available to meet emergencies caused by the influenza epidemic[43]. In other words, volunteers could be used to aid families which could not receive help from paid employees of the local authorities under existing legislation. Several specific schemes were established by branches of the main voluntary organisations as a result of these developments. A major scheme was being planned for Oxford in the period 1943/44 by the WVS[44] while the Berkshire branch of the BRCS established a home help scheme in Windsor. The 1945 Annual Report of the BRCS made perhaps rather inflated comments about the overall impact of this latter scheme:

> **It is interesting that the new Defence Regulations giving powers to Local Authorities to provide domestic help to households suffering hardship owing to sickness or emergency, covers precisely those contingencies which the Voluntary Home Help Scheme, at present operating in Windsor, under the Red Cross now covers. It is a fine example of voluntary initiatives and experiment being followed later by state action.(BRCS, 1946, p 27)**

The politics of this increased state action, however, was more complex than suggested by the above quotation.

By early 1944, Ernest Bevin and senior officials from the Ministry of Labour and National Service were pressing the Minister of Health (Willinck) for an extension of the home help service to include sick and frail elderly people. Officials at the Ministry of Health were far from convinced about this[45]. The initial objection was that there were not enough applicants for home help posts to meet the needs of expectant mothers, so there was little point in extending the scheme to other client groups. The Ministry of Labour replied that a new mother needed 24-hour care but the elderly only needed a couple of hours' support. In the end, the Ministry of Health seemed to have decided that if the Ministry of Labour could find the women, then local authorities should be willing to organise and employ them. However, despite this, some officials at the Ministry of Health were less than wholehearted in their enthusiasm for such a service. For example, an Assistant Secretary produced a report for her Minister on possible home help provision. She stressed it would be no good relying on the voluntary organisations since "we could not hope to make the service anything like complete except by means of local authorities"[45]. She ended the report by suggesting a reply from Willinck to Bevin:

> **I do indeed know of the consideration which you have been giving to the question of domestic help to institutions and individuals in urgent need and I have heard from my officers of the discussions they have had with yours about possible means of meeting the most urgent need of private households. The matter is, as you will have appreciated, full of difficulty. Local authorities are over-burdened with urgent work and already feel they are asked to do the impossible with depleted staffs. I am, however, intending to consult the Association of Local Authorities to see how much help they can give.**[45]

The suggested reply was sent off by Willinck on 9 May 1944 and Bevin's response, received on 18 May, was that a new deal for the sick and aged "will make a lot of difference to morale"[46]. The Ministry of Labour wished to see the new scheme operating for the coming Autumn and Winter.

The next stage for the Ministry of Health was to approach the local authority associations. In June 1944 the Metropolitan Boroughs' Standing Joint Committee replied that they would support the extension of the home help scheme to the aged and sick only on the clear understanding that the necessary legislation authorising the councils to undertake the work in question was obtained, that the whole of the cost was reimbursed by the government, and that the Minister of Labour would guarantee that the necessary administrative staff would be made available to the borough councils[47]. The Ministry was not slow to respond to the issue of reimbursement since the Treasury was contacted about the need for direct financing of the scheme on the grounds that "the position has now been reached where our Minister and the Minister of Labour are satisfied that definite action to remedy this unsatisfactory state of affairs must be taken without delay if service and civilian morale is not to suffer during the coming autumn and winter"[48]. This letter stressed how the new scheme of domestic help was separate from the existing scheme of home helps for maternity cases.

In June 1944, the CCA had been contacted by a letter which pointed out that they may have "seen a good deal in the press in the last month about the supply of domestic help to households that are in special straits" and "the Ministry of Labour is very anxious to have some scheme to meet this trouble on foot not later than the autumn of this year and has been pressing on our Minister the view that the best way to do this is with the assistance of the local authorities"[49]. In August 1944, officials from the Ministry of Health and the Ministry of Labour met representatives from the local authority associations[50]. All agreed on there being 'a real need' but some of those present expressed reservations about how easily the scheme could operate in rural areas. A week later the CCA wrote to the Ministry of Health stating they would support any scheme put forward but that they had grave doubts whether such a scheme would get off the ground because of lack of staff[51].

The Ministry of Health now lost little time. They decided new legislation was not required but that the Defence Regulations needed to be amended. A new clause 68E was inserted into the 1939 Defence (General) Regulations which stated that:

> **Any authority which is a welfare authority for the purposes of Part VII of the Public Health Act, 1936, or Part XII of the Public Health (London) Act, 1936, may, subject to the general approval of the Minister, make arrangements for providing domestic help for households where the provision of such help appears to be necessary for the prevention and mitigation of hardship, and may, if it appears necessary or desirable so to do, themselves to employ women to provide such help.**

The regulation went on to give welfare authorities power to delegate to urban and rural districts if they wished. A draft circular was prepared and sent to the local authority associations and other interested bodies. On 18 November 1944, the War Cabinet approved the proposed changes and *Circular 179/44* was issued in December.

Circular 179/44 was entitled 'Domestic help' (Ministry of Health, 1944)[52] and so the new scheme was distinguished from the existing provision of home helps for maternity cases. The 'reasonable expenses' incurred in the running of the new scheme would be reimbursed by the Ministry of Health unlike the home help cases where costs had to be met by the local authority. Domestic help cases were seen as likely to come from households:

- where the housewife falls sick or must have an operation;
- where the wife is suddenly called away to see her husband in hospital and arrangements have to be made to look after the children;
- with elderly people who are infirm, or one of whom suddenly falls ill;
- where several members are ill at the same time, for example, during an influenza epidemic.

The task of the local authority under the scheme was three-fold. First, they needed to appoint, and maintain a register of domestic helpers available for work at any time, and to arrange for their payment. Second, they would have to determine which were the most urgent of the applicants known to them. And lastly, they had to assess what part of the cost of the help provided should be recovered from each household, and to secure its payment. The Ministry of Labour had allowed the local authorities to appoint extra administrative and clerical staff to run the schemes. Finally, it was stressed that the need for this new service was greater in urban than in rural areas and it was suggested that an organised service should be established in the latter only after consultation with the Minister.

How quickly were domestic help schemes started by local authorities? It is not easy to answer this in detail, although by February 1945, the Ministry of Health had received 45 enquiries and 19 authorities were known to be establishing schemes (*Hansard*, House of Commons, vol 407, 8 February 1945, col 2245; speech by Sir Henry Willinck). This was not seen as satisfactory by the Ministry of Labour who persuaded the Ministry of Health of the need to carry out a general review of progress combined with a detailed investigation of six schemes, since such schemes had "not been introduced in many areas, but also that many schemes started have proved inadequate to meet local needs, owing mainly to inability to recruit sufficient helpers" (Ministry of Health, 1946b).[53] The resultant report[54], produced by the Deputy Chief Nursing Officer from the Ministry of Health and an official from the Ministry of Labour, praised the schemes at Lewisham and Oxford but were highly critical of the other four. The two 'successful' schemes had both invested considerable time in administration; in Lewisham this was carried out by a local authority employee, but in Oxford this was done by the WVS.

Circular 110/46 was issued in June 1946 and stressed this finding by stating that "in both cases the success achieved was attributed largely to the fact that those responsible for the scheme gave their whole time to it and to the enthusiasm and resource of the organiser in overcoming the difficulties inherent in the overall shortage of woman-power". More specifically, it was suggested that the home help and domestic help schemes should be run as one and known as the 'Home Helps Service'. Helpers should be used for clients from either service although separate records would have to be kept for accounting and grant purposes. The organiser needed to maintain a close link with clients and helpers. Helpers needed to be treated as part of a public service, while rates of wages, hours and conditions of employment should be clearly specified.

The Circular also stressed the potential value of the contribution of the WVS to the development of both the home help and domestic help services. A capable full-time organiser was essential to success and "the main advantage to the Welfare Authority of delegating the organisation of the scheme to a voluntary body is that the authority's own staff are relieved of the burden which may be particularly heavy in the early stages, when much outdoor visiting is generally involved". The Circular said all WVS regional officers now had a dossier on the Oxford scheme and local branches would consider establishing a similar scheme if paid to do so by the welfare authority.

Negotiations over this took place in February 1946. An Assistant Secretary from the Ministry of Health met two representatives of the WVS, including their Chief Administrator, and stated that "the Ministry is being pressed by the Minister for Labour and National Service to take some immediate action to impress welfare authorities with the genuine public need for the service"[55]. He went on to mention the success of the WVS scheme in Oxford and he asked the Chief Administrator whether she could inform the Ministry of Labour that the WVS would be willing to undertake similar work in other areas on behalf of welfare authorities and whether she thought welfare authorities would welcome their cooperation. As a result of this request, WVS must have sounded out opinions among their senior organisers since on 16 February 1946, the

Chief Administrator wrote back that "the general feeling of WVS at the moment is that they are prepared to help when directly asked by a local authority but that people are far too tired to go out and ask for work with the possibility of a rebuff into the bargain"[56].

This apparent reluctance to become more involved may have been tactical. It could have been a case of 'playing hard to get' in order to emphasise the importance and value of WVS organisers to local authorities with their staff shortages. This was crucial to WVS at the time because the continued existence of the organisation had been questioned by the Labour government (see below). Certainly as early as January 1946, the Oxford organiser had written to Lady Reading:

> **I am itching to get on with helping other areas to get Home Helps established, for until it becomes a National Uniformed Service, one will meet the kind of difficulty of customers enticing the Helps into private service which is contemptible but a constant temptation.**[57]

Also, in May 1946, the WVS sent a circular to all its senior organisers which called upon branches to follow the Oxford initiative of helping local authorities with the home help schemes since "any such plan of co-operation would have the full support of the Ministry of Health which is shortly issuing a circular to local authorities suggesting that they might approach WVS for co-operation"[58]. In April 1947, WVS headquarters sent a progress report to regional administrators on developments during the eight months following the issue of Circular 110/46. Out of the first 110 enquiries received, 55 were from local authorities, 45 from WVS organisers and 10 from various voluntary agencies. Of the 34 schemes that resulted from these enquiries, 24 were administered by WVS on behalf of the authorities concerned[59].

By this time, of course, the 1946 National Health Service Act had already passed through Parliament (see Chapter Four), including Section 29 which gave local authorities a permissive power to provide domestic help "for households where such help is required owing to the presence of any person who is ill, lying-in, an expectant mother, mentally defective, aged, or a child not over compulsory school age". On the appointed day, the old arrangements for reimbursing welfare authorities the whole of their expenditure under Defence Regulation 68E would cease; there would no longer be separate schemes of home helps and domestic help necessitating separate records and accounts, but instead a consolidated scheme of domestic help, which would be grant-aided on the same basis as other local authority health services.

To some extent, this was only a consolidation and clarification of existing legislation; the home help service had always been associated with child and maternity welfare and so its inclusion in Part III of the 1946 Act was hardly surprising. And yet certain interesting questions do remain to be answered. Were the local authority associations keen to see an expansion of this service? Were they upset at the loss of financial reimbursement obtained under the defence regulations? Above all, did the Ministry of Health need to be persuaded of the value of this service for households with sick and frail elderly members? There is some evidence that doubts remained, and this may have been reflected in the decision to make the service permissive rather than mandatory. Certainly S.F. Wilkinson, Assistant Secretary at the Ministry of Health, appeared to express doubts about the appropriateness of the service for elderly people at a major home help conference in 1947:

> **The needs of the ill, nursing and expectant mothers were obvious, provided they had no one on whom they could call. The aged should not be considered as having an automatic claim, but their circumstances should be investigated. The period of need should also be carefully watched and the amount of help to be given. Public funds must be protected. (Wilkinson, 1947)**

The needs of frail and sick elderly people were again to be given a lower priority than other dependent groups.

Health services to be provided by local authorities under the 1946 Act were outlined in *Circular 118/47* (Ministry of Health, 1947b). The main difficulty in the home help service was a shortage of 'woman power' to do the work in individual homes. The view was expressed that the National Institute of Houseworkers, set up as a result of the 1945 Ministry of Labour report on private domestic employment (Markham/Hancock Report; Ministry of Labour and National Service, 1945, p 4) would overcome the problem in the long run. In the meantime a good organiser could still find helpers with the appropriate skills so that:

> **The appointment of an able and energetic organiser seems, therefore, to be an essential first step in the inauguration of a scheme. She may be appointed directly by the authority, or**

seconded by a voluntary body (eg Women's Voluntary Service) on reimbursement terms.

Such organisers were seen as being in need of induction training and the circular suggested this could best be achieved through two-week courses to be run by the WVS. The first of these took place in February 1948 and the course was funded by the Ministry of Health[60]. Two months earlier, 400 delegates, most of them from local authorities, had attended a two-day WVS conference on the home help service in London. The WVS claimed the conference was "to provide an opportunity for Home Help Organisers to discuss some of their problems and pool ideas, as well as to enable Authorities who have not yet appointed Organisers to obtain information from those who are already operating a satisfactory service"[61]. Local authority delegate expenses were paid by the Ministry of Health. It was, also, of course, an ideal chance for the WVS to stress their potential role in the future growth of the service[62].

The 'welfare state reforms' of the late 1940s are often seen as a replacement of voluntary social provision by state services. The development of the home help service shows a more complex picture. The extension and development of the service during wartime was agreed reluctantly by the Ministry of Health; considerations of civilian morale in general rather than the needs of the potential clients proved the deciding factor. Even after the war, some senior officials at the Ministry of Health retained doubts about the justification of the service for groups such as elderly people. There was also uncertainty about the respective roles of voluntary agencies and local authorities in the home help service. The WVS proved adept at arguing their own potential contribution as they attempted to establish their role and function within the 'welfare state' after the war.

The meals on wheels service

A mobile meals service also developed during the 1940s. The Ministry of Health had no doubts that this was a service that should be run by voluntary organisations rather than local authorities. What is less clear is which voluntary organisation initiated the scheme. Roberts, in *Our future selves,* stressed how OPWCs began to set up lunch clubs for elderly people in the 1940s. The Woolwich OPWC went further than this and set up a mobile unit which took meals to housebound old people "so, in 1943, modestly enough, meals on wheels began" (Roberts, 1970, p 42). This is denied by Walker who claims "in Britain the service was inaugurated by

Women's Voluntary Service" since "as long ago as 1943 a total of five meals was produced and carried to housebound people" (Walker, 1974).

It is clear, however, that the WVS soon became the dominant provider of such meals. From the beginning of the war, they had been heavily involved in food cooking and distribution for those whose lives had been disrupted by the war. At first, this was mainly in terms of helping to feed evacuated children. Later mobile canteens were provided for residents and civil defence staff after mass bombing raids on London. Graves has remarked how:

> **The need for canteens seemed endless. Civil Defence personnel at work in clouds of acrid dust cheered as a canteen bumped towards them over the debris, and men who could not have worked much longer without a hot drink went back with strength renewed. (Graves, 1948, p 122)**

Such work was also developed in other major cities as the bombing raids spread; 15,000 meals a day were supplied in Coventry in the week after the November 1940 raids. As a result of the Coventry experience, the Ministry of Food established food convoys and the WVS were largely responsible for staffing them (Graves, 1948, pp 128-30).

As the danger from bombing raids receded after the middle of 1942, the WVS decided to make more flexible use of its capacity to produce and distribute food on a mass scale. The logic of this has been explained by Walker in the following way:

> **The whole purpose of WVS was to keep a keen lookout for human need in the context of a nation embattled, rationed and in the midst of every kind of shortage and privation, and to devise or improvise, and at least to try to do something practical to meet whatever need they saw. The spectre of malnutrition was appearing despite rationing, and WVS was involved in attempts to provide easily accessible sources of ration-free food, which by 'collective' cooking made the most of our limited supplies. (Walker, 1974)**

Three main schemes evolved from this. The system of British Restaurants which was the responsibility of the Ministry of Food but used 17,000 WVS volunteers; these were based on the old Communal Feeding Centres set up during the early bombing raids. The Agricultural Pie Scheme attempted to produce cheap nutritious food for farmworkers. And finally the meals on wheels scheme developed in urban areas for those too frail or sick to use the British Restaurants. By 1947, 6,000 meals were being supplied through "family cooking on the family stove, or sometimes on improvised stoves at WVS centres, extended by supplies from commercial and industrial canteens" (Walker, 1974).

As already indicated, other organisations were interested in the impact of food rationing upon sick and frail elderly people. The OPWC sent a questionnaire to their local committees on this issue in late 1943 and this elicited the following complaints:

- that old people do not readily adapt themselves to using alternative foods such as dried egg powder, dried milk;
- that old people cannot stand about in queues in order to obtain non-rationed food such as fish;
- that old people need more tea and milk than the rationing scheme allows;
- that many old people cannot get to Communal Restaurants and/or cannot afford the cost of the meal served there[63].

However, OPWC did not feel these complaints were sufficient to justify a deputation to the Ministry of Food while the Ministry of Health was not seen as relevant to the issue. There was a "suggestion that Mobile Meal Services for old people should be developed" although this does not seem to have generated any great enthusiasm. In the mid-1940s, the OPWC and its local committees seemed more interested in developing clubs and lunch clubs for elderly people rather than meals on wheels services[63]. Many of these clubs were funded by the Lord Mayor's National Air Raid Distress Fund (1954, p 31) (see below).

Most of the meals on wheels schemes in the period 1943-47 were based in London. As late as August 1947, only 23 schemes could be traced from outside that area in a survey carried out by Assistance Board officers. Even in London, there was found to be 'no regular pattern' and "where services exist, they cater for different categories, emphasizing a variety of methods"[64]. The Assistance Board had become interested in meals on wheels schemes because of the question of whether they should increase benefit levels for recipients; the eventual decision was that this could be done on an individual hardship basis but not as a general rule[65]. However, the Assistance Board seemed less than convinced by the value of the schemes:

> **It is noticeable that where there is a well organised Home Help Service, the categories covered by that service are not considered to be in need of the Mobile Meals Service. It is, however, unlikely for a long time that the supply of Home Helps will be sufficient to provide a service to cover all the categories.**[66]

Such lack of enthusiasm seems to have been shared by the Ministry of Health prior to early 1947. There appeared to be little evidence of interest in the early meals on wheels schemes from civil servants in that Ministry. Early drafts of the 1948 National Assistance Act made no mention of the service. However, Section 31 of the eventual Act stated that "a local authority may make contributions to the funds of any voluntary organisations whose activities consist in or include the provision of recreation or meals for old people". Why did this change of opinion occur?

In January 1947, Lord Amulree (geriatrician and part-time medical officer at the Ministry of Health) made a speech to the LCC in which he claimed that many elderly people did not get enough food because of rationing – what they needed was "extra cake and a glass of sherry". This had been reported in the press as 'Doctor champions the old people' (*Sunday Express*). This argument did not convince everyone. One official from the Ministry of Health complained in a handwritten comment that "I can't see how a daily glass of sherry and a piece of cake can be financed and I doubt whether the Assistance Board could supplement the OA pension to meet the cost"[67]. However, the issue did not go away and several press stories followed which focused on how difficult it was for elderly people to wait in queues for rationed and non-rationed food. The *Evening Standard* claimed in September 1947 that "old people go short of food" while the *Yorkshire Evening News* went even further by stating "Many Leeds aged on brink of starvation". The *Daily Mail* called for "a new deal for the old people" in December 1947 while the *Daily Express* asked "how are the old folk on the rations?" Such stories continued to be published in early 1948 and several of them seemed to have been inspired by OPWC branches. For example on 30 January 1948, *The Times* ran a story on "Helping the aged: old people – our proposals" in which Holborn OPWC called for an end to food queuing, a hot meal service, chiropody facilities and cheap wireless licences[68].

By December 1947, officials were responding to such publicity by arguing the case for "the Ministries of Health and Food [to] take action to alleviate the position" through "the provision of a personal service to those who need it"[69]. The two ministries decided to call a conference[70], inviting representatives from the NOPWC, the WVS, the BRCS, the National Federation of Women's Institutes and the National Union of Townswomen's Guilds. The Chief General Inspector of the Ministry of Health said that the conference had been called to discuss methods of helping old people get their share of non-rationed food. A medical officer said the problem had grown since the introduction of bread rationing in 1946; elderly people found it hard to supplement their rations, since it was difficult for them to walk miles for food or to queue at shops for hours. The voluntary organisations were asked to extend the scope of their meals on wheels operations; the possibility of direct provision by local authorities does not appear to have been considered. The NOPWC reported 20 mobile meals services in operation, while the WVS said they had 97 schemes with 9,000 meals delivered per week. The Red Cross indicated they had started only a few schemes because they were so expensive to set up. The need for a series of regional and local conferences to coordinate and promote developments was agreed.

In March 1948, the NOPWC sent a Circular to their regional officers and committees on *Old people living alone and adequate food supplies*[71]. This asked them to "urge upon the Local Old People's Welfare Committees the urgent importance of expanding visiting schemes and trying to promote mobile meals services and clubs". The Chief General Inspector sent a letter out to his inspectorate on *Meals on wheels and allied services*[72] which pointed out:

- voluntary organisations are setting up meals services;
- there is a need to expand and get this service coordinated;
- the 1948 National Assistance Act will give local authorities the power to allocate grants;
- general inspectors should be willing to organise the chairing of local conferences on this subject.

The WVS also sent out a Circular to their regional officers on 22 March 1948[73]. This told members to set up local and regional conferences on mobile meals through OPWCs, where these existed. If not, they should use Ministry of Health General Inspectors. They were informed that "at these conferences WVS should report in full the work being done and should be prepared to undertake further work where it is still needed". During the rest of 1948 a series of regional and local conferences on mobile meals took place[73].

The meals on wheels service thus emerged from concern about the impact of food rationing upon sick and frail elderly people. However, the cause of this concern in central government was again not the actual suffering of those people but the impact that suffering might have on the perceptions of others. The sick and frail were no longer perceived as a troublesome burden in a war torn country but a group that needed to be seen to be treated with sympathy in the context of the overall reconstruction plans. However, a later government study threw considerable doubt upon the belief that rationing had created queuing problems for elderly people. Bransby and Osborne took a one in 30 sample of women over 60 and men over 65 from the food office register for Sheffield. Fieldwork was carried out from January 1950 to March 1951. Some allowance must be made for the fact that some frail respondents may not have completed the research but the findings did conclude:

> **When asked whether they had any particular difficulties in getting food, less than 1% mentioned physical difficulties such as queuing. The remainder who mentioned some difficulty spoke of the shortage of rations, the lack of variety or the high prices; as high a proportion, however, as 63% said they had no particular difficulty in getting food (Bransby and Osborne, 1953, p 164).**

The survey concluded that "the operative factor in most instances in the amounts of different foods taken was the size of their income" (Bransby and Osborne, 1953, p 169).

Voluntary organisations and service provision for elderly people after the Second World War

This chapter has repeatedly made the point that voluntary organisations argued the need to extend social provision for elderly people in a way that often emphasised their own potential role as actual providers of those services. The extent of this was indicated by John Moss, Chairman of the NOPWC, at their 1947 Annual Conference. He noted developments in the number of voluntary residential homes in the past 12 months:

> **The Salvation Army was one of the pioneers in the establishment of Eventide Homes and Darby and Joan Homes and had opened five more Homes. The Church Army had opened two and two**

more were being adapted. Local Old Peoples Welfare Committees had opened nine Homes. WVS had opened eight Homes and more were nearly ready. The British Red Cross Society had opened two Homes and two more were nearly ready. The Methodists had opened three Homes and more were being prepared. The National Union of Teachers had opened two Homes. The Church Army Housing Society had eleven houses open in flatlets and seventeen more in process of adaptation. In addition, the Soroptimists, Rotary, the Free Churches and others were opening Homes for old people every month. (Moss, 1947, pp 44-8)

He also mentioned the major expansion of recreation clubs and lunch clubs for elderly people run by the churches, WVS, the BRCS and the OPWCs. In the same period, the Assistance Board was encouraging voluntary organisations to develop visiting schemes to lonely elderly people in the community[74], while visiting schemes for those in institutional care were also being expanded (see for example, BRCS, 1948, p 53). This chapter has also illustrated how voluntary organisations became involved in home help and meals on wheels provision.

How can this growth of service provision for elderly people be explained? Part of the answer lay in the availability of funds from a variety of sources. It was not a period of unlimited money for voluntary organisations. The NOPWC had frequent arguments with the NCSS over lack of finance[75]. The WVS was being asked to reduce its costs by central government[76]. At the same time, various charitable funds from countries such as South Africa, Canada and Australia were being offered to voluntary organisations for 'reconstruction' work.

Much of this money was channelled through the Lord Mayor's National Air Raid Distress Fund and the Nuffield Foundation. The Lord Mayor's Air Raid Distress Fund was opened in September 1940 and closed in June 1946. The Fund continued to distribute money until January 1954 and final receipts were £4,980,223. Most of this money came from the USA and from countries who were "Dominions and Colonies" (Lord Mayor's National Air Raid Distress Fund, 1954, p 11). The original aim of the fund during the bombing raids:

... was to fill any gaps appearing in the official provision for the relief of distress, and to furnish help promptly ... by supplying food, clothing, and any immediate necessities, often

meeting payments towards the cost of funerals, removal of furniture, cost of storage ... indeed, anything which would help quickly to make the lot of bombed-out people a little easier. (Lord Mayor's National Air Raid Distress Fund, 1954, p 11)

At the end of the war, the fund still contained a large amount of money. It was decided to develop schemes to help both young people and elderly people whose lives had been disrupted by the war. On 16 January 1946, an Old People's Homes Committee was formed and this helped to establish 153 homes to be run by voluntary organisations as well as numerous recreation and lunch clubs. The WVS alone received £184,973 to help with the establishment of residential homes (Lord Mayor's National Air Raid Distress Fund, 1954, p 31).

In 1947, the Fund provided £500,000 to help in the creation of the National Corporation for the Care of Old People; the Nuffield Foundation also supplied £500,000 (p 31) .Earlier in this chapter, the financing by the Nuffield Foundation of the survey into the social conditions being experienced by elderly people was described. The OPWC had encouraged this in the hope that it would lead to them receiving Nuffield funding for the establishment of a national advisory service on the availability of residential care in voluntary and private homes. The Nuffield report, however, concluded that:

There is need for a centre of research and reference, of guidance and encouragement, of co-ordination and leadership in all matters affecting the aged. Considerations such as these have led the Committee to examine very seriously the desirability of recommending that a new and central body be set up, to study the changing conditions and needs of the aged; to undertake or stimulate research; to advise on, and where necessary to co-ordinate and support, the activities of local authorities and voluntary organisations. Since much of the activity on behalf of the aged must and should continue to be carried out by local voluntary bodies, it has been represented to the Committee that such a central body shall be in a position to make loans or grants ... for local organisations. (Rowntree, 1980, pp 104-5)

The Nuffield Foundation was already beginning to make grants to voluntary organisations to establish residential homes, but was concerned that this might overlap with the Lord Mayor's National Air Raid Distress Fund (NCCOP, 1948, pp 3-4). The two organisations decided to establish the National Corporation for the Care of Old People (NCCOP) although the air raid fund money had to be used "for the benefit of persons suffering distress as the result of air raids" (Lord Mayor's National Air Raid Distress Fund, 1954, p 31). The NCCOP became a major grant provider to voluntary organisations wishing to establish a wide range of residential and domiciliary services for elderly people. During its first year it received 250 applications for financial assistance and paid out grants totalling of £257,620 (NCCOP, 1948, p 6).

The availability of finance was not the only stimulus to voluntary organisations in the period 1945-48. The BRCS and the WVS were large national organisations that had controlled vast numbers of volunteers to help in the running of the country during wartime. What would happen to these organisations in peacetime? Did they have a role to perform in the postwar settlement? The Labour government of 1945 had doubts about the WVS. In September 1945, the Home Office issued a Circular which indicated that the activities of the WVS would "continue to be necessary on its present general lines during the transitional period following the end of the war – perhaps for about two years" (Home Office, 1943)[77]. Suspicion of the WVS existed in the Labour Party during this period. Caerphilly Labour Party wrote to the Prime Minister, attacking the WVS as Tory dominated, and claiming they campaigned against the Labour Party in the general election. As a result, they demanded that the WVS should be excluded from the work of reconstruction. Lady Reading discussed the situation with senior officials from the Home Office: "could we not say that the WVS is non-political, that women from every walk of society were invited to join in it, that its membership is open to all, and that certain changes are being made in the higher offices?"[78].

The WVS responded to the threat to their future in several ways. The core of their argument was that "one of the most obvious advantages of WVS is its availability in times of national emergency and for this it is of infinite advantage that it forms a national network, organised on a local authority pattern" (Beveridge and Wells, 1949, p 138). This network was to be maintained in peacetime through its welfare functions such as the provision of home help services, old people's clubs and visiting schemes.

The WVS reorganised itself onto a peacetime footing as early as 1945. By then, there was a separate Old People's Welfare Department[79] (responsible for clubs, meals on wheels, residential homes and visiting schemes) while by 1949 there was also a Health Department[80] (support for hospital patients, provision of home help services). These developments strengthened support for WVS among senior civil servants. (Lady Reading seems to have been very effective in using such influential friends and contacts. See, for example, WRVS, 1978, pp 13-16 (Dame Mary Smieton) and pp 17-19 (Dame Enid Russell-Smith)). The war had brought them influential 'friends' in the Home Office who were probably sympathetic to the national emergency argument. By July 1946, the argument being put by Lady Reading to the Home Secretary (Chuter Ede) was that:

> **I am constantly being put in a very bad predicament by my own staff and local authorities who feel that if the life tenure of this organisation is merely September 1947 many forms of work should not be undertaken and enterprises must automatically wane.... It places the undertaking of national projects of real importance in a predicament as to their fulfilment.**[81]

The 'deal' made was that the preferential funding of the WVS would have to end; they could no longer be the only voluntary organisation that had all its administrative costs met by central government. WVS would have to negotiate with the National Council of Social Service over the creation of a central organisation that would prevent overlap, increase efficiency and provide value for money within the voluntary sector; this organisation would distribute all the funds from central government[82].

As a result, a Circular was issued to local authorities asking them

> **... to make full use of the Womens Voluntary Service when they feel that their service would be useful, and that they will take an early opportunity for discussing with the appropriate local office of the Service how best the Service can give help in present circumstances, and will give them every facility for carrying on their work. (Home Office, 1947)**[83]

Lady Reading proved adept at 'spinning out' negotiations with the NCSS[84] despite her protestation to the Home Secretary that she was "deeply distressed that this state of impasse should have been reached"[85]. By early 1949 meetings at the Home Office between the NCSS and the WVS were dominated by discussions about preparations for civil defence[85]. The cold war had begun, provoking fresh fears of world conflict. The continuation of the WVS as a separate organisation with preferential central government funding was ensured.

The BRCS was not dependent on central government funding in the same way as the WVS and so its continuation after the war was not in question. However, this voluntary organisation did have to decide what role it was to perform in 'reconstruction' after the war. To this effect, a major conference on the postwar work of the BRCS was held in September 1946. The opening address by the Countess of Limerick stressed that membership had risen from 33,598 in 1938 to 175,994 in 1944. Their task at the conference was "to find out if there is a place for the British Red Cross in peace-time". However, she was already developing a logic similar to that of the WVS:

> **We must, of course, always remember that our primary function is to supplement the Medical Services in times of war. But to carry out that role we must have an active, virile and efficient organisation in time of peace.**[86]

The BRCS had already established a Welfare Department in May 1946, with separate sections for Disabled Civilians, Physically Handicapped Children and the Aged Infirm (BRCS, 1947, p 59). In the following year, this last section was renamed the 'Old People's Section" (BRCS, 1948, p 50), a sign of the changing terminology used in describing elderly people. By 1947, there were eight BRCS residential homes, 100 clubs and numerous visiting schemes in local authority homes (BRCS, 1948, p 53). The overall task was "to build up an efficient Welfare Office in every County Branch, under the care of a trained and experienced Welfare Officer, and open at all times for the reception of calls and dispatch of visitors" (BRCS, 1947, pp 59-60).

The NOPWC did not have to face the same issue of defining its peacetime role. It had been established in 1940 to promote the welfare of elderly people, a task that obviously needed to continue after 1945. At the same time, the policies and mechanisms for achieving this had to be decided. Local committees were seen as having a key role to play in this process, but were these meant to include:

- advice on service developments within their localities;
- provision of services such as clubs and meals on wheels;
- coordination of services provided by voluntary organisations;
- coordination of all welfare services, whether provided by voluntary organisations or local authorities.

Such complex issues were not to be resolved before July 1948 and the continuing debate is examined in later chapters. From the beginning, local OPWC committees were received with hostility by the WVS, who wished to be accountable only to their own headquarters and to local authorities[87]; they also felt that existing OPWCs should be advisory, and should not provide any direct services[88]. Service provision should be left to voluntary organisations with more reliable volunteer resources such as the WVS and the BRCS.

Despite these conflicts, it is possible to identify certain assumptions shared by central government and the key voluntary organisations about the role of the voluntary sector in the post-1948 arrangements; assumptions that later chapters show were not always shared by local authorities. The assumptions included an acceptance that, in the words of the report on *Voluntary action* prepared by Lord Beveridge, "the State cannot see to the rendering of all the services that are needed to make a good society" (Beveridge, 1948, p 304). Shortages existed and priorities for government action needed to be established. Violet Markham (Deputy Chairwoman, Assistance Board) gave an indication of what these might be at the BRCS Welfare Conference in September 1946:

> **So you see, though we want to do everything we can to make our old people happy and comfortable, give them the proper means of livelihood, their claims have to be seen in relation to these other claims, primarily the claims of the children and those of the other social services that the country has to carry out.**[89]

As a result she argued "no Government Department can run a club or ought to run a club" for old people; "it is not the sphere of Government". Under these circumstances, it was perhaps not surprising that the WVS and the BRCS joined the NOPWC in becoming major providers and coordinators of services for elderly people. Central government would be responsible for pensions and supplementary pensions. Local authorities would develop residential care. The NHS would offer medical services. The voluntary organisations would be expected to develop visiting schemes and other services for those in hospital and residential care as well as a wide range of domiciliary services for those people who remained in their own homes, especially where they were lonely and isolated.

This emphasis was not in conflict with the post-1945 growth of residential homes run by voluntary organisations. These homes were not usually intended for low income elderly people. The focus of the Homes Advisory Service of the OPWC on the needs of 'better off' elderly people seeking residential care has been outlined. The WVS and the BRCS homes followed a similar pattern. Graves wrote how

> **... admittance to these WVS homes was to be restricted to those with an income up to £200-£250 but, while the financial stability of the scheme demanded that the contributions of the residents should vary from old age pensioners paying twenty-eight shillings weekly to those who could afford two and a half guineas weekly, a definite effort was made to select residents of approximately the same educational standard". (Graves, 1948, p 245)**

The 1947 Annual Report of the BRCS argued that the substance of what was to become the 1948 National Assistance Act did not lessen the need for BRCS residential homes; they were "both for short-stay inmates who need to be looked after during convalescence from illness or during the absence of their own relatives, and also for the permanent accommodation of those who would never feel at home in a state institution" (BRCS, 1948, p 53).

After 1948, central government was to see voluntary organisations as providing a useful addition to the overall availability of local authority residential care facilities; and they were to be seen as central in the provision of domiciliary services for those elderly people who remained in their own homes. This was a reflection of the main provisions of the 1948 National Assistance Act. The detailed politics behind this act form the subject of the next chapter.

Notes

[1] See, for example, the Reconstruction Leaflets of the British Red Cross Society (BRCS); copies of these are available from the archives at the BRCS Training Centre, near Guildford.

[2] See DHSS 99063/10/1, *WVS social welfare: Organisation and administration of civil defence by WVS.*

[3] WRVS Archives: Box A1/38, *WVS outline of policy and terms of reference, 1938-42*, memorandum from Mr Johnston (Ministry of Home Security) to Miss Smieton, 28 April 1940.

[4] DHSS 99063/10/1, memorandum, 27 July 1940.

[5] WRVS Archives: Box A1/38, *WVS outline of policy and terms of reference, 1942-51*, the 1942 Annual Report, published in June 1943.

[6] Graves claims these financial arrangements were agreed in early 1940 (see p 47). However, DHSS 99063/10/1 and WRVS archive files suggest that the Ministry of Home Security remained uncertain for some time after that on the extent it wished the Women's Voluntary Service to develop its welfare responsibilities.

[7] NCVO Archives: File C47/17, *Broadcasts for old people, 1942-52*, letter from George Haynes to BBC Director of Talks, 5 August 1942.

[8] DHSS 94014/1/142, *Relief, general: Circular 2105*, memorandum dated 27 April 1940.

[9] Age Concern Archives; Box Files 1 to 4, *Historical and early activities*; DHSS 99063/11/1A, *Social welfare: National Council of Social Service: General correspondence and Executive Committee 1940-1946*.

[10] See various memoranda in DHSS 99063/11/1A.

[11] DHSS 99063/11/1A, memorandum from Puxley to Samson, 21 October 1941.

[12] DHSS 99063/11/1A, memorandum from Turner to Puxley, 21 October 1941.

[13] Age Concern Archives: Box Files 1-4. Figures supplied in report dated 7 December 1942.

[14] Ibid; see report on 'Placing of old people in homes', 31 March 1943.

[15] Ibid; see report on 'The future of the advisory sub committee' by Dorothea Ramsey, 4 April 1944; also, memorandum from D. Keeling, 17 July 1944.

[16] Age Concern Archives: Box Files 1-4. Publicity pamphlet on LCC Rest Homes, November 1941.

[17] PRO AST7/557, *Welfare: Homes and hostels,* memorandum, 6 August 1941.

[18] Ibid; see correspondence between Barter and Stuart King, and between Reid and Maude.

[19] DHSS 99063/11/1A, Minutes of meeting with representatives of the OPWC, 26 March 1942.

[20] The Public Assistance Officer for Kent was John Moss. Despite being a leading member of OPWC, he was a fierce critic of the 30 shilling hostels – see correspondence in PRO AST 7/557.

[21] DHSS 99063/11/1A, minutes of meeting, 24 April 1942.

[22] Ibid; memorandum from Lindsay, 2 June 1942.

[23] Ibid; see correspondence from Hill to Brown (29 August 1942) and from Brown to Rathbone (10 December 1942).

[24] Ibid; letter from Lindsay to OPWC, 23 September 1942.

[25] Ibid; memorandum from Turner, 28 January 1943.

[26] Age Concern Archive: Box 8A; report on 'Old people's welfare' to Emergency Committee of National Council of Social Services, 8 July 1943.

[27] DHSS 94001/8/14, *The Nuffield Foundation: Ageing and the care of the aged,* memorandum, 3 September 1943.

[28] These clippings are collected in DHSS 99063/3/2, *Social welfare: Aged and infirm: General correspondence.*

[29] DHSS 99063/3/5, *Accommodation for and care of the aged,* contains copy of CGI 115, 4 September 1945.

[30] DHSS 99063/3/9, *Hostels for the aged,* letter from National Association of Administrators of Local Government Establishments, 18 March 1946.

[31] DHSS 99063/3/2, *Social welfare: Aged and infirm: General correspondence*, memorandum from AMC, 12 April 1946.

[32] Ibid; memorandum from National Association of Local Government Social Welfare Officers, 7 October 1946.

[33] These are collected together in DHSS 99063/3/2 and 99063/3/17, *Social welfare: Aged and infirm: Aged policy during interim period.*

[34] DHSS 99063/3/17, letter from Fred Messer, 24 October 1946.

[35] Ibid; minutes of meeting between Ministry of Health and the NOPWC, 29 November 1946.

[36] A copy of this can be found in DHSS 99063/3/2.

[37] DHSS 99063/3/17, memorandum from Boucher to Symon, 4 February 1947.

[38] DHSS 99063/3/17, minutes of meeting, 9 October 1947.

[39] DHSS 99063/3/ CGI 115 from Howell James to Senior Regional Officers, 4 September 1945.

[40] DHSS 99063/8/1A, *Social welfare: Domestic help to householders*, letter from Ministry of Health to Joint Committee, 14 June 1944.

[41] Much of the material in this paragraph draws on a 20-page report on *WVS and the home help service*. We have not been able to trace an author or date, although it was clearly produced for one of the short courses for home help organisers run by the WVS in the late 1940s and early 1950s. A copy of this can be found in WRVS Archives: Box File, *Miscellaneous memoranda*: *WVS wartime activities, 1938-45 (home helps etc)*.

[42] WRVS Archives: Box File A1/38, *WVS outline of policy and terms of reference*; this information is contained in WVS Industrial Welfare Leaflet No 7, 'A woman's job', July 1942.

[43] This quotation is taken from *WVS and the home help service*.

[44] Ibid; see also letter from Lady Reading to Mrs Dunbar, 15 August 1962 in the same box file.

[45] DHSS 99063/8/1A, report prepared by Puxley for Lindsay, 6 May 1944.

[46] Ibid; memorandum from Bevin, 18 May 1944.

[47] Ibid; letter from Metropolitan Boroughs' Joint Standing Committee, 20 June 1944.

[48] Ibid; memorandum from Ministry of Health to E. Hale (Treasury), 10 June 1944.

[49] Ibid; letter to CCA, 16 June 1944.

[50] Ibid; minutes of meeting, 1 August 1944.

[51] Ibid; letter from CCA to Lindsay, 8 August 1944.

[52] A copy of this can be found in DHSS 99063/8/1A.

[53] A copy of this can be found in DHSS 99063/8/1A.

[54] DHSS 99063/8/1A, *Report on enquiry into emergency domestic help services*, 17 December 1945.

[55] Ibid; minutes of meeting on 6 February 1946.

[56] Ibid; letter from Miss Halpin to Wilkinson, 16 February 1946.

[57] WRVS Archives: Box File, *Miscellaneous memoranda: WVS wartime activities, 1938-45 (home helps etc)*; letter from Macdonald to Lady Reading, 14 January 1946.

[58] WVS Circular CC8 M6/45, dated 30 May 1946; a copy is in DHSS 99063/8/1A.

[59] This information comes from *WVS and the home help service.*

[60] See various correspondence in DHSS 99063/8/18, *Social welfare: Domestic help to householders.*

[61] This information was obtained from *WVS and the home help service*.

[62] A 52-page conference report was produced by the WVS: 'Conference on Some Aspects of the Home Helps Scheme' held at Caxton Hall, London on 11 and 12 November 1947.

[63] Age Concern Archives: Box Files 1-4, Report of 'Second enquiry regarding hardships which old people may be suffering owing to the present food restrictions', 21 February 1944.

[64] PRO AST 7/851, *Mobile meals and allied services*, Report on meals on wheels services, 15 August 1941.

[65] Ibid; memorandum, 31 March 1949.

[66] Ibid; report on meals on wheels, 15 August 1947.

[67] This information has been abstracted from DHSS 99063/3/39A, *Social welfare: Aged and infirm: feeding of aged: Meals on wheels*.

[68] These newspaper clippings are collected in DHSS 97063/3/3919.

[69] Ibid; memorandum from Bransby to Magee, 22 December 1947.

[70] Ibid; minutes of Conference, 26 February 1948.

[71] Ibid; NOPWC Circular, 13 March 1948.

[72] Ibid; memorandum from Howell James, 16 March 1948.

[73] Ibid; WVS Circular, 22 March 1948.

[74] PRO AST 7/664, *Welfare and the visitation of old people; Cooperation with voluntary organisations*.

[75] NCVO Archives: NCSS File C.47/1/Finance: *Finance of Old People's Welfare Committees*.

[76] WRVS Archives: Box File A1/38, *WVS outline of policy and terms of reference, 1942-51*; see letter from Sir Alexander Maxwell (Home Office) to Lady Reading.

[77] A copy of this can be found in WRVS Archives: Box File A1/38.

[78] WRVS Archives: Box File A1/38; see letter from Caerphilly Labour Party, 29 September 1943 and letter from Lady Reading to Home Office, 3 November 1945.

[79] WRVS Archives: Box File, *WVS Annual Reports 1940-53*; see report on 'WVS old people's Welfare Department, August to December 1945'.

[80] Ibid; see WVS Annual Report for 1949.

[81] WRVS Archives: Box File A1/38; letter from Lady Reading to Chuter Ede, 31 July 1946.

[82] Ibid; draft paper from Home Office on the Future of the WVS, March 1947; author unknown; it was discussed by the Home Secretary and senior officials from the Home Office and the Ministry of Health.

[83] A copy of this can be found in WRVS Archives: Box File A1/38.

[84] This represents an interpretation of numerous documents in Box File A1/38. The NCSS certainly did feel frustrated by the tactics of the WVS and in June 1948 they asked the Home Office for an independent chair for their negotiations: see letter from Deedes to Maxwell, 22 June 1948.

[85] Ibid; letter from Reading to Chuter Ede, 5 August 1948.

[86] BRCS Archives: File on *BRCS headquarters training course on the post war work of the BRCS at home*; opening address by Countess of Limerick to Welfare Conference, September 1946.

[87] WRVS Archives: File OP5, *Old people's welfare policy, 1946-50*.

[88] DHSS 98063/3/39A, minutes of meeting on 26 February 1948 from Ministry of Health about establishing meals on wheels services indicates considerable conflict on this point between representatives of the WVS and NOPWC.

[89] BRCS Archives: File on *BRCS headquarters training course on the post war work of the BRCS*; speech by Violet Markham on 'The care of old people' at the BRCS Welfare Conference, September 1946.

FOUR

The 1948 National Assistance Act and the provision of welfare services for elderly people

Introduction

Chapters Two and Three considered in detail government responses to the needs of sick and frail elderly people in the period 1939-48. The 1948 National Assistance Act has been mentioned, but as yet no attempt has been made to outline any of the detailed negotiations which took place between civil servants, politicians, representatives of local authority associations and of pressure groups, and which helped to decide the eventual content of this legislation, in so far as it influenced local authority welfare provision for elderly people. Section 21 of the 1948 Act stated that "it shall be the duty of every local authority ... to provide residential accommodation for persons who by reason of age, infirmity or any other circumstances are in need of care and attention which is not otherwise available to them". Other sections of the Act dealt with how such residential accommodation was to be financed (exchequer contributions, charges, and so on), contributions to voluntary organisations, the registration of old people's homes and the compulsory removal of old people from the community.

Why did the legislation take this form and what alternatives were excluded? Did this legislation provide real gains for elderly people? Or should one accept the view, argued by Brown, that the welfare services in Part III of the Act "were not the product of clear thinking on the needs of the groups they were to serve so much as the almost casual outcome of the tidying-up of the social service scene after the major reorganisation had taken place"(Brown, 1972)?

Aneurin Bevan (Minister of Health, 1945-51) had been more positive than Brown about the 1948 National Assistance Act. He described it as "a coping stone" placed on previous legislation (*Hansard*, House of Commons, vol 443, 24 November 1947, col 1063). It is therefore necessary to consider in the first instance the relationship of the more 'famous' Acts to the 1948 Act insofar as they were also concerned with government intervention into the lives of elderly people and their families.

The 1946 National Insurance Act and the 1946 National Health Service Act

Background

There are numerous descriptive accounts (Fraser, 1973; Bruce, 1961) of the growth of social policy in Britain which chart the growth of factory and public health legislation, state education, council housing, the social security system, health service provision and the personal social services in the period prior to 1939. These accounts also show how such developments were greatly speeded up by the impact of the Second World War, so that the 1940s saw three major pieces of social legislation enter the statute book.

The 1944 Education Act established a comprehensive educational system which provided free education for all children between the ages of five and fifteen. The 1946 National Insurance Act followed through the main proposals of the Beveridge Report by establishing a compulsory system of insurance which guaranteed flat rate benefits for all workers during periods of sickness, unemployment and after retirement; these benefits were to be based on contributions deducted from wages and a safety net system of national assistance was to be provided for those who failed to meet these contribution conditions or who had exhausted their entitlement to insurance benefits. The 1946 National Health Service Act created a system of healthcare that was to be financed from general taxation rather than from payment at the point of treatment.

The last two Acts were passed by a Labour government, the first by the Conservative-dominated wartime coalition. The Conservative Party did not attempt any major dismantling of any of this legislation when it returned to office in 1951 and stayed in power for the next 13 years. The services established and extended by the legislation of the 1940s came to be known as 'The welfare state' and, as Titmuss pointed out, many commentators came to "see the development of 'The welfare state' in historical perspective as part of a broad, ascending road of social betterment provided for the working class since the nineteenth century and achieving its goal in our time" (Titmuss, 1961, p 34).

Such a 'social rights' perspective on social policy developments has since been challenged by numerous authors writing from a variety of perspectives. Macnicol, for example, has underlined the extent to which the major reforms of the Second World War and early postwar period were far less 'radical' than they first appeared. The schemes of social security, health service and education 'reform' had their origins in earlier legislation, and so can be seen as often little more than a 'tidying up' exercise. He goes on to argue that not only were they a logical development of what had gone before, but that they were specifically designed to exclude more radical alternatives from discussion:

> **Education policy-making provides a good example of this. Ostensibly, the 1944 Education Act granted what the labour movement had been demanding for thirty years – 'secondary education for all'. However, the new education system envisaged by the Board of Education was one that was to be divided on class lines, with only a limited, strictly-controlled crossing of the boundaries by 'bright' working-class children. (Macnicol, 1981, p 6)**

Macnicol's conclusion about the major social policy legislation of this period was that "the exaggerated rhetoric within which the reforms were packaged achieved its objective of engineering consent and minimising social upheaval" (Macnicol, 1981, p 8).

Social insurance

However, this does not address the narrower issue of what provision was actually made for elderly people by the legislation of this period, particularly in terms of pensions and medical care. The Beveridge Report saw elderly people as a problem because of their growing numbers[1] although the biography of Beveridge by Harris (1977, pp 409-11) indicates that it would be unfair to suggest that Beveridge himself fully shared this view. His original proposals had envisaged a system of pensions available to retired men and women that would be equal in amount to benefits payable for sickness and unemployment. However, this was criticised by Sir George Epps (Government Actuary) and Edward Hale (Treasury) on the Inter-Departmental Committee. They felt that subsistence-level old age pensions should be introduced gradually over an extended period, during which time the pension received would be related to the contribution records of the applicant, including contributions made since 1926.

Similar concern was expressed by the Economic Section of the War Cabinet Office in their discussions with the Beveridge Committee. The pension proposals were seen as requiring a level of taxation unacceptable in peacetime and might seriously hamper postwar investment; it was suggested that the pension plan should be developed in gradual stages. At a private meeting in June 1942, Keynes urged Beveridge to accept the above advice and reduce the cost implications of his pension plans since these were the least interesting and least essential of the whole.

The Beveridge Report reflected this advice and stressed from an early stage that:

> **The plan is based upon a diagnosis of want. It takes account of two other facts about the British community, arising out of past movements of the birth rate and the death rate, which should dominate planning for its future. The first of these two facts is the age constitution of the population, making it certain that persons past the age that is now regarded as the end of working life will be a much larger proportion of the whole community than at any time in the past. The second fact is the low reproduction rate of the British community today.... The first fact makes it necessary to seek ways of postponing the age of retirement from work rather than of hastening it. The second fact makes it imperative to give first place in social expenditure to the care of childhood and to the safeguarding of maternity. (Beveridge Report, 1942a, para 15)**

In other words, elderly people were seen as a problem; concern about the cost implications of the growing elderly population was spread throughout the report. This led Beveridge to propose a transitional system of contributory pensions that would be gradually introduced over a 20-year period from 1945-65, in which 1965 would be the first year when such pensions would become payable as a right irrespective of means at the full provisional rate of 40 shillings for a married couple or 24 shillings for a single person. Such pensions were to be payable only on retirement from work, unlike previous schemes (see Chapter Two), and considerable incentives were to be offered for those who delayed such retirement for as long as possible. During the transition period the incomes of the retired would be brought up to subsistence level by the National Assistance Board which would pay assistance pensions based on a means test rather than contributions.

Those qualified under the previous contributory scheme were to be given a 25 shilling joint pension or a 14 shilling single pension; thus the report followed its own advice that "it is dangerous to be in any way lavish to old age, until adequate provision has been assured for all other vital needs, such as the prevention of disease and the adequate nutrition of the young" (Beveridge Report, 1942a, para 256). This harsh approach to older people was criticised by a number of groups. Samson (1944, pp 17-20) outlines how various pressure groups such as the NFOAPA, Political and Economic Planning and the OPWC complained about the low level of the proposed retirement pensions, and the unfairness of the transitional concept when compared to arrangements for the sick and unemployed. The White Paper on social insurance reflected these criticisms in part, and abandoned the concept of a transitional scheme. At the same time, it was argued:

> **The Government recognise the general desire of the country that proper provision should be made for old age, and they share it. But the steady prospective increase over a period of years in proportion of pensioners to people of working ages makes it of particular importance to take a prudent view. In the result, the Government find themselves unable to adopt permanent rates of 40s joint and 24s single and propose rates of 35s joint and 20s single to take effect from the commencement of the new scheme. (Ministry of Reconstruction, 1944)**

In other words, pensioners were still to receive a lower rate of benefit than the sick and unemployed. The 1946 National Insurance Act of the Labour government, however, was to go further than this by offering standard rates of benefit (26 shillings per week for a single recipient and 42 shillings per week for a couple) for sickness benefit, unemployment benefit and retirement pensions. This immediate provision of full level retirement pensions enabled Griffiths, the Minister for National Insurance, to claim at the 1947 annual conference of the Labour Party that the government had legislated for a scheme infinitely better than the one contemplated in the Beveridge Report (Heb, 1981).

How is this shift to be explained? There may have been a greater understanding of the financial plight of many elderly people within the

Labour Party than in the Conservative Party. Chapter Three indicated that there was sympathy for elderly people in this period; many civil servants recognised that this group had had a difficult time during the war and needed special help. The whole package of reforms represented a postwar settlement between capital and labour and so the 'kind' treatment of elderly people represented an important act in ideological terms. Such concessions could always be clawed back at the implementation stage. Research by Phillipson (1977, pp 27-40) underlines how the late 1940s and early 1950s was a period of labour shortage, and shows how the government responded to this by emphasising the delaying of retirement; an elderly person could only avoid mental and physical deterioration if they remained in work and did not take up his 'generous' pension. Finally, the generosity of benefit levels proved to be limited. Benefit rates made no allowance for rent and so many of those on sickness benefit, unemployment and retirement pensions still needed to apply for a supplementary allowance from the National Assistance Board.

However, the most crucial point for this chapter is that state provision for elderly people was dominated by the issue of pensions. Pensions were of interest to nearly all elderly people; they were expensive to provide and they had high visibility as a political issue. All political parties had a policy on pensions and continued to do so throughout the postwar period. Local authority welfare provision, on the other hand, was concerned with only a small segment of the elderly population, and it was not a major political issue. This was reflected in the negotiations on the 1948 National Assistance Act.

The Beveridge Report was not only concerned with insurance schemes:

> **Social insurance fully developed may provide income security; it is an attack upon Want. But Want is one only of five giants on the road of reconstruction and in some ways the easiest to attack. The others are Disease, Ignorance, Squalor and Idleness. (Beveridge Report, 1942a, para 8)**

More specifically the Report called for both a system of family allowances and a national health service. It is the second of these major reforms which is considered in the next section of this chapter.

The national health service

The politics of the creation of the national health service are immensely complex, and numerous authors have attempted to unravel the various strands from a variety of perspectives (see, for example, Lindsay, 1962, pp 3-98; Eckstein, 1959; Honigsbaum, 1979; Pater, 1981). These arguments lie beyond the purpose of this section, which aims merely to outline how the 1946 National Health Service Act affected the provision of medical services for elderly people on its implementation in July 1948. The situation before 1948 was briefly outlined in Chapter Two. The new system divided the health service into three entirely separate parts: the hospital sector, the executive council sector and the local health authorities. Doyal (with Pennell, 1979, p 181), has argued that consultants gained most from the scheme, because hospitals were to be removed entirely from local authority control and put under regional hospital boards and hospital management committees, on which consultants were granted a high level of representation. General practitioners favoured the scheme because they avoided the status of salaried employees through having contracts with the executive councils which replaced the old insurance committees. She concludes that:

> **In terms of power and resources the hospital sector was dominant in the new NHS, followed by the executive council sector which provided primary medical care. The local authorities were left with a residual collection of environmental health services, midwives, health visitors, home helps and district nurses. The lack of resources awarded to the local authority sector, combined with the failure to provide an industrial health service, was the final nail in the coffin of preventative medicine. It was a clear illustration of the declining prestige of public health in the twentieth century, and reflected the fact that these caring and background services offered the least scope for tangible profitability, either to capitalist industry or to the medical profession. (Doyal, with Pennell, 1979, p 182)**

Medical staff from the hospital sector, however, did not show equal enthusiasm for all types of patient; and, in particular, the treatment of elderly people was perceived as being of low status and priority.

As seen in Chapter Two, this bias against elderly patients influenced the development of the hospital service before 1948. Three types of hospital then existed. The voluntary hospitals were run on a charitable basis and concentrated upon those defined as the 'acute sick'. Public health hospitals were those that had been removed from the Poor Law system by the 1929

Local Government Act, and these also tended to focus on patients with acute healthcare needs. The 'chronic sick', which included most sick elderly people, tended to be catered for in those hospitals that were still administered by public assistance committees.

It has already been shown how the Second World War treated the 'chronic sick' as a problem – they blocked scarce hospital beds. The late 1940s did see 'reforms' in the medical care of elderly people, and a growth of interest from the medical profession in the specialism of geriatrics. The economic argument for better treatment was well put by Fairfield in an article in *The Lancet*:

> **Problems raised by chronic sickness are important but have been neglected in most schemes for medical reorganisation. Chronic sick patients are numerous, especially in the higher age groups, and their long occupancy of beds holds up a high percentage of the total accommodation. (Samson, 1944, p 52)**

At the same time, the medical profession was becoming aware of the excellent results that were being obtained in one or two large municipal hospitals, notably the West Middlesex Hospital at Isleworth, where the 'chronic sick' were classified and treated. It was found that a large number of patients were capable of a considerable degree of rehabilitation even though they had been bedfast for a number of years (Lord Amulree, 1951a, p 38).

The extent to which most hospitals failed to offer effective treatment to their 'chronic sick' patients was underlined by the government hospital surveys of the 1940s. Ten survey teams were appointed in 1941, some by the Minister of Health and some in conjunction with the Nuffield Provincial Hospitals Trust to cover both voluntary and public hospitals (see, for example, Gray and Topping, 1945; Easton et al, 1945). The aim of the surveys was to gather information about existing hospital facilities as a basis for future planning. The findings were drawn together in *The hospital surveys: The Domesday Book of the hospital services* which stressed how the surveys outlined the haphazard growth and lack of planning within existing hospital services. The Domesday Book showed how care for the 'chronic sick' received the bitterest comments from the investigators:

> **All are agreed that the 'reproach of the masses of undiagnosed and untreated cases of chronic type which litter our Public Assistance Institutions must be removed'. Without proper**

> **classification and investigation, at present young children and senile dements are 'banded together' in these institutions, along with many elderly patients whom earlier diagnosis and treatment might have enabled to return to their homes.... 'The great essential is that every patient should be thoroughly examined and treated with a view to restoration to a maximum degree of activity. Only if treatment is unsuccessful or is clearly useless, should [he] be regarded as chronically sick', and 'even then [he] should be subject to periodic review'. (Nuffield Provincal Hospitals Trust, 1946, p 16)**

All the investigators called for hospital services and accommodation to be completely divorced from PAIs.

The Ministry of Health[2] appeared convinced of such arguments because of concern about the high cost of 'blocked' beds. This was reflected in its Annual Report for 1945-46:

> **With an ageing population, it is important to ensure that people are kept on their feet and able to live happy and useful lives for as long as possible. Anything which tends to keep patients, and especially aged patients in bed unnecessarily is bad for them and, in these times of shortage of hospital beds and of staff, it is essential that it should be avoided. (Ministry of Health, 1947, p 81)**

The proper classification of patients and accurate diagnosis was seen as essential. The 'chronic sick' suffered from a variety of diseases such as cardiac disease and arthritis. Such people could be helped by medical treatment. Similar arguments were presented in the report of the Chief Medical Officer. This indicated that 70,000 beds were occupied by 'chronic sick' patients in England and Wales so that "it is obvious that more could and should be done to rehabilitate a large proportion of these patients at least to such an extent that they no longer occupy hospital beds" (Ministry of Health, 1948b, p 89).

The British Medical Association (BMA) did not ignore this growing interest in geriatric medicine and the 'chronic sick'. In July 1946 the Representative Body of the BMA decided that a committee should be set up to consider the inadequate provision that was being made for the treatment and care of the elderly and/or infirm. The 21 members of the committee were chaired by Dr Greig Anderson and included several doctors associated with the emerging specialism of geriatrics, such as Marjorie Warren, L.R. Cosin and Lord Amulree. The resultant report was called *The care and treatment of the elderly infirm* (Anderson Report, 1947) and provided the following classification of elderly people:

- the elderly
- the elderly and infirm
- the elderly sick:
  - senile sick
  - long-term sick (potentially remediable)
  - irremediable
- elderly psychiatric patients
- other special groups.

The first category comprised those healthy enough to manage in their own homes. The second category of 'the elderly and infirm' were composed of those "who suffer from the disabilities of age but not from extreme frailty or from chronic disease" (Anderson Report, 1947, p 8). Such people needed to be in residential homes. The elderly sick needed treatment in hospitals and it was argued that the most urgently needed reform was the provision of a full diagnostic investigation of these cases before they were classified as 'chronic'. Such diagnosis should take place in special geriatric departments to be established gradually in selected general hospitals. Those considered irremediable would be admitted to long-stay annexes, closely associated with the hospital.

At the moment, the report argued, there were too few facilities for rehabilitation and often an atmosphere of defeatism. This lack of treatment condemned many elderly people to be confined to bed for long periods so that they soon "drift into the 'infirmary decubitus' with its avoidable contractures and deformities" (Anderson Report, 1947 p 17). In other words, elderly patients were becoming bedfast because of the deficiencies of the existing hospital system. The introduction of more appropriate medical treatment would eliminate waiting lists and bed blockages. According to the BMA report, 40% of all new geriatric admissions could be discharged from hospital, 40% would die, leaving 20% of patients who, after failure to respond to treatment, would require permanent nursing care in a long-stay annexe.

Two points need to be made about this growth of interest in the 'chronic sick'. First, the various reports from central government and the BMA assumed it was possible to distinguish between the frail in need of general care and attention and the sick in need of medical and nursing support.

The NHS was to concern itself with the sick; the 1948 National Assistance Act was to establish a system of local authority residential care for those in need of care and attention. Second, high discharge rates from hospitals were seen as dependent upon the availability of such residential accommodation. The 1945-46 Annual Report of the Ministry of Health spoke of:

> **... patients, who have been admitted with a chronic disease, but have improved so much that they could go home if they had some care and attention available there. This last class is the type for which the specially arranged home or hostel is so useful. (Ministry of Health, 1947c, p 81)**

The apparent intention of Part III of the National Assistance Act was to make such homes more readily available through replacing the large old public assistance institutions by 30-40 bed residential homes that would impose no loss of social rights upon residents.

The National Assistance Bill: early proposals

Beveridge consulted the local authorities about the powers they should retain in terms of cash and institutional provision; he also asked what special provision should be made for old people. The AMC agreed that all cash needs should be met by central government but that:

> **... persons, [who] require assistance in kind by way of treatment or training, personal help or care and attention and other similar welfare services either in an institutional establishment or in their own home, should be dealt with by the local authority, who for this purpose should have powers to direct and co-ordinate all the activities of welfare work within the area. (Beveridge Report, 1942b)**

The CCA took a different position. It felt that many people in financial need would fall outside any extended scheme of national insurance, and that financial assistance to such cases should remain with the local authority. However, it agreed with the AMC that institutional provision should remain a local authority responsibility, although it still seemed to reflect a Poor Law outlook with the comment that "'facilities' should be available for a reasonable scheme of classification, regard being had to character and habits" (Beveridge Report, 1942b, p 199). The LCC argued that all financial benefits, apart from special petty cash payments, should be made by central government whether inside or outside the insurance scheme. On the other hand, the LCC was of the opinion that "personal services (eg hospital and mental hospital treatment, school meals, and so on) should be administered by local authorities" (Beveridge Report, 1942b, p 216). This included small residential homes for elderly people that would be "associated as far as possible with the life of the district in which the homes are situated" (Beveridge Report, 1942b, p 216).

To what extent Beveridge was influenced by such evidence is not known, although Harris (1977, pp 378-418) suggests that the main outline of his plan was written at a very early stage in the review process. The following two paragraphs from his report dealt with the potentially complex relationship between the work of the Assistance Board, the local authorities and the new NHS:

> **The abolition of the Poor Law will still leave in the hands of Local Authorities the important and growing task of organising and maintaining institutions of various kinds for treatment and welfare. In view of the increasing number of old persons, there is probably considerable scope for experimentation with and development of Services concerned with the recreation and welfare of the old, including special housing facilities. The domiciliary Poor Law Medical Service will presumably be merged into the comprehensive health service which is Assumption B of the Report, and in which Local Authorities will continue to play a very important part .... The Poor Law Code will, it is proposed, be abolished....**
>
> **The proposal in the report, in accord with the views expressed by the English Local Authorities, is that responsibility for Assistance should be transferred to the Ministry of Social Security while provision for institutions will in general remain with Local Authorities who will be empowered to give cash payments which are incidental to institutional treatment. The precise dividing line, and the details of the transfer, including the consequential financial adjustments, will have to be worked**

out in consultation with the Local Authorities. (Beveridge Report, 1942a, paras 164-5)

The various committees established as a result of the Beveridge Report tended to focus on social insurance and little attention was given to institutional care for elderly people. However, in October 1943, the Cabinet Committee on Reconstruction Priorities supported the abolition of the poor law code but resolved that:

... Local Authorities should continue to undertake the duty of providing indoor accommodation for the aged, either as a public health, or as a housing function.

As a result of this resolution, an Assistant Secretary from the Ministry of Health was asked to prepare a paper on 'The break up of the Poor Law and the care of children and old people' which was ready by February 1944. The passing of legislation on this issue was seen as awaiting final discussions on social insurance but still of great urgency because of the position of evacuees after the end of the war.

District councils in reception areas and individual householders wanted to be relieved as soon as possible of the responsibility of caring for evacuees. Unless early legislation was introduced, it would fall to the public assistance authorities (county borough and county councils) in the reception areas to meet the needs of children and old people, if parents and relatives could not or would not provide for them. Such an eventuality "would be intolerable to public opinion because of the stigma attached to the Poor Law".[3] At the same time, the likely length of time for establishing the new system of care indicated that it would be necessary to establish some kind of transitional arrangements for evacuated children and old people that would keep them outside existing Poor Law provision (see Chapter Two).

The internal Ministry paper suggested that the key legislative task was not difficult:

... at first sight ... the proposed Bill need do no more than take out of the Poor Law all the functions of lodging and caring for children and old people not otherwise provided for, and transfer them to a new organisation (perhaps a statutory 'Children and Old People Committee' or 'Social Welfare Committee') ... within the councils of counties or county boroughs....

Some consideration was given to the definition of those elderly people who should benefit from the new arrangements. The paper argued that need rather than age should be the selection criterion. This led to the suggestion of a concept of those "in need of care and attention, not being constant medical or nursing attention" as being "sufficiently precise for the craftsman to use as a basis". This wording was, of course, eventually incorporated into Section 21 of the 1948 National Assistance Act.

The paper concluded by considering the question of finance for the new services. It pointed out that some form of special Exchequer assistance to support local authority funding from the rates would counter any complaint that the Bill was merely continuing Poor Law practice under another name. Such special assistance would also help poorer counties and county boroughs to bring their institutional provision up to the level of the more progressive and prosperous of the public assistance authorities. At the same time:

> **The service is not, however, a new service, though in the less progressive areas it may need to be administered in a new spirit. Nor is it easy to see how the precedent of making an Exchequer grant towards 'additional' expenditure could be followed, since in the areas where standards are already high no additional expenditure is likely to be involved.**

In other words, the issue of finance was left open by this paper. It was to become a major issue of contention between the local authority associations and central government.

Soon after this, doubts began to be expressed in the Ministry of Health about whether the proposed Bill was elaborate enough in relation to elderly people. In May 1944, the civil servant primarily responsible told Sir Arthur Rucker (Deputy Secretary, Ministry of Health) how he had "learnt during the last few days that the Nuffield Foundation [Rowntree, 1980] some months ago set up a Sub-Committee which is surveying the needs of old people and the defects in the present means of meeting those needs", a sub-committee that included the Chief General Inspector of the Ministry of Health as an adviser. He had also been informed by other civil servants of growing public interest in elderly people so that "we should watch this question carefully lest we be met with the criticism when we introduce our Bill that we have dismissed the old far too summarily"[4].

However, this concern for the needs of elderly people was not very apparent in a February 1945 paper about the proposed Bill. It abandoned the idea of a Social Welfare Committee on the grounds that "the needs of the children differ so much from those of old people that separate arrangements seem to be desirable"[5]. Instead, a Children's Committee was proposed so that welfare staff experienced in the needs of children could be employed and these would be financed partly from Exchequer grant. At the same time:

> **There seems no reason why such a staff should not concern itself with the welfare of the old people, as well as of the children, covered by the Bill, or, indeed, with general welfare problems. It is not, however, thought necessary to set up a statutory 'Old Persons' Committee.**

The paper also argued that no provision for Exchequer grant should be made in the bill, except in respect of the employment of welfare staff, but that it should be recognised that the county and county borough councils would probably make a case for such assistance and that this case might have to be met.

The emphasis on services for children seems to have been a defensive response from the Ministry of Health[6] to the development of a childcare lobby that was calling for separate legislative provision for this group (for a detailed account of the build-up of pressure for childcare reform, see Heywood, 1959, pp 94-149). This lobby was especially keen for a unification and simplification of central government control since, at the time, responsibility for children deprived of a normal home life was divided between the Ministry of Health, the Ministry of Education, the Ministry of Pensions and the Home Office.

Parker (1983) has produced a detailed account of the gestation of the 1948 Children Act. On 4 December 1944, the Reconstruction Committee of the Cabinet approved the setting up of the Curtis Committee (Curtis Report, 1946) to consider existing methods of providing for children deprived of a normal home life. However, its terms of reference specifically precluded any consideration of the sensitive issue of the allocation of central responsibilities. The Reconstruction Committee had decided to refer this specific issue to the Machinery of Government Committee[7]. This was another Cabinet committee under the chairmanship of Sir Alan Barlow (Treasury) charged with advising on the various issues of departmental boundaries which the mass of new legislation created. Both the Home Office and the Ministry of Health argued to this committee that their departments should have overall control of childcare services. The Barlow committee decided in March 1945 in favour of the Home Office. Responsibility for the administration of the Factory Acts had just been taken from it and it was felt "contrary to the public interest for the Home Office to be shorn of too many functions not purely repressive in character" (Parker, 1983, p 206). The Ministry of Health claimed that this had badly damaged them in the eyes of local authorities who felt that the Ministry was losing its power and influence. Sir Arthur Rucker felt "the process of bleeding us should be brought to an end"[8].

Parker (1983)[9] indicates that this decision by the Machinery of Government Committee did not bring the matter to an end. The general election victory of the Labour Party in July 1945 allowed the Ministry of Health and later the Ministry of Education to reargue their cases for control of these services. The issue had still not been resolved by the time of the publication of the Curtis Report in September 1946 and it was not until a Cabinet meeting in March 1947 that Home Office responsibility was finally confirmed. Of more relevance to this chapter, however, is that from the appointment of the Curtis Committee, it became certain that the final break up of the Poor Law legislation would contain two elements, a children's bill and a bill dealing with any other remaining issues, including state welfare provision for elderly people.

The Rucker Report

The new Labour Cabinet set up a Social Services Committee[10] to supervise social policy reform. At its first meeting, James Griffiths (Minister for National Insurance) raised the issue of the break up of the Poor Law:

> **... the last stage in the legislative process required to introduce the new scheme would be the final break-up of the Poor Law and the distribution of public assistance functions between the Assistance Board and other committees of the local authorities. When other Bills had made satisfactory progress, it would be necessary to open discussions with local authorities on this final stage with a view to the preparation of the legislation.**[11]

In other words, developments on the bill to end the Poor Law and the children's bill would be delayed until legislative progress had been made on the key bills for national insurance and the NHS. An internal memorandum from the Minister of Health and Minister of National Insurance in March 1946 confirmed the need for a National Assistance

Bill that would determine how and by whom assistance would be given for those presently dependent on the Assistance Board and those who "have no recourse but to the Poor Law or are dealt with under special schemes that need to be integrated"[12]. The memorandum went on to explain how:

> **The Bills now before Parliament are primed to bring the system into simultaneous operation in early 1948. It has always been assumed that the final step, breaking up the remnants of the Poor Law, would be taken at the same time. Politically, this seems essential [since it is] ... impossible to contemplate an uneasy interregnum when the insufficiently protected are compelled to turn to the outmoded and dying Poor Law. The argument applies with special force to ... the old.**

It was crucial that the break up of the Poor Law did not get out of step with the rest of the social services programme. Preparation of the bill needed to occur without delay and, consequently, it was proposed to set up a small interdepartmental committee of senior officials to prepare proposals. The Break Up of the Poor Law Committee first met in April 1946 with Sir Arthur Rucker (Deputy Secretary, Ministry of Health) as chairman and representatives from the Ministry of Health, the Department of Health for Scotland, the Ministry of Education, the Ministry of Labour, the Ministry of National Insurance, the Home Office and the Assistance Board.

The committee met eight times between April and July 1946 and a draft bill was ready by the seventh meeting. The report of the Break Up of the Poor Law Committee (the Rucker Report)[13] was considered by the Social Services Committee of the Cabinet on 12 July 1946. The report assumed that Poor Law legislation would be totally repealed. It would be replaced by new legislation that would become operative on the same day as the national insurance scheme and NHS, and would reflect the following guiding principles:

- the Assistance Board will be responsible for assisting any persons living in their homes whose needs are not fully met by the National Insurance and allied services, and for providing such persons and their dependants with the kind of general welfare service which the Board already provide for old people and other applicants; and
- local authorities will be responsible, except in a few special cases, for

> providing institutional care for those who need it and specialised welfare services for certain defined classes of persons.

The committee thought that this could be achieved in one bill (apart from children's services) and that 'National Assistance Bill' would be a suitable short title. Local authority services under this bill would be provided by counties and county boroughs.

A major section of the report dealt with maintenance in institutions although an earlier draft had spoken of the need to find an alternative word for institutions[14]. The White Paper on Social Insurance indicated that institutional provision for elderly people should remain a local authority responsibility but that the Assistance Board should have the duty of "making suitable provision for those, other than the sick, the young and the old, for whom assistance in cash is not appropriate".

The Rucker Report agreed with the recommendations on elderly people but argued that local authority responsibility should be extended to include other groups unable to live a normal life (for example, physically disabled people, people with learning difficulties) as well as those rendered homeless through such factors as eviction, fire or flood. In terms of institutional provision, the Assistance Board should retain full responsibility only for "able-bodied persons, either homeless wanderers (the 'casuals') or 'work-shy' persons on whom every other possible persuasion has been tried without success". The report made no recommendation as to which committee of the local authority should supervise institutional provision although it did suggest that the health committee might be best for this purpose.

This section of the report went on to propose two important changes in local authority institutional care. The first of these was that local authorities were to be encouraged to move away from large general institutions and to develop specialised accommodation suited to the varying needs of the persons under their care, particularly small homes for the old and infirm. Second, the report considered payment for residential care. Previously, accommodation in PAIs for reasons other than medical need led to a loss of pension rights. However, the report argued that:

> **... as a further step towards breaking away from the old association of parish relief and in particular the conception of an institution for 'destitute persons', we think that a resident in a local authority's Home should keep charge of whatever income or other resources he may have and pay the authority for his accommodation and maintenance.**

This "conception of a 'hotel' relationship" would work for most pensioners by them paying to the local authority 21 shillings a week from their 26 shilling pension and keeping five shillings for 'pocket money'.

The next issue considered was that of possible central government financial support for new local authority residential provision. It has already been seen how earlier drafts of the bill had suggested that this should be opposed despite possible objections from the local authorities. This view was supported by the Rucker Report which pointed out how the White Paper on Social Insurance (Ministry of Reconstruction, 1944, para 160) gave no grounds to expect any financial assistance from central funds for this service. It was also stressed how "our proposal under which such an old person will be put into a position to contribute 21s to the cost of his maintenance is therefore in this respect more favourable to local authorities than anything they have been given reason to expect"[15]. However, this view was not held by all members of the committee. The representative from the Department of Health for Scotland[16] argued for some form of central government subsidy but was over-ruled by other members. However, it will be seen later that local authorities did complain about this treatment and that they did receive in the event the support of the Minister of Health.

In terms of financial maintenance, the report stressed the need to abolish the law of settlement and removal under which public assistance authorities disputed which of them was responsible for the maintenance of destitute people. Such people could be removed from their 'place of settlement' or have a charge raised against the authority of their 'settlement' in respect of maintenance costs (see Chapter Two). It was hoped that the minimum contribution of at least 21 shillings a week for each resident would persuade local authorities to accept that the responsibility for providing institutional care would 'lie where it falls' that is, on the authority in whose area the person was residing at the time, although the report did accept that in practice "some residential qualification may be necessary".

The next section of the Rucker Report was concerned with 'Special provision for certain handicapped persons'. The theme of this section was the need to avoid overlap between the work of local authorities and the 'welfare' function of the Assistance Board as laid down in the 1940 Old Age and Widows Pension Act. This led the report to argue:

> **We think, not only that the specialised services now provided for the blind should be continued and should remain the responsibility of local authorities, but that the service should**

> **be extended and adapted to cover other handicapped persons. There seems to be no logical reason why there should be special welfare provisions for the blind and not for cripples or for the deaf and dumb. We recognise that there are difficulties in defining the class of 'handicapped persons'. If the definition is drawn too wide the class might be held to include all old and infirm people. This will lead to an unnecessary overlap with the Ministry of National Insurance and the Assistance Board and would almost certainly result in local authorities appointing Social Welfare Committees and staff to administer a general welfare service. The outcome would be likely to be not only a duplicated and consequently extravagant system of administration, but also the perpetuation of the Public Assistance Committees and their staffs under a new name (in fact, the name Social Welfare Committee has already been adopted by some authorities).**

This long extract underlines how the Rucker Committee perceived local authorities as having only a limited role in the care of frail elderly people apart from the provision of institutional care. Those left in the community would depend upon help from the officers of the Ministry of National Insurance and the Assistance Board unless they could be categorised as suffering from one of a limited number of physical or sensory impairments.

The 1930 Poor Law Act stated that "it should be the duty of the father, grandfather, mother, grandmother, husband or child, of a poor, old, blind, lame or impotent person, or other poor person, not able to work, if possessed of sufficient means, to relieve and maintain that person". In other words, the cost of relieving an elderly person could be reclaimed by a local authority from a wide range of relatives. These rules had come under increasing attack. Ford (1939), for example, argued in 1939 that there was little justification for the complex existing arrangements. This view was shared by the Rucker Report which argued that:

> **... the present extensive liabilities under the Poor Law should be brought to an end, and that for the purposes of assistance under the Bill, whether assistance by the Assistance Board or maintenance in a local authority institution, there should be a simple liability of spouses in respect of each other, and of parents in respect of their children under sixteen.**

Finally, in a section entitled 'Miscellaneous', the Rucker Report dealt with two other local authority powers with regard to elderly people. The first of these was compulsory removal to institutions. This concerned the problem of "the old or infirm person who is living in a state of filth and neglect which cannot be remedied because of his own incurably unclean habits or eccentricity or because domestic help cannot be found". In such a case, the report felt that removal to an institution might be the only solution, but the elderly person might not be willing to enter on his or her own accord. This suggested the need for a power to enforce a person's removal to an institution in such circumstances. The report pointed out that such a proposal was supported by the AMC and that over 70 English and Welsh authorities had such powers through local Acts (for an initial account of the background to the growth of local authority powers of compulsory removal see Muir Gray, 1981). These Acts "empower the medical officer of health to apply to the Courts, subject to giving adequate notice to the person concerned, for an order to remove to an institution a neglected person suffering from chronic disease or 'aged' infirm or physically handicapped, who is living under insanitary conditions"; such orders are usually made for a limited period of three months.

The second power concerned the registration and inspection of private and voluntary residential homes which was felt necessary because "there is ... nothing to prevent an individual or private body setting up a Home for old people which may be and sometimes is run on undesirable lines". Nursing homes were already registered under the 1936 Public Health Act which defined such homes as "any premises ... for the reception of, and the providing of nursing for, persons suffering from any sickness, injury or infirmity". As Woodroffe and Townsend (1961, pp 7-16) have pointed out, the Act made no distinction between maternity homes and homes specialising in the nursing of elderly people and it was riddled with definitional problems over such issues as what "the providing of nursing" really meant.

Despite these weaknesses, the NOPWC had been trying to persuade the Ministry of Health since May 1944[17] of the need to extend this system of registration to old people's homes where no nursing care was offered. The NOPWC felt that all such homes should be registered and in March 1945 it sent evidence of 'bad' homes to the Ministry of Health with a resolution "that legislation is desirable requiring the registration with its consequent implications for all Homes which receive persons suffering from the infirmities of age"[18]. In June 1946 Sir Arthur Rucker met Dorothea Ramsey (Secretary) and John Moss from the NOPWC about this issue and this led to a request that NOPWC should come up with a definition of an old people's home. The following definition was communicated to Sir Arthur Rucker on 19 July 1946:

> **Any Home, other than one administered by a Local Authority, which is stated by the Medical Officer of Health to be maintained with the primary object of providing, for more than one month, care and attention, over and above accommodation, food and normal service, for 4 or more people of pensionable age – not being relatives.[19]**

This definition came too late to be considered for inclusion in the report. Instead, the report noted local authority support for powers of registration and inspection and stated that those local authorities responsible for the provision of accommodation for old people would be the natural registration and inspection authorities. However, the report concluded "there are certain difficulties, including the difficulty of defining an 'Old People's Home' and we propose that this question also should be discussed with representatives of the authorities". No preliminary definition was offered by the Rucker Report.

The eventual definition chosen for the 1948 Act was that a home for disabled or old people meant "any establishment the sole or main object of which is, or is held out to be, the provision of accommodation, whether for reward or not, for persons to whom section 29 of this Act applies, or for the aged or for both". Future events were to show this definition to be less than watertight.

The 1948 National Assistance Act

The Social Services Committee of the Cabinet considered the Rucker Report in July 1946, and it received a favourable response. Indeed the main concern seemed to have been over the title National Assistance Bill which the Minister of Health "was not entirely satisfied with"[20]. The next stage was to allow the full Cabinet to consider the main proposals and then to open up discussion with the local authorities. However, these discussions had to be fairly brief; the bill was not thought to be controversial, but it would take time to draft. It had to be through Parliament in time to come into operation on the same day as the NHS and the national insurance schemes.

The local authority associations were invited to discussions about the bill by Rucker just two weeks after his report had been passed by the Cabinet Social Services Committee. His memorandum stressed that:

> **The provision of institutional treatment for the sick will in future be made under the National Health Service. As regards other persons it is proposed that local authorities (counties and county boroughs) shall have a duty to provide accommodation in institutions for any person in need of it.[21]**

Rucker chaired the subsequent meeting at the Ministry of Health on 26 July 1946 where members of the Break Up of the Poor Law Committee met representatives from the CCA, the AMC and the LCC. Members of the Rucker Committee met to consider the issues raised in this discussion in early September 1946, and they then reported back to the Cabinet Social Services Committee. The local authority associations raised several points of detail, but the general lines of the scheme were acceptable apart from two major issues.

The first objection was that local authorities should be free to allocate functions concerning the provision of institutions and other services to such committees as they thought appropriate, and that the bill should not prescribe which committees should undertake the duties[22]. The civil servants felt that there was no very strong reason why local authorities should not be required, as in the case of analogous services such as education, to administer the proposed services through specified committees; this was seen as a mechanism to ensure, as far as possible, that when public assistance committees were abolished, no loophole was left for their revival in another name[23]. The local authority associations, however, were prepared to accept a duty to submit administrative schemes for the approval of the Minister, without the bill providing that their functions should be discharged by a specified committee. This was agreed by the Cabinet Social Services Committee and subsequently drafted into the 1948 National Assistance Act.

The second major obstacle to agreement with the local authority associations proved much more difficult to solve. It concerned the issue raised as early as 1944 over whether expenditure on institutions and specialised welfare services should attract a direct government grant. The local authority representatives had submitted that, as the Minister would have power under the scheme to make institutional and specialised welfare services a duty of local authorities and to impose standards, expenditure on such services should attract a direct grant from central government.

The advice of the Break Up the Poor Law Committee was that "the claim for direct grant should be resisted on the grounds that proposals had been approved in principle (but not yet announced to local authorities) under which the existing block-grant system would be placed on a new basis providing for grants directly related to the rate-borne expenditure of local authorities"[24].

However, it was noted that the Curtis Committee (Curtis Report, 1946, p 141) had recommended direct grant in the development of services for children in the care of local authorities. Nevertheless, the Cabinet Social Services Committee agreed with Rucker that the proposals in the Curtis Report would place substantial new duties on local authorities, whereas the proposals under the National Assistance Bill were concerned with duties which, with some exceptions, already fell to local authorities. The Social Services Committee agreed to resist the claim of the local authorities for direct grant.

The National Assistance Bill was, therefore, drafted without any provision for direct grant aid to local authorities. However, in July 1947, it was confirmed that a separate Children's Bill was to be passed and that the Chancellor of the Exchequer had agreed to pay 50% of approved expenditure incurred by local authorities on those aspects of childcare which were not already the subject of specific grants from the Exchequer. This led senior civil servants to conclude that the lack of such grants under the National Assistance Bill would "be difficult to defend now that there is to be grant-aid for the child care service as well as for local authority services under Part III of the National Health Service Act"[25].

A major rethink appears to have occurred in the Ministry of Health. In the past, grant aiding had been frequently discussed and always dismissed as unnecessary. Now, Ministry officials began to argue that services under the National Assistance Bill were as much in the nature of new services as those to be established under the Children's Bill or Part III of the National Health Service Act[26]. It was also pointed out that the absence of grant necessarily limited the degree of control which the Minister could exercise over the administration of the services, and the extent to which he could influence their development.

It would appear that these arguments proved convincing within the Ministry of Health. The Treasury were contacted about possible grant aiding. Their response was curt:

> **The direct grant proposal was discussed at the Social Services Committee on 25 September 1946 and resisted. The distinction**

> **between children's and other services was recorded, so there is no need to reverse the decision.**[27]

Ministry of Health officials decided that "if the matter is to be taken further it must presumably be done at Ministerial level[28].

On 3 September 1947 Bevan wrote to Hugh Dalton (Chancellor of the Exchequer) and argued for a reversal of the decision by the Cabinet Social Services Committee. He claimed that:

> **It would be a serious mistake to present the Bill in a form which made the Local Authorities' services in relation to old people, and the blind and other handicapped classes, stand out among comparable services as the only ones which are to have no claim on the help of the nation as a whole.**[29]

Dalton was not impressed. His reply[30] reiterated the arguments of the September meeting of the Social Services Committee. Many of the services for children were new, and others already received grant aid. The new block grant system would favour poorer authorities. The elderly residents of the new accommodation would contribute at least 21 shillings per week to the cost. The financial burden of outdoor relief had been removed from the local authorities. He concluded that "we have got to draw the line somewhere, if the Exchequer is to be protected against demands which sometimes become quite shameless", and he asked Bevan not to raise the matter again.

Bevan, however, wrote back immediately, stressing that it was wrong to treat services for children and old people differently. He went on to stress that "as a matter of mere expediency, the plain fact is that without the inducement of grants we shall not get the local authorities to put their backs into the new scheme and, as time goes on, produce the better kind of hostels and services which we want"[31]. Dalton's reply remained the same and he stressed how generously the local authorities were being treated and the need to "protect the sorely tried taxpayer"[32].

By this time, senior officials at the Ministry of Health seem to have accepted that the Treasury would not back down on grant aiding. Instead they were developing ideas about alternative forms of subsidy from central government that would represent 'lesser demands'[33]. Two alternative proposals were developed:

- grants should be paid on local authorities' capital expenditure on new building, adaptations of existing premises and equipment for residential accommodation they have to provide under the bill;
- new building under this head should attract housing subsidy pro rata to that payable for ordinary dwelling houses under the 1946 Housing (Financial Provisions) Act.

It was argued that "we must get (the second proposal) at least to persuade Parliament and the country that we are in earnest in trying to get better accommodation for the old and others needing care". By this time, the issue had been further considered by the Lord President's Committee[34] (of the Cabinet) and Bevan had been asked to have further talks with the Chancellor.

Bevan and Dalton met on 20 October 1947. Dalton again rejected the possibility of grant aiding but he did concede the establishment of some form of subsidy for new residential accommodation along similar lines to that available for new council housing[35]. As a result, the Ministry of Health was able to contact the Parliamentary Draftsman about a 60-year subsidy system in which:

> **The annual contribution is to be: in respect of a bedroom designed for one – £7.10s in England and Wales and £11.0.0. in Scotland; in respect of each other bedroom a sum not exceeding £6.10s in England and Wales and £9.10s in Scotland, multiplied by the number of residents for whose accommodation the room is designed.[36]**

Details of this subsidy system appeared in the National Assistance Bill (Ministry of Health, 1974d) when it was presented to Parliament on 31 October 1947. Pressure was brought to extend the subsidy system further. The AMC[37] argued that the subsidy should be backdated to 7 March 1947, which was the date of issue of *Circular 49/47*. This Circular had urged local authorities to improve their institutional provision for elderly people. The NOPWC[38] argued that the subsidy should apply to adaptations to old buildings as well as the construction of new ones. In the end, the Treasury agreed to the subsidy being backdated to 31 October, and for it to be extended to adaptations. Bevan[39] wrote to Cripps, the new Chancellor of the Exchequer, making a further argument for a backdated time of 7 March, but this was rejected on the grounds that "we must avoid creating the impression that the issue of this kind of circular gives a claim for retrospective assistance"[40].

Apart from the introduction of the subsidy arrangements, the National Assistance Bill broadly followed the proposals of the Rucker Report with regard to local authority provision for elderly people. Two important additions were introduced about the role of voluntary organisations. A clause was introduced which gave counties and county boroughs the power to use voluntary organisations to provide residential accommodation for any of the various groups covered by the bill, and also the power to make financial contributions to them. This was not a controversial clause. Chapters Two and Three underlined the growth of voluntary run hostels for elderly people, and the gradual reduction of hostility from the Ministry towards this development. There was a general acceptance that the capital building programme would be very 'tight' in the immediate period after 1948, and so homes run by the WRVS, Red Cross and others could provide a valuable extra source of accommodation.

The second change concerned the power given to counties and county boroughs to make contributions to voluntary organisations that provide recreation and meals facilities for old people. The Break Up of the Poor Law Committee had considered some form of general grant making power for local authorities, since Section 67 of the 1930 Poor Law Act enabled public assistance authorities to subscribe to voluntary bodies which provided various welfare services. The Committee seemed unsure whether the Assistance Board should have power to make such grants but did seem to agree that "local authorities should have power to subscribe to associations giving services which the authorities will have a duty to provide"[41]. Despite this, the Rucker Report made no mention of giving local authorities such a power under the new arrangements.

The need for such powers was raised, however, by Dorothea Ramsey (Secretary, NOPWC)[42] in a June 1947 letter to the Ministry of Health in which she stressed how the 1930 Poor Law Act was being used by local authorities to finance OAP clubs and to help with the cost of mobile meal canteens. Such views were also supported by a representative of the LCC at a meeting with Ministry officials in August 1947[43]. This raised again the issue of whether the Assistance Board should make such grants. However, their position remained that they did "not want to pay subscriptions to a thousand different concerns"[44], so that the only solution was to give local authorities the power to continue such subscriptions if they thought fit to do. The response of the Ministry of Health to this reply was that:

> **The generality of the poor law provision to which you refer is tempered by a clear limitation to services for which the local authorities themselves are responsible.... I am afraid we shall have to follow the same line in the Bill and limit the local authorities' power to pay subscriptions in respect of activities which are related to their own services.[45]**

This seems to have been interpreted to mean grants for residential accommodation and grants for recreation and meals services. The choice of the second can be explained by a general desire to limit the extent of this power; Ramsey had originally asked specifically about meals services and there was, at the time, a desire to develop meals services for elderly people because of the difficulty they found in queuing for food that was both rationed and often scarce (see Chapter Three).

However, the NOPWC were not happy with the wording of Clause 30 with regard to contributions to voluntary organisations that provided meals. They argued that district councils should have the power to make grants as well as county and county boroughs[46]. This was conceded by Ministry of Health officials:

> **On reconsideration, however, I think that the minor Authorities are better able to judge the merits and needs of such organisations than the Counties. Indeed Mr. Moss[47] of the County Councils Association told me that the Counties regarded the tasks of considering applications from such bodies, whose needs often involve quite trivial sums, as exceedingly irksome, and would much prefer the County Districts to handle the matter.[48]**

A suggestion from Somerville Hastings MP, that local authorities should have the power to develop their own clubs and meals services was opposed by Ministry officials:

> **... it would be more satisfactory ... if we concentrated for the time being on stimulating the local authorities to encourage the voluntary bodies and assist them financially where necessary.[49]**

This Ministry 'advice' seems to have been accepted because the relevant clause was amended to enable both tiers of local government to make such grants, but no power was given for them to develop direct local authority provision.

The media reaction to the publication of the bill on 31 October 1947 was one of considerable enthusiasm and the theme of 'hotels for the old folks' was almost universally taken up[50]. The *Daily Mirror* spoke of "state to build hostels for the old folk", while *The Star* spoke of "hot and cold rooms for 21 shillings". However *The Times* warned that "the new welfare services to be promoted under this Bill can only be paid for by diligent work and an expanding national income". The *Glasgow Herald* was even more specific:

> **... the proposals in the Bill will remain no more than proposals until the present period of financial stringency is past. The new services and new buildings which will replace the old Poor Law system and institutions will make heavy demands on finance, building construction, and manpower, all of which are not only subject to restrictions but are needed for projects of more immediate importance.**

Such worries were only partially reflected in the speech by Bevan which introduced the second reading of the National Assistance Bill in the House of Commons. His main message was that "the workhouse is to go" (*Hansard*, House of Commons, vol 443, 24 November 1947, col 1608), and be replaced by special homes for up to 30 residents who would be composed of "the type of old person who are still able to look after themselves ... but who are unable to do the housework, the laundry, cook meals and things of that sort" (col 1609). Access to these homes would be available on demand by an old person. Bevan went so far as to claim that "the whole idea is that welfare authorities should provide them and charge an economic rent for them, so that any old persons who wish to go may go there in exactly the same way as many well-to-do people have been accustomed to go into residential hotels" (col 1609).

However, Bevan did warn that "the extent to which these new hotels for old people could be established would depend upon the overall development of the building programme" (*Hansard*, House of Commons, vol 443, 24 November 1947, col 1611). The whole tone of the subsequent debate on the bill reflected pleasure from both main political parties at the ending of the Poor Law, and Brown feels this created a situation in which "they welcomed the new National Assistance Board and the welfare departments which were to replace it in a markedly uncritical way" (Brown, 1972, p 17).

Nevertheless, there were several speeches, especially from Conservative MPs, during both the second and third readings, which picked up the theme that the building of fresh residential accommodation for elderly people would be dependent upon economic recovery after the war. Richard Law, for example, in his winding up speech for the Conservative opposition at the end of the third reading stated that:

> **This is a very good Bill, but I cannot help reflecting as it leaves the House, that its effects will not depend entirely on what is written into it. It will not depend even upon the spirit with which it is administered. Its results will depend, above all, upon the degree of economic recovery of this country for which we can hope. (*Hansard*, House of Commons, vol 448, 5 March 1948, col 752)**

The period after 1948 did not see a major expansion of small homes for elderly people. Consequently, many elderly people remained in former PAIs, a situation condemned by Townsend in his detailed and penetrating research on *The last refuge* (1964). The reasons for such building delays and their implications for frail elderly people are the subject of the next chapter.

Between the second and third reading of the bill, some changes did occur; two of these have already been specified. First, the subsidy arrangements for new buildings came into operation from October 1947 rather than July 1948, and these subsidies were also made available for adaptations of old buildings. Second, district councils were given the power to make contributions to voluntary organisations that provided recreational or meals services.

Two other changes are also worth a brief mention. Local authorities were given 12 months rather than 6 months from the appointed day to get their administrative schemes approved by the Minister; this was changed because it was realised that negotiations with the new hospital authorities over which PAIs would be classed as hospitals and which as Part III accommodation (residential homes) could be quite complex and lengthy[51]. Each institution was to "be treated as a single unit, the future ownership and management being determined by its predominant user" (Ministry of Health, 1947e)[52]. Even then, some residential homes would on the appointed day continue to house sick people and some hospitals would continue to contain those in need of care and attention because of an inability to transfer them. Such accommodation became known as joint user institutions, and they were seen as a temporary expedient.

Lastly, the wording of the clause on the compulsory removal of elderly people into an institution was amended. The final clause read:

> **The following provisions of this section shall have effect for the purposes of securing the necessary care and attention for persons who:**
>
> **(a) are suffering from grave chronic disease or, being aged, infirm or physically handicapped, are living in insanitary conditions, and**
>
> **(b) are unable to devote to themselves, and are not receiving from other persons, proper care and attention.**

The amendment had added "and are not receiving from other persons" to ensure, in the words of John Edwards (Parliamentary Secretary to the Minister of Health), "that action will not be taken to remove persons, if proper care and attention are available to them from persons who are not residing with them, but are living nearby" (*Hansard*, House of Commons, vol 448, 5 March 1948b, col 704). Only one speaker in the House of Commons queried the principle of the clause that the decision to remove such an old person should be decided solely between the medical officer of health and the magistrates' court (*Hansard*, House of Commons, vol, 444, 24 November 1947, cols 1622-3). Norman has since claimed that "there can be no better indication of the very low status which the disadvantaged elderly occupy in society than this very cursory treatment of their fundamental liberty" (Norman, 1980, p 32; a detailed account of this part of the 1948 National Assistance Act together with the more general background is provided by Muir Gray, 1981).

The dissenting MP was criticised during the second reading by another member for "the worst carping speech I have ever heard" (Norman, 1980, p 32). However, as already indicated, this was an exception to the general tone of the speeches and *The Times*[53] claimed that "the atmosphere in the House of Commons was entirely friendly". Most of the press coverage of the second and third reading reflected this friendliness. Some doubts about the economic implications of the new measures were expressed, but most papers concentrated upon Bevan's apparent inability to find a name for this new type of accommodation for elderly people. Speakers in the House of Commons had suggested 'Eventide Homes' (*Hansard*, House of Commons, vol 443, 24 November 1947, col 1068) or 'Churchill Homes' (col 1707). The *Daily Mail* spoke of "Wanted – name for old folks' hotels" while the *Daily Graphic* said "Homes for aged to be named like small hotels".

Royal assent for the National Assistance Bill was given on 13 May 1948. Local authorities were officially informed of the contents of the new act by *Circular 87/48* (Ministry of Health, 1948b)[54] which was sent out on 7 June 1948. This had already been sent to the local authority associations for suggested amendments, many of which were accepted by the Ministry of Health. Queries from these associations included concern over what the 5 shillings pocket money should be used to buy and what should be provided by the local authorities[55]. Another doubt was whether sick bay facilities should be provided in new residential homes[56]. A reference in the Circular to the use of rules for the repression of residents under the previous system found little favour with the CCA because "this rather infers that public assistance authorities have been repressive, which is open to argument"[56].

The Circular that emerged from these negotiations began by stating that the appointed day for the new provisions would be 5 July 1948, although Sections 37-40 which dealt with the registration of disabled persons' and old age persons' homes would not be brought into operation until later. The Circular pointed out how the main functions of local authorities were imposed by Part III of the Act and that "responsibility for these functions is placed on the councils of counties and county boroughs acting under the general guidance of the Minister, who is empowered by Section 35(2) of the Act to make regulations for this purpose" (Ministry of Health, 1948b). These functions were to be exercised in accordance with schemes submitted and approved by the Minister. With regard to their schemes for residential accommodation for old people, the local authorities were asked to have:

> **... particular regard to what is said in paragraphs 4 and 5 of Circular 49/47 of the 7th March, 1947, concerning the need for establishing small homes for the aged, accommodating 30 to 35 residents.... The Act charges local authorities with the duty of providing residential accommodation only for those who are in need of care and attention, and requires them to provide different types of accommodation for different needs.... The authority's scheme should specify how these varying needs are to be met (a) in existing accommodation provided by or on behalf of the authority, and (b) in the authority's long term plan.**

The fate of these schemes and of the hopes for a new form of residential accommodation for elderly people run "with a simple code of rules designed for the guidance, comfort and freedom of the residents" is the theme of the next chapter.

Concluding comments

Few social policy academics have had a kind word to say about the 1948 National Assistance Act. Authors such as Brown (1972, pp 11-28), Townsend (1964, p 10) and Parker all stress the inadequacy of the Act in terms of its 'obsession' with residential care. Parker, for example, summed up the situation in the following way:

> **The concern to maintain and foster family life evident in the Children Act was completely lacking in the National Assistance Act. The latter made no attempt to provide any sort of substitute family life for old people who could no longer be supported by their own relatives. Institutional provision was accepted without question. (Parker, 1965, p 106)**

Why did this heavy emphasis upon residential care exist within the Act? How is the 1948 National Assistance Act perceived by the authors of this book?

One explanation for the contents of this Act is that they were a reflection of the low priority of elderly people in terms of social policy provision, although it is important to remember the cost to the state of the post-Beveridge concessions made to elderly people over pensions. However, in terms of local authority welfare provision, there is no doubt that they were treated in a very different way from other client groups in terms of both residential and domiciliary care. Most frail elderly people were not considered to be in need of the new 'special welfare services' that local authorities were allowed to develop for certain narrowly defined groups of the physically and sensorily impaired under the 1948 Act. Outside residential care, the 1948 Act gave local authorities only very limited powers to make contributions to certain types of voluntary organisation. There was no power to provide directly meals services, clubs, chiropody facilities or counselling help. The only balance to this was in the 1946 National Health Service Act, which did give local authorities the power to provide district nursing and home help services.

The low priority of elderly people for welfare services is seen even more clearly when comparison is made with children in care. The latter group were to have a statutory Children's Committee in each county and county borough to supervise their interests. The proposal of the Rucker Report that residential care for other groups should be the responsibility of the Health Committee was rejected by the Cabinet Social Services Committee because of pressure from the local authority associations. Each county and county borough was given freedom by the 1948 Act to locate responsibilities for these services where they liked in terms of committee supervision. The new children's services obtained a direct government grant to aid their speedy development. However, the establishment of such a grant system for client groups under the 1948 National Assistance Act was opposed first by the Ministry of Health and then by the Treasury.

As has been outlined, a subsidy system for new completions and adaptations of residential homes was eventually conceded by the Treasury. It can be argued that this involved an acceptance of the claim from the Ministry of Health that such a subsidy system was needed "to persuade Parliament and the country that we are in earnest in trying to get better accommodation for the old and others needing care"[57]. Other examples have been provided in Chapters Two and Three which suggest that the treatment of elderly people in residential care was a subject of public concern. It was perhaps not the same scale of concern generated about children by the evacuation experience (see, for example, Women's Group on Public Welfare, 1943; Isaacs et al, 1941), but there had been pressure and publicity about various aspects of state services for elderly people. This included the debate over pensions, the exposure of bad conditions in PAIs and press stories about elderly people queuing for food.

These various threads of concern may not have represented a major issue, apart from pensions, but in the context of the reconstruction debate of the 1940s they did suggest the need for further expenditure by government on this group. In other words, there were countervailing forces to the general tendency to make elderly people a low priority for local authority welfare provision. This could be seen in the new form of residential care proposed: to be available on demand, to be run like hotels and with a system of payment from pensions rather than any loss of civil rights. Whether such models of care were to be turned into reality for frail elderly people in terms of implementation of the Act is, of course, a different story.

This suggests an alternative approach to the 1948 Act. It can be seen as a genuine attempt to address a major social problem, namely conditions within PAIs. Perhaps there has been a tendency to minimise the potential change of status accorded to those living in such institutions by the 1948 Act. At the same time, the Act did little that was positive to destroy the old Poor Law tradition of institutional care. No consideration was given to the staffing of residential homes and the need to retrain those used to the regimentation and authoritarian ethos of many public assistance institutions.

The Ministry of Health could not claim ignorance of the need to influence such attitudes. As early as 1943, the Standing Joint Advisory Committee of Officers' Associations[58] within public assistance administration had expressed reservations to senior officials[59] about various aspects of the Beveridge Report. In August 1943 a member of their deputation had suggested "the unfit should be graded by institutions according to their merit"[60]. In March 1944, the Treasurer of the National Association of Administrators of Local Government Establishments in a publication approved by their Executive Council had spoken of how "there are ... many facilities and amenities that can be provided in the large home which cannot be easily provided elsewhere" so that small homes should only be used as "an annexe to the main institution" (Morgan, 1944, p 5). This document had argued that hospitals should remain under local authority control. Nearly four years later the same organisation had accepted the division between the 'sick' and those in need of 'care and attention' but warned the Ministry of Health that this would leave a residue of the "infirm aged (those whose physical impairments or defects of character, require constant supervision, thus rendering them unfit for accommodation in hostels)"[61]. Located in such comments were Poor Law attitudes to those in residential care that were still present when Townsend surveyed staff attitudes in the late 1950s (Townsend, 1964, pp 37-46).

It is, therefore, more appropriate to perceive the 1948 Act as representing the self-interest of the Ministry of Health. Criticism of PAIs had to be 'bought off'. Labour government politicians needed to be satisfied that frail elderly people were being 'looked after'. The 'bleeding process' exemplified by the loss of childcare services to the Home Office had to be brought to an end, if the status of the Ministry was to be maintained. There was little evidence of reforming zeal among those who took the major responsibility for drafting the contents of Parts III and IV of the 1948 National Assistance Act. Their conversion to a belief in the need for a central government subsidy system seemed to have been a desire as much for equity with the Home Office as for developing services for elderly people.

However, if senior civil servants in the Ministry of Health were concerned with departmental self-interest, why did they show so little interest in the development of domiciliary rather than residential services for elderly people? It is possible to address this issue in terms of the broader functions of residential care within society. Townsend has argued:

> **The failure to shift the balance of health and welfare policy towards community care also has to be explained in relation to the function of institutions to regulate and confirm inequality in society, and indeed to regulate deviation from the central social values of self-help, domestic independence, personal thrift, willingness to work, productive effort and family care. (Townsend, 1981, p 22)**

In other words, residential care is only available to a minority; and it is meant to be perceived as an unpleasant experience. It encourages the bulk of low income, frail elderly people to struggle on with life in their neighbourhoods despite the lack of support from domiciliary services. The policy is cost effective and reinforces the central values of society.

There are, however, problems of applying this analysis directly to the 1948 Act. The article by Rackstraw (1944), the Rucker Report[13] and the speech by Bevan (*Hansard*, House of Commons, vol 443, 24 November 1947, cols 1608-11) seemed to reflect an optimism about the quality of life that could be provided within a residential setting, if it was made available on demand to all income groups. Such a system may still have been bedevilled by the limitations of residential life, but this is unknown because this model of care has never been attempted. However, the model of care proposed by Bevan would have been extremely expensive. If such small 'hotels' had proved popular, they would hardly have encouraged personal thrift and family care.

And yet there was still lack of imagination about the forms of government support which could be developed for frail elderly people, other than residential care. This was partly a reflection of the dominant belief that the very frail could not manage in their own homes unless living with other members of their family; domiciliary services provided by the state and voluntary organisations could not offer sufficient support for the very dependent. For example, the Nuffield Provincial Hospitals Trust funded a meals on wheels scheme in Essex and the Assistance Board were informed of the groups the service was to cover. One of them was 'feeble old people, living alone' but the Trust stressed that "the ideal solution in such cases will be admission to a residential home, but in view of the lack of such accommodation a mobile meals service would be of value as a preventative measure"[62]. Meals on wheels was seen very much as a second best alternative. The Nuffield Foundation report was even more firm on this point:

> **If sufficient Homes can be provided, and if the homelike atmosphere found in some of them is introduced into all Homes, many old people will prefer no doubt to enter them rather than to continue living in unsatisfactory conditions in private houses. This will lessen the need for extensive plans of home help, home nursing, visiting, and home meals service for old people who would be better off in a Home or Institution. The right sphere for such domiciliary services is in helping able-bodied old people in cases of temporary illness or during convalescence. (Rowntree, 1980, p 96)**

Not all members of the committee agreed with such sentiments. Roger Wilson (personal correspondence, 10 May 1983) had been associated with the evacuation hostels of the Quaker Relief Organisation and he warned that residential care was full of difficulties, both architectural and in terms of personal relationships; such care was also incapable of meeting future demographic pressure. This appears to have been a minority view in the late 1940s.

The material in this and the previous chapter indicates that most senior officials in the Ministry of Health were also pessimistic about the potential of domiciliary care. Domiciliary care was not effective for the very frail. It was a useful method of helping the lonely and temporarily ill who lacked family support. It was an 'extra frill' and so should be provided by voluntary organisations. Any attempt to challenge this consensus was attacked by the Ministry of Health. In 1948-49, certain Labour controlled authorities (Liverpool, York and Blackburn) were pressing for permission to establish services for elderly people in their own homes, especially visiting schemes[63]. In April 1949, Barbara Castle (MP for Blackburn) asked Bevan if the 1948 Act could be used to establish such services, and he agreed to look into it[64]. In July 1949, the Association of Directors of Welfare Services wrote to the Ministry of Health that they were "strongly of the opinion that there is an urgent need for legislation to authorise the provision of welfare services for aged persons unable or unwilling to enter residential accommodation provided by local authorities"[65]. In August 1949, an

Assistant Secretary from the Ministry of Health wrote to a senior official from the Assistance Board and argued that:

> **My own view is that, quite apart from the unlikelihood of legislation amending the National Assistance Act in the foreseeable future, the job is essentially one for voluntary rather than local authority effort. I am inclined to ask the National Old Peoples Welfare Committee to come and see us here shortly to discuss the problem and consider what more they can do to encourage their local units to undertake this work on a large scale.[65]**

The product of this meeting was *Circular 11/50* on the 'Welfare of old people' (Ministry of Health, 1950a) which argued that the experience gained since the 1948 Act came into force "has shown an urgent need for further services of the more personal kind which are not covered by existing statutory provision and which indeed can probably best be provided by voluntary workers activated by a spirit of good neighbourliness". The Circular argued that local old people's welfare committees should be used to coordinate such voluntary effort. The Circular was an attempt to ensure that direct provision of welfare services for elderly people by local authorities remained focused on residential care; it was not, as Brown (1972, p 39) has claimed, "the first real evidence" of a shift to concern with issues of community care from the Ministry of Health.

Lastly, a common feature of the early debates about the 1948 National Assistance Act from civil servants, politicians, academics, voluntary organisations and local authorities was that it tended to focus on the needs of lonely and isolated elderly people. Implicit within this was a belief that those with nearby children had less need of either residential or domiciliary services. In fairness, the Act did reduce the financial obligations through abandonment of the concept of liable relatives in terms of residential care. Against this, Elizabeth Wilson has spoken of how the reforms of the 1945–51 Labour government were based upon a "depoliticised, cosy family version of socialism" (Wilson, 1980). The dependent position of women was reinforced by many of these reforms. The correct place for the woman was in the home, and one of her roles was to be a supporter of elderly parents. An important theme of the following chapters will be the consistent emphasis of the centrality of the 'family' in the care of frail old people.

Notes

[1] Committee members used population projections later issued as Ministry of Health (1942b). This overestimated the furure growth of the elderly population.

[2] See PRO MH77/18; this includes various reactions to the hospital surveys. It also has a copy of the report on 'Hospitals services' from the Hospital Almoners Association, which spoke of how "chronic patients ... are condemned to a life spent almost entirely in bed".

[3] PRO MH 80/47. This early processing of Beveridge's proposals on local authority institutional care was outlined in a paper from S.F. Wilkinson (Assistant Secretary, Ministry of Health) on 'The break up of the Poor Law and the care of children and old people', February 1944.

[4] PRO MH 80/47, memorandum from S.F. Wilkinson to Sir Arthur Rucker, 11 May 1946.

[5] PRO MH 80/47, draft Bill on 'The break up of the Poor Law and the care of children and old people', February 1945.

[6] PRO MH 80/47. It is clear that the Ministry of Health was aware of this pressure from the document entitled 'Care of children and old people: Points for discussion and decision', 1 April 1944.

[7] PRO MH 80/47, memorandum by the Minister of Health on 'Enquiry into the methods of providing for homeless children: Central administrative machinery', 8 December 1944.

[8] PRO MH 80/47, memorandum from Sir Arthur Rucker, May 1945.

[9] We would like to acknowledge information supplied by Kenneth Brill on the background to the Curtis Committee and childcare reform.

[10] The Social Services Committee was chaired by A. Greenwood (the Lord Privy Seal) and functioned from 1945 to 1947.

[11] PRO CAB 134/697, minutes of First Meeting of the Social Services Committee, 29 August 1945.

[12] PRO MH 80/47, *National Assistance Bill: Memorandum of the Minister of Health and the Minister of National Insurance*, March 1946.

[13] PRO CAB 134/698. A copy of the Rucker Report is attached to the Minutes of the Seventh Meeting of the Social Services Committee, 12 July 1946.

[14] PRO MH 80/47, *Welfare Bill: Possible outlines*, dated 7 February 1946.

[15] PRO MH 80/47, note by S.F. Wilkinson prior to meeting with Mr Stuart King and Mr Fieldhouse (Assistance Board) on the Break Up of the Poor Law.

[16] PRO MH 80/47, comment from Henderson (Department of Health for Scotland), 27 April 1946.

[17] Age Concern Archives, Box 3, *Historical and early activities*. Correspondence begins with minutes of OPWC Meeting, 17 July 1944 in which a resolution from Somerset County Council on registration was recorded, to a letter, 21 July 1949 from S.F. Wilkinson to Dorothea Ramsey (Secretary) on new provisions for registration in the 1948 National Assistance Act.

[18] Ibid; resolution from NOPWC to Ministry of Health, March 1945.

[19] Ibid; letter from Dorothea Ramsey to Sir Arthur Rucker, 19 July 1946.

[20] PRO CAB 134/697, minutes of the seventh meeting of the Social Services Committee, 18 July 1946.

[21] DHSS 94018/1/12, memorandum to local authority associations, 25 July 1946.

[22] PRO CAB 134/698, minutes of the tenth meeting of the Social Services Committee, 25 September 1946.

[23] PRO MH 80/48, minutes of tenth meeting of the Break Up of the Poor Law Committee, 12 September 1946.

[24] PRO CAB 134/698, tenth meeting of Social Services Committee.

[25] PRO MH 80/49, memorandum from W.H. Boucher to S.F. Wilkinson, 4 July 1947.

[26] Ibid; see paper headed 'National Assistance Bill Memorandum: Should local authority services be grant aided?', 9 July 1947.

[27] DHSS 94018/1/3, memorandum from Hale (Treasury) to H.H. George (Accountant General, Ministry of Health), 29 July 1947.

[28] Ibid; memorandum from H.H. George to S.F. Wilkinson, 12 August 1947.

[29] Ibid; letter from Aneurin Bevan (Minister of Health) to Hugh Dalton (Chancellor of the Exchequer), 3 September 1947.

[30] Ibid; letter from Dalton, 8 October 1947.

[31] Ibid; letter from Bevan, 9 October 1947.

[32] Ibid; letter from Dalton, 17 October 1947.

[33.] Ibid; memorandum from S.F. Wilkinson to J.M.K. Hawton (Under Secretary, Ministry of Health),10 October 1947.

[34] Ibid; memorandum from Wilkinson to Hawton, 10 October 1947.

[35] DHSS 94018/1/3, letter from Dalton to Bevan, 21 October 194t. PRO CAB 80/49 is also a useful source of information about the grant aiding arguments.

[36] Ibid; memorandum from Wilkinson to Parliamentary Draftsman, 23 October 1947.

[37] DHSS 94018/1/24; see correspondence between Banwell (AMC) and S.F. Wilkinson from 26 November 1947 to 19 January 1948.

[38] Ibid; letter from Dorothea Ramsey (Secretary, NOPWC).

[39] DHSS 94018/1/3, letter from Bevan to Stafford Cripps (Chancellor of the Exchequer), 28 January 1948.

[40] Ibid; letter from Cripps to Bevan, 16 February 1948.

[41] PRO MH 80/48; see minutes of the seventh and eighth meetings of the Break Up of the Poor Law Committee, 18 June 1946 and 19 July 1946.

[42] DHSS 94018/1/18, letter from Dorothea Ramsey (Secretary, NOPWC) to S.F. Wilkinson, 7 June 1947.

[43] DHSS 94018/1/11, note of meeting at Ministry of Health to discuss with local authority association officers government proposals on the National Assistance Bill, in so far as they affected local authorities, 7 August 1947.

[44] DHSS 94018/1/18, memorandum from Bullard (Assistance Board) to W.H. Boucher (Ministry of Health), 7 August 1947.

[45] Ibid; memorandum from Boucher to Bullard, 8 August 1947.

[46] DHSS 94018/1/24, letter from Dorothea Ramsey (Secretary, NOPWC) to S.F. Wilkinson, 5 December 1947.

[47] John Moss was also a leading member of the NOPWC.

[48] PRO MH 80/51, memorandum from W.H. Boucher to S.F. Wilkinson, 27 January 1948.

[49] Ibid; memorandum from W.H. Boucher to S.F. Wilkinson, 30 January 1948.

[50] These press comments are collected in DHSS files, 94018/1/23, *Break up of the poor law: Public (sic) Assistance Bill: Press comments.*

[51] PRO MH 80/52, memorandum from Boucher to Wilkinson, 18 February 1948.

[52] A copy of this can be found in DHSS 94018/1/24.

[53] As already indicated, press coverage of the second and third readings can be found in DHSS 94018/1/23.

[54] A copy of this can be found in DHSS 94018/1/24.

[55] DHSS 94018/1/24, letter from Sir Sidney Johnson (CCA) to W.H. Boucher, 12 May 1948. Also, letter from Thigh (LCC) to Boucher, 14 May 1948.

[56] Ibid; letter from Johnson to Boucher.

[57] DHSS 94018/1/3, memorandum from Wilkinson to Hawton, 10 October 1947.

[58] Among the organisations in the Standing Committee were the Association of County Borough Public Assistance Officers, the National Association of Rehousing Officers, the National Association of Administrators of Local Government Establishments and the Society of Public Assistance Officers of Scotland.

[59] DHSS 94001/8/7, *Post war public assistance administration: Recommendations by Standing Joint Advisory Committee of Officers Associations.*

[60] Ibid; minutes of meeting between Ministry of Health officials and Standing Joint Advisory Committee, 6 August 1943.

[61] DHSS 94018/1/24, NAALGE Memorandum on possible effects of legislation in connection with the National Assistance Bill and the repeal of the Poor Law Acts upon the administration of Local Authority Welfare Service Establishments, 8 January 1948.

[62] PRO AST 7/851, *Mobile meals and allied services*; letter from Nuffield Provincial Hospitals Trust, 26 September 1947.

[63] PRO AST 7/710, *Welfare of the aged: Old people living in their own homes.*

[64] Ibid; report of House of Commons speech on 28 April 1949.

[65] Ibid; this quotation is contained in a memorandum from Wilkinson to Bullard, 10 August 1949.

FIVE

Issues in residential care

Introduction

Reference was made in the last chapter to the optimism in both central and local government associated with the passing of the 1948 National Assistance Act. The 1949 Ministry of Health Report claimed that the workhouse was doomed and that local authorities were busy planning and opening small, comfortable homes, where old people, many of whom were lonely, could live pleasantly and with dignity. The report claimed "the old 'master and inmate' relationship is being replaced by one more nearly approaching that of a hotel manager and her guests" (Ministry of Health, 1950b, p 311). Similar views were expressed by a public assistance officer from Middlesex County Council:

> **The old institutions or workhouses are to go altogether. In their place will be attractive hostels or hotels, each accommodating 25 to 30 old people, who will live there as guests not inmates. Each guest will pay for his accommodation – those with private income out of that, those without private income out of the payments they get from the National Assistance Board – and nobody need know whether they have private means or not. Thus, the stigma of 'relief' – very real too, and acutely felt by many old people – will vanish at last. (Garland, 1945, p36)**

This chapter discusses some of the reasons why such hopes were never realised. The first half is concerned to explain how bed shortages in residential homes and hospitals led to a constant questioning of the boundaries between NHS and local authority provision. What was meant by in need of care and attention? Did it include those with physical and mental impairments? The second half of the chapter explores issues about the quality of life in residential homes, including the general criticism which emerged of all forms of institutional provision. Why did such criticism fail to lead to a reassessment of the priority given to residential care as opposed to domiciliary services for elderly people?

The organisation of welfare services

Before developing a detailed analysis of residential care for the period, it is important to outline briefly the main organisational arrangements that emerged during this period for welfare services. The Ministry of Health was responsible for local authority services under the 1946 National Health Service Act (for example, home helps, home nursing) and the 1948 National Assistance Act. The Ministry has been seen as having a laissez-faire attitude towards local authorities, which Griffith has defined as "a positive philosophy of as little interference as is possible within the necessary fulfilment of departmental duties" (Griffith, 1966, p 515). Brown has stressed that the Ministry seemed to send circulars only on matters of detail but failed to specify the objectives and overall direction of the welfare services (Brown, 1972, p 246). Townsend complained about lack of consistency in advice over the size of residential homes (1964, pp 23-4). Parker spoke of a welfare service suffering from comparatively little interest from ministry officials (Parker, 1965, p 174). The division that dealt with local health and welfare services was the GP, Nursing and Local Health Services Division which was amalgamated in 1952 with the National Assistance, Blind, Deaf and Dumb Division. This spread of responsibilities would seem to reflect the lack of priority accorded to services under the 1948 Act by the Ministry of Health. An important influence on service development was that provided by the Welfare Division of the Ministry, established in 1941 to supervise the work of welfare workers in reception areas (interview with Dame Geraldine Aves, 3 March 1983). The Division was retained in 1948, and was seen as responsible for 'professional aspects' of the new services; it had a regional inspectorate that attempted to encourage backward local authorities to move away from Poor Law attitudes (interview with Elspeth Hope-Murray, 14 April 1983), although this division had few sanctions to draw upon.

The organisation of services at the local authority level was even more complicated. The 1948 Act did not specify which committee should run welfare services. Some local authorities established welfare committees and departments that were separate from health committees and departments. In these authorities the chief welfare officer was, in theory at least, of equal status to the chief medical officer. Other local authorities subsumed their welfare responsibilities within health departments and the medical officers of health were made responsible for these services. Some authorities took a middle position and formed a welfare subdepartment/ subcommittee as part of overall health provision. A small postal questionnaire in 1953 found a considerable spread of arrangements (see Table 3).

Brown argued from her four local authority case studies that "the administration of welfare services by a separate department rather than alongside health led to better overall standards of social care" since "a separate committee and chief officer had more time to devote to the special issues of welfare services" (Brown, 1972, p 237). Later research by Davies and his colleagues indicated that variation in service development was the product of a far more complex set of factors, such as political control, inherited stock and size of authority (Davies et al, 1971).

Table 3: The administration of welfare services

Part III services	County councils	County borough councils
Welfare Departments	33	42
Health Departments	9	13
Clerks Departments	1	3
Housing and Welfare Departments	-	1
Not stated	-	2
Total	**43**	**61**

Source: Higham (1953, pp 201-3)

During the 1950s and 1960s, local authorities fed information about welfare services into their local authority associations which in turn negotiated over policy issues with central government. The county councils were organised into the County Councils Association (CCA) and the county borough councils into the Association of Municipal Corporations (AMC). The LCC tended to be included in these central government negotiations as a separate yet equal partner. There is little agreement about the importance and influence of these organisations during the 1950s and 1960s. Griffith has claimed that "it is difficult to exaggerate their importance in influencing legislation, government policies and administration, and in acting as co-ordinators and channels of local authority opinion" (Griffith, 1966, p 33). However, this view has been challenged by Gyford and James who have stressed how the local authority associations were dominated by officers and not councillors during this period, and that they "concentrated on fulfilling an essentially protective role, defending the interests of their corporate members, but rarely if ever generating new ideas about the role of local government" (Gyford and James, 1982, p 23). As indicated in Chapter One, the central task of this book is not to answer questions about the relative influence of different groups in the policy-making process, though the data presented in this chapter does suggest a more complex situation than allowed for by either of these two positions. The AMC and CCA had different conceptions of the role of local government. Both could be effective in blocking policy but they had less success in attempts to persuade the Ministry of Health of the need for innovation.

The elderly sick and the elderly 'infirm': boundary arguments about hospital and residential care, 1948-65

The 1946 National Health Service Act and the 1948 National Assistance Act created confusion over the distinction between elderly people who are sick and others who are 'in need of care and attention'. This chapter illustrates how competing professional, local authority and voluntary groups engaged in a debate with the Ministry of Health over how they might contribute to a resolution of this problem and how boundary disputes should be solved. The Ministry of Health responded as a section of government sensitive to issues of cost (hospitals are more expensive than homes) but reluctant to expand the variety and depth of local authority provision (that is, to offer domiciliary services as well as residential homes).

Chapter Four described the early growth of geriatric medicine in England and Wales and its link with concern to reduce bed blockage by the so-called 'chronic sick'. The BMA committee on *The care and treatment of the elderly and infirm* (Anderson Report, 1947) played a major part in establishing interest in this issue within medical and government circles. The main argument of the report for more geriatric facilities has already been outlined, but one further point needs to be made. Coordination between healthcare services and local authorities was seen as a major problem area. The committee asked how it could be guaranteed that residential homes would admit only persons considered suitable by geriatric medical staff and would retain them only so long as they continued to be suitably housed in these establishments. The warning was given that:

The scheme may well fail unless, through the establishment of standing liaison committees, means are found to bring about such close co-ordination of the functions of the various authorities as will ensure the free passage of elderly people, under the expert guidance of the geriatric department, from home to hospital and from hospital to home in accordance with their changing needs. (Anderson Report, 1947, p 12)

In other words, a strong case was being made for the medical control of any future system of local authority residential care for elderly people. This aspiration was, of course, denied by the 1948 National Assistance Act.

A number of commentaries appeared in 1946 and 1947, arguing the case for the development of geriatric units as the main solution to the problem of 'chronically sick' elderly patients, a problem which had been exposed by hospital surveys (summarised in Nuffield Provincial Hospitals Trust, 1946). The main argument for such units was that they increased bed turnover; a secondary theme in many of the articles was that medical staff should control access to local authority residential homes. Howell attacked the lack of interest in geriatric medicine and claimed that such units could classify different types of elderly patient. Several of these groups could then be placed in 'homelike institutions' but it was stressed that "these institutions should preferably be attached to a general hospital with proper facilities for all necessary investigations"(Howell, 1946, p 399). Lord Amulree and E. Sturdee, in their remarks to the Parliamentary Medical Group, stressed that:

The provision of some sort of accommodation for old persons who are not entirely capable of looking after themselves will have to be undertaken, and in providing this there is a medical responsibility which must not be overlooked. Proper classification of patients and accurate diagnosis are essential, which means that the expert diagnosis and treatment obtainable in a general hospital must be available for chronic cases and aged, sick and infirm persons. (Amulree and Sturdee, 1946, p 617)

Warren claimed that the creation of a geriatric unit within a general hospital "would raise the standard of work done, shorten the time of stay in hospital and avoid the unnecessary blocking of beds by patients who could be treated sufficiently to return to their own homes or enter a home" (Warren, 1946, p 843). She argued that residential homes should in every case be attached to general hospitals and that residents should enter such homes only after classification by staff at the geriatric unit. Cosin expressed the opinion "that improved care of the aged sick must depend upon the organisation of a geriatric department in the hospital system" (Cosin, 1947, p 1046). Such views were supported by a leading article in *The Lancet*, which claimed that geriatric units could carry out a proper classification of patients and so avoid the present mess in which 'chronic cases' were mixed in with other types of patient to create "the great dumpheap institution" (*The Lancet*, 1946, 'Infirm and old', 6 June, pp 857-8).

The passing of the National Health Service and National Assistance Acts did not end the debate about the care of frail and sick elderly people, which Macleod (Minister of Health) described in 1953 as "perhaps the most baffling problem in the whole of the National Health Service" (*Hansard*, House of Commons, vol 552, 14 December 1953, col 167). The NOPWC described such care in the same year as "a serious blot on our modern social services" (NOPWC, 1953a, p 13). Much of this debate focused on the difficulties created by the division of responsibility between hospital authorities and local authorities. Who should take charge of those who were "partly sick and partly well" (*Hansard*, House of Commons, vol 476, 29 June 1950, col 2631; speech by Arthur Blenkinsop, Parliamentary Secretary to the Minister of Health)?

The most obvious starting point is to ask what constituted being 'in need of care and attention' as opposed to being in need of medical treatment. Godlove and Mann, for example, feel that it is impossible to make a clear distinction and that this had led to a multitude of problems requiring "much time, effort and concern on the part of British professionals, politicians, and administrators" (Godlove and Mann, 1980, p 3). The implications of this for the relationships between the hospital service and the welfare service recur throughout this chapter. At this stage, it is important to stress that:

> **It seems fairly clear that the authors ... of the Act, which brought what came to be known as 'Part III homes' into being, did not envisage this type of care as being adequate for people suffering from incontinence, serious loss of mobility, or abnormal senile dementia. A 'Part III home' was to be a home rather than a hospital or a nursing home. (Godlove and Mann, 1980, p 4)**

What is clear from the study of this issue over time is that it is not possible to provide unambiguous definitions of such terms as 'chronic sick', 'infirm', 'frail', 'care and attention' and 'able-bodied', and then to allocate them either to residents in homes or patients in hospitals. The meanings of such terms have shifted over time as has the frequency of their usage. However, the general point can be made that residential homes have increasingly accepted elderly people with greater degrees of illness and disability than originally intended. The reasons for this change are explored throughout the chapter.

Bed shortages?

During the 1950s, there were frequent complaints about bed shortages in both hospitals and residential homes. This was seen as a major factor in the conflict between health authorities and local authorities over their respective responsibilities to those elderly people seen as in need of institutional care.

Local authorities complained that there was a shortage of hospital beds for elderly people, and that consequently they were having to look after residents who were in need of medical treatment rather than just care and attention. This issue was taken up by the local authority associations in the early 1950s. Parker provides a detailed account of early complaints from Surrey and Hampshire to the CCA over this issue. A working party was set up by the CCA and AMC in 1953 and:

> **The evidence received from sixty-one county councils and eighty-two county boroughs emphasised the shortage of hospital beds. Estimates suggested that three per cent of old people in welfare homes needed hospital care as well as 4,578 living in the community. The position was so bad, the local authorities claimed, that many general practitioners had ceased to apply for hospital beds for non-acute cases since prospects of admission were so slight. (Parker, 1965, p 115)**

The LCC was also concerned with this issue. A special committee on provision for elderly people argued that "it is found that beds in hospital are not available for persons in welfare homes who have become chronic sick and there are now between 400 and 500 such persons in the Welfare Committee homes" (*Hospital and Social Service Journal*, 1952, 'Provision for the aged in London', 21 November, p 1264). Such views received support from politicians. For example, Barnett Janner moved an adjournment debate in the House of Commons in March 1953 which stated "that this House expresses its concern at the shortage of hospital beds for the chronic and aged sick" (*Hansard*, House of Commons, vol 512, 6 March 1953, col 706).

What solutions were suggested to meet this problem of an apparent shortage of beds in hospitals? One proposal was for the development of hospital annexes to be controlled by the geriatric unit. Graham, for example, spoke of the need for "some extra-hospital accommodation" for the group that "are not up to the physical standard required by residential homes" (Graham, 1954, p 304), while Geffen and Warren argued that:

> **By and large, most hospital staffs are not anxious to accept patients who need little surgical or for that matter medical care, for whom little can be done, and who may occupy a bed for some very considerable time.... The cases we are considering are not cases that could alternatively be sent to an institution, for their condition is such that they need a degree of nursing and medical care that can only be provided in a hospital or hospital annexe. (Geffen and Warren, 1954, p 289)**

The local authority associations were also calling for increased annexe and nursing home provision.

However, in many of the large hospitals turnover rates for geriatric patients were increasing. Amulree et al carried out a survey of 340 elderly patients admitted to a geriatric unit of a large London hospital over 12 months. They found that 300 stayed in hospital for less than six months while the average length of stay for the 300 was 40.2 days. They concluded that "the stay in this hospital of the great majority of elderly sick is not much longer than that of younger medical patients" (Amulree et al, 1952, p 191). However, the geriatric service was expanding. Lindsay points out how the hospital service by 1959 was able to increase the number of staffed beds for the chronically ill by 14% above the total in 1948 while 46% more chronically ill patients were accommodated in 1959 than eight years earlier. The number of geriatric outpatients had increased four-fold during the same period (Lindsay, 1962, p 297). At the same time, other authors have correctly stressed that medical provision for elderly people in hospitals remained a 'Cinderella' service in many regions (see, for example, Ham, 1981, pp 98-109). It was a low priority for resource allocation and there was a continuing debate about whether a separate medical specialism of geriatrics should be encouraged (for a useful discussion of the arguments for and against geriatrics as a medical specialism see National Labour Women's Advisory Committee, 1964, p 23).

What was the response of central government to complaints about bed shortages? At first, Ministry of Health officials tended to stress the limited funds and the shortage of staff (Parker, 1965, p 117). The Phillips Committee, on the other hand, in *The economic and financial problems of the provision for old age,* emphasised the high cost of hospital care relative to provision by the local authorities (Phillips Report, 1954, p 74). Worries about the cost of the NHS were a major political issue in the early 1950s (Seldon, 1981, p 263) and the Guillebaud Committee was established to investigate this issue. This Committee's report not only stressed the value for money offered by the NHS but described the growth of provision for the 'chronic sick'; it claimed "striking results can be achieved by an efficient geriatric unit where there is enthusiasm for the work and determination to see that the three branches of the service are made to work harmoniously and constructively together" (Guillebaud Report, 1956, p 218).

However, by this time, the Ministry of Health had decided that a more general review of provision was required. In 1954, C.A. Boucher (Senior Medical Officer, Ministry of Health) was asked to organise a survey:

> **... of the services available to old people throughout England and Wales in order to obtain a more accurate assessment of the quantity and quality of the hospital and local authority services available to the chronic sick and elderly than was given by the statistical information available to the Department and in order to reveal in what areas and in what respects it could be improved". (Boucher Report, 1957, p 1)**

The Boucher Report on *Services available to the chronic sick and elderly 1954-55* concluded that the main shortage of provision was in local authority residential provision rather than hospital beds:

> **The number of beds for the chronic sick in England and Wales is thought to be about sufficient in total if they are properly used and better distributed. The efficient use depends on the strength of the rehabilitation services, the sufficiency of welfare accommodation for the infirm, and the adequacy of the local**

health services and of the voluntary services. (Boucher Report, 1957, p 51)

At the same time, "4,500 patients in chronic sick wards were considered no longer to need hospital care and treatment" and that "the majority would be suitable for welfare accommodation only if more staff were available and more ground floor accommodation or its equivalent, provided" (Boucher Report, 1957, p 51).

This perspective had long been supported by many doctors working with other people. As early as 1948, some members of the BMA were arguing that "unless sufficient residential homes are provided for old people ... hospital beds will inevitably become 'blocked' and the whole service will break down" (BMA, 1948). The Ministry of Health received frequent complaints on this issue during the late 1940s and early 1950s from both individual hospital authorities[1] and medical pressure groups[2]. The Medical Society for the Care of the Elderly had been formed in 1947 to represent all those who, as one geriatrician put it, "had made the care of the aged sick their life work" (Howell, 1948, pp 23-7). In October 1949, the Society complained to the Ministry of Health about the lack of residential homes and how this blocked hospital beds. A similar complaint from a hospital management committee in August 1950 received the reply that "the solution of the problem is, of course, the provision of sufficient Part III accommodation, by local authorities to meet the needs in their areas"[3]. The basic argument from the hospital authorities tended to be two-fold. First, the NHS had inherited many patients who had been admitted for social rather than medical reasons. These needed to be returned to the local authorities as soon as possible (see, for example, McEwan and Laverty, 1949, p 96). Second, new methods of treatment meant that many elderly patients were ready to be transferred back to the community and some of these needed places in residential homes; a failure to provide these would create a discharge 'bottleneck' (McKeown and Lowe, 1950, p 323).

At first glance, the development of such a 'bottleneck' seemed unlikely given the five-year plans submitted by local authorities to the Minister of Health under Section 34 of the National Assistance Act. A total of 52,000 extra places in residential accommodation for old people by 1954 was forecast (Douglas, 1950, p 12), with many authorities using the bed ratio suggested by the 1947 Nuffield survey on *Old People* (this is suggested by Davies, 1968, p 92). What happened in practice can be seen from Tables 4 and 5. These underline the failure of such new places to emerge and the extent of continued dependence on former PAIs that still existed into the early 1960s.

Table 4: Number of institutions and homes of various types (1 January 1960)

Type of institution	Number of home institutions	Number of beds
Former public assistance	309	36,934
Other local authority	1,105	36,699
Voluntary	815	25,491
Private	1,106	11,643
Total	**3,335**	**110,767**

Source: Townsend (1964, p 24)

Table 5: Council homes opened for old and handicapped persons in England and Wales (1948-60)

Year	Number of homes opened	Of which newly built
1948	97	0
1949	103	0
1950	138	1
1951	112	5
1952	130	5
1953	119	17
1954	99	15
1955	57	13
1956	73	22
1957	72	29
1958	53	26
1959	55	27
1960	76	47
Total	**1,184**	**207**

Source: Townsend (1964, p 22)

The years after the Second World War have been characterised as an age of austerity (Sissons and French, 1963) in which there were restrictions on many aspects of public expenditure. Britain – and many other parts of the world – were undergoing the strains of moving from a war to a peacetime economy. With respect to capital projects, there was a shortage of labour and building materials[4], and this drastically affected plans to build new residential homes for elderly people. As early as June 1949, the Minister of Health was warning the NOPWC that "considerations of finance, materials and labour will continue to restrict operations for some time yet ... I cannot extend any hope that it will be possible to give approval in very many cases"[5]. The implications of this were spelled out by the Ministry of Health in its annual report for 1949 in the following way:

> **The aim is gradually to close down large and obsolete premises formerly used for Poor Law purposes. Owing, however, to pressure on existing accommodation for the aged and infirm which the wider responsibilities of local authorities have undoubtedly stimulated, it will obviously be necessary to continue to use existing buildings for some years to come. (Ministry of Health, 1950b, p 314)**

However, the closedown of the older property proved much slower than suggested by this quotation. This was a consequence of the desire to limit the size of the capital investment programmes of most government departments. Highest priority was given to what was seen as productive investment, for example, industrial estates, new towns, housing for families – the economically active of the present and the future, or to national security. The expansion of the defence programme in 1951 further worsened the situation. The Principal Regional Officers of the Ministry of Health were informed that:

> **We are moving into serious difficulties in connection with the Capital Investment Programme for 1951. Though a final decision has not yet been taken it is probable that following the review that has taken place by reason of the accelerated defence programme the amount we shall be authorised to spend in the current year on capital works of adaptation etc on accommodation provided under the National Assistance Act will be only £600,000 or only two-thirds of what we have been envisaging.[6]**

All capital projects over £4,000 were deferred. The annual report of the Ministry of Health for that year confirmed this "would entail a temporary slowing up in the construction and bringing into use of new small homes" (Ministry of Health, 1952, p 101).

Few new residential homes for elderly people were built in the early 1950s. The meagre funds that were available were spread thinly and focused on the conversion of existing premises and upgrading of former PAIs, rather than the provision of new buildings. By the end of 1954, only 43 new buildings had been provided and 755 existing premises had been converted (Sumner and Smith, 1969, p 25). The overall picture was 29,342 people in PAIs (20,675 of whom were elderly) and 39,820 (28,838 elderly) in small homes (Ministry of Health, 1955a, pp 133, 238). The increase in the number of places between 1948 and 1955 was 21,000 compared with the forecast of 52,000 for the 1948-54 period (Davies, 1968, pp 68, 42).

By this time, the mechanism of control had ceased to be general schemes for provision; loan sanction now had to be obtained from the Ministry of Health for each individual project. Hepworth has argued that "the loan sanction system was first introduced to prevent the debt of individual local authorities from becoming too large, but now the system is primarily a way of regulating local authority capital expenditure to keep it in line with national economic plans" (Hepworth, 1976, p 137). Others have claimed that a loan sanction system discourages thought about objectives and long-term planning (see, for example, Bosanquet, 1978, p 109). Davies, for example, has argued that the stop-go nature of capital investment programmes in the 1950s "shortened rather than lengthened local authorities' time horizons, made fundamental thought about the pattern of development less likely and possibly reduced the efficiency of expenditure decisions" (Davies, 1968, p 101). As already indicated, some attempt at forward planning had been made by the Ministry of Health in late 1954 when it asked local authorities for a list of schemes likely to be started in the next two financial years (Ministry of Health, 1954a). However, local authorities were never allowed to implement these schemes fully.

Instead, the middle years of the 1950s saw a continued limitation on capital expenditure by local authorities. In July 1955 the Chancellor of the Exchequer stressed that restrictions on loan sanction would continue (Davies, 1968, pp 101-2). This was followed in October 1955 by a request to local authorities to keep their capital expenditure within the same limits as 1954-55. Actual cuts in capital expenditure in selected services were announced in February 1956 (Ministry of Health, 1956a) and this "restriction continued until the Bank Rate went up to 7% in 1957, when the government stated its intention to stabilise total capital investment at its current level in money terms during the financial years 1958-59 and 1959-60" (Davies, 1968, p 102). As a result, certain local authorities cancelled projects for which loan sanction had already been promised by the Ministry of Health.

A relaxation of capital restrictions on health and welfare projects was finally announced at the end of the 1950s. In November 1958, the government brought forward into the following 12 months some capital expenditure which would otherwise have to be incurred later. Local authorities were invited to consider projects which could be considered for loan sanction within three months (later extended to six months) and which could be completed by the end of 1959. This move led to the approval of additional capital expenditure amounting to £3.6m, divided roughly between health and welfare. Sumner and Smith explain this had the following effect:

> **Loan sanctions for welfare homes in England and Wales totalled £5.5 million in 1959-60, £8.3 million in 1960-61, and £9.0 million in 1961-2. This compares with an average of £4.2 million for health and welfare projects together in the five years preceding 1960-61. (Sumner and Smith, 1969, p 41)**

On 15 September 1959, the Ministry of Health again asked (as it had in 1954) for building programmes to be forwarded by local authorities for the next two financial years (1960-61 and 1961-62). The Ministry hoped that this procedure would be repeated each year and "in the light of experience" to settle future programmes longer in advance (Ministry of Health, 1959a).

By this time, the central government subsidy system had been changed. On 1 April 1959, the small Exchequer subsidy which, since 1948, had been paid towards the capital expenditure incurred in providing new (or adapted) residential accommodation was absorbed within the new general grant, provided for under the 1958 Local Government Act (Ministry of Health, 1959b, p 253). A Labour Party research report criticised the new arrangements on the grounds that:

> **It can hardly be disputed that including expenditure by local authorities on residential accommodation for the elderly in the General 'Block' Grant under the Local Government Act 1958 ... is unlikely to encourage the less progressive authority**

> **to mend their ways.... Not only did the general grant remove the incentive effect of the specific grants and the central Government's ability to encourage the expansion of certain local authority services, the way in which the amount was calculated did not bear any relationship to the state and number of existing institutions that were to be replaced. (National Labour Women's Advisory Committee, 1964, p 10)**

The local authority associations were equally unhappy. They proposed that, in computing the annual aggregate amount of the general grant, there should be included the equivalent of a 50% grant on all welfare services provided under Part III of the 1948 Act. The Minister of Health had replied that the government felt financial circumstances "did not permit of the Exchequer shouldering the substantial commitment involved" (*Municipal Review Supplement*, 1958, 'Local Government Finance', Report No 4 of General Purposes Committee, July, p 125). It was accordingly the intention that, for these particular services, the amount to be included in the general grant – and the allowance for further development – should be on the basis of the existing small capital subsidy. The local authority associations continued to complain about this situation throughout the early 1960s (see, for example, *Municipal Review Supplement*, 1961, 'Residential care of old people: increased expenditure', Report No 3 of Welfare Committee, February, p 51; *Municipal Review Supplement*, 1965, 'Eighty Fifth Annual Report of the AMC', October, p 225; *CCA Gazette Supplement*, 1964, 'Seventy Forth Annual Report of the Executive Council', March, p 50).

At the end of 1960, 207 new buildings had been provided since July 1948 and 914 converted premises were still in use (Townsend, 1964, p 23). However, as Shenfield pointed out, there were still "nearly 34,000 beds, about half of those which local authorities have at their disposal, in large old institutions most of which everybody would like to see replaced" (B. Shenfield, addressing the 1960 Conference of NOPWC, quoted in Roberts, 1970, p 103). Criticism was developing about this "blot on the conscience of the nation". The publication of Townsend's *The last refuge* (Townsend, 1964) in 1962 created a much wider appreciation of the extent of what some called "the workhouse legacy" (Ryan, 1966, pp 270-1). Townsend's incisive critique of all forms of residential care for elderly people is examined towards the end of this chapter. Central government responded, however, by stressing the need to replace former PAIs with new residential homes.

This situation raised issues about the quality of life offered by local authority residential accommodation which will also be explored later in this chapter. However, the gap between demand for places and their availability also challenged the apparent intention of Aneurin Bevan when Minister of Health (see Chapter Four) that such accommodation should be available on demand for the relatively 'able-bodied'. In 1951, Amulree had felt able to claim:

> **... the staff of a Home for the able-bodied need not be large, for most of the residents will be able to keep their own rooms clean and tidy, and may even be able to help with some of the general work of the household and grounds. (Amulree, 1951a, p 76)**

Russell-Smith, when Deputy Secretary at the Ministry of Health, reflected how "in the early days those we thought of as needing a place in an old people's home were active old people whose overriding need was for accommodation, both comfortable and suitable" (Russell-Smith, 1960, p 47). As late as 1961, Margaret Hill stated that "the time is probably not far distant when any old people who find it impossible to go on living at home will find acceptance in some type of communal residence provided they are fairly able bodied" (Hill, 1961, p 15). Such views were not without opposition. Shenfield, for example, argued in 1957 that shortages of residential accommodation meant that "such care should only be provided for the really frail and infirm elderly who must have a substantial degree of care" (Shenfield, 1957, p 164).

Townsend's evidence in *The last refuge* was that many residents in both new properties, converted properties and old institutions were frail. In converted and new properties, for example, he found that:

> **One and a half per cent are permanently and 6 per cent temporarily bedfast; a further 13 per cent required at least some help in dressing. Altogether 37 per cent are unable to walk outside the Home unaided. Approximately 59 per cent are stated to require help in bathing, 8 per cent are incontinent and 2 per cent required assistance in eating. (Townsend, 1964, p 66)**

Townsend correctly pointed out that many other residents lacked any major physical and mental impairments; they had no need of residential care, if sufficient financial and domiciliary service support was available.

However, the relevant issue at this point is that the idea of residential care available on request for the relatively active, elderly person was abandoned under the overall pressure of demand for such care.

The 'partly sick and partly well'

The abandonment of any idea of open access to residential care for 'able-bodied' elderly people did not signify the emergence of a consensus about how to define 'in need of care and attention'. Were local authority residential homes intended for the 'able bodied' or the 'infirm'? Was there an intermediate group that fell between residential and hospital provision who were 'partly sick and partly well'?

As already described, the expansion of new and converted residential homes was slow in the early 1950s. There was also a feeling that such property should only take elderly people who were considered able bodied. The Parliamentary Secretary to the Minister of Health made it clear in a 1951 adjournment debate that the small homes were "intended mainly, if not entirely, for the healthy old" (*Hansard*, House of Commons, vol 488, 6 June 1951, col 1187). Others argued that former PAIs were equally inappropriate for the frail. Andrews and Wilson looked at a new geriatric service in West Cornwall in which a central active treatment unit was linked with a number of peripheral long-stay annexes. They found that:

> **Of the patients discharged from the geriatric unit during the period under review, about a third went to hostels or old people's homes: more could have been discharged had the vacancies been available. But the greatest need was for a more sheltered type of hostel for the frail old person, not in need of hospital care yet incapable of climbing flights of stairs – often difficult stone steps in the older institutions. These perforce had to remain in a hospital bed. (Andrews and Wilson, 1953, pp 785-9)**

Such perceptions led to numerous calls for an intermediate institution between a hospital and a residential home; this was called usually a rest home or halfway house.

Huws Jones, for example, claimed that the provision of such homes would help those old people who "are stranded in the no man's land between the Regional Hospital Board and the local welfare department – not ill enough for one, not well enough for the other" (Huws Jones, 1952, pp 19-22). Warren expressed the problem in the following words:

> **There is unfortunately a wide gulf between the aids given by the Regional Hospital Board and those administered by the Local Authority. Hence the needs of the elderly frequently fall between the two bodies – the individual being not sick enough to justify admission to a hospital and yet too disabled or frail for a vacancy in a Home. (Warren, 1951, p 106)**

An MP used almost the same terminology in an adjournment debate in March 1957. He spoke of the 'no man's land' between the National Health Service Act and the National Assistance Act so that "there are old people who, because they are not sick enough for hospital and yet need more care and attention than can be given to them in their own homes – or would normally be given to them in a local authority home – are not receiving the attention they require" (*Hansard*, House of Commons, vol 512, 6 March 1957, col 710).

In 1950-51, the trustees of the King Edward's Hospital Fund for London set aside £250,000 to establish a series of rest homes in London to be administered by the Regional Hospital Boards. Each 25-35 bed home would, according to Amulree, contain the following two types of client:

> **The first will include elderly persons who have been rehabilitated far enough to make them at least able to fulfil the three criteria of being able to be up for most of the day, to feed themselves and to proceed unaided, either on foot or in an appropriate wheeled chair, to the w.c.... They will, in all probability, stay in the Home until they become mortally ill, when they will be transferred to the parent hospital. The other type of resident in these Homes will be the patient who has recovered sufficiently to leave hospital, is not yet well enough to go home and yet who is not a suitable candidate for admission to a Convalescent Home because still requiring a certain amount of skilled treatment. (Amulree, 1951b, p 8)**

King Edward's was not the only voluntary organisation interested in financing the development of such accommodation. The NCCOP was arguing that "there is, in practice, a gap between the Acts and it is the Corporation's intention to place these Rest Homes, as it were, across the gap"[7]. To enable such homes to be started the Corporation agreed to provide the necessary capital and suggested that the maintenance costs should be shared between the hospital and welfare authorities in proportions to be agreed from time to time according to the number of residents which each authority was prepared to accept as its responsibility. Access to these homes was to be through geriatric assessment units only (NCCOP, 1950, p 8; 1951, p 9). Eventually the NCCOP established four such homes: Clydeneuk, Glasgow in 1949; Springbok House, Stanmore, Middlesex in 1952; Seapark, in Belfast in 1952; and Hurdis House, Oxford in 1958.

Rest homes or halfway houses were faced with certain difficulties that hampered their development. First, local authorities were often unhappy with the idea that access to such homes should be controlled by medical consultants. A proposed home in the LCC area was abandoned by NCCOP because of the proposition from the chief welfare officer that "the home should be under lay control and not medical control"[8]. Second, there was the problem of how to decide who should pay maintenance costs. Amulree had foreseen this might be a problem:

> **This experiment, which was warmly greeted by the Minister of Health and all other interested bodies, may get into serious difficulties because of the rigidity of administration between the National Health Service and the National Assistance Acts.... In 'Half-way Houses' some of the residents may become rightly the responsibility of the local authority as subjects for Welfare rather than of Regional Hospital Boards as subjects for hospital care. (Amulree, 1951b, p 9)**

The NCCOP certainly did find this to be a problem. It took two years of negotiation over the issue before they were allowed to proceed by the Ministry of Health with their Middlesex home. Even then it was difficult to persuade local authorities and regional hospital boards to agree who should pay maintenance costs for each resident/patient. Local authorities were reluctant to pay when they had no control over entry. Hospital boards were keen to reserve as many beds as possible for their own patients. As a result a 1960 review of NCCOP rest homes (NCCOP, 1960, Appendix, pp 30-9) found that "in Springbok House, although some residents have been paid for in the past by the Middlesex County Council, only one was so paid for at the date of this review in spite of the fact that a fair proportion of the residents there must be regarded as welfare cases" (NCCOP, 1960, Appendix, p 32). The review concluded that the name 'rest home' was misleading and that "recovery unit is a nearer description of the function of the Homes" (p 37). In other words, they differed in practice very little from an ordinary convalescent home run by the hospital authorities.

Rest homes and halfway houses also suffered from the opposition of the Ministry of Health. At first, ministry officials complained about the administrative complexity of the arrangements for maintenance costs. There was also a feeling that by mixing the sick and the frail, the rest home "might soon become something like the old mixed Public Assistance Institutions"[9]. The NCCOP[10] tried to undermine this opposition by arguing the case for rest homes to the Phillips Committee on *The Economic and Financial Problems of the Provision for Old Age.* The Phillips Report was sympathetic to rest homes since it admitted "the elderly infirm present a special problem" as they are often "not receiving the type of care or treatment which they require because they do not fit the categories defined by the Acts" (Phillips Report, 1954, p 73). The report then outlined how certain voluntary organisations had set up intermediate homes to meet the needs of this group but did warn that "the question of administrative and financial responsibility for the day to day running of establishments which are jointly used clearly requires serious consideration" (p 74). The 1956 Guillebaud Report's *Enquiry into the Cost of the National Health Service* was far less sympathetic. It dismissed the value of such accommodation in the following words:

> **The term 'half-way house' is used here to denote a special type of accommodation where old people would be cared for as long-stay patients. In our view, the provision of such accommodation would only add to the existing confusion by creating yet another category of aged patient and adding to the difficulties of defining borderline cases. (Guillebaud Report, 1956, p 214)**

The report goes on to stress that these strictures do not apply to convalescent homes that are called halfway houses. These provided temporary accommodation for elderly patients on their way from active treatment to their own homes or to local authority welfare homes and were seen as "a proper part of the hospital service" (Guillebaud Report, 1956, p 214).

This view had already been taken by the Ministry of Health in *Circular 3/55.* It stated quite bluntly that "it is generally recognised that the type of old person for whom residential accommodation under the National Assistance Act is needed is nowadays found increasingly to be the very infirm person often requiring periods of care in bed" (Ministry of Health, 1955b); the Circular went on to outline the implications of this for the size of newly built homes, the facilities of such homes and for staffing ratios. The partly sick and partly well were no longer in no man's land. They would increasingly be directed to local authority residential accommodation despite fears that this would recreate "the old 'infirmary' ... in modern garb" (*The Medical Officer*, 1954, 'Institutions for ailing and frail old people', 3 December, p 283).

Institutions, dementia and mental health problems in later life

Circular 3/55 helped to clarify the debate about the most appropriate institutional location for elderly people who were 'infirm'. And yet it provided no definition of 'infirmity', nor identified who should diagnose and assess individual cases. Should there be ground rules for deciding whether borderline cases needed hospital or residential home care? Did 'infirmity' as a concept cover those with dementia and other mental health problems as well as physical impairments?

In her book on mental illness in old age, Norman stressed the need to distinguish between the main psychiatric disorders, such as acute confusional states, depression, emotional disorders and dementias (Norman, 1982, pp 6-16); this must be achieved in a way that allows elderly people the same right as others to be "sad, bad-tempered, unsociable or eccentric without being labelled as 'mentally infirm'" (p 6). However, this did not occur in the 1950s. Instead, there was a tendency to talk loosely of the 'mentally infirm' as a group who were seen as 'confused', 'senile' or 'awkward'. Social provision for this group was frequently seen as inadequate because they were certified under the Lunacy Acts and forced to live in mental hospitals. (For the background to the legislation and how it operated see Jones, 1972.) Looking back, it is impossible to assess the real needs of elderly people labelled in this way. How many were just expressing legitimate anger at their overall social situation? How many were depressed? How many were suffering from dementia? What we do know is that those labelled as 'mentally infirm' were another source of conflict between local authorities and hospital authorities in the 1950s. Should they be placed in a mental hospital or a local authority residential home?

Many of the complaints came from officers involved in the operation of the mental health legislation. For example, early in 1951, a duly authorised officer was complaining in the *Hospital and Social Service Journal* (letter from 'Old timer', 19 January 1951, p 61) that there was no accommodation in general hospitals for the 'chronic sick' who "by the natural order of life have lost their mental grip". Such clients needed a 'haven' but were offered only mental hospitals, often after certification. One of the most persistent critics of this situation was Russel Reeve when President of the National Association of Local Government Health and Welfare Officers. He argued:

> **During recent years there has been much criticism of the lack of suitable accommodation for cases of senile infirmity. These persons, mostly 70 years of age and over, have in many areas during the past four years had to be dealt with by using the procedure and machinery of the mental hospital in order to secure beds for them. In some cases it has been found necessary to resort to mental certification of the patient to obtain accommodation. This has caused much distress to the relatives and, because of the age and condition of the patient has been most unfortunate for them. (Reeve, 1953, p 394)**

The NOPWC, the National Association of Mental Health, the Magistrates' Association and the NCCOP all expressed concern over this issue (NOPWC, 1954, p 31). In July 1953, the NOPWC met representatives from the Board of Control who were responsible for overseeing certification at that time. Among the points agreed at this meeting were, first, that an extension of geriatric assessment services would ensure that only the really mentally ill, who could not be nursed in the geriatric wards of a general hospital, were admitted to mental hospitals. Second, it was wrong to certify elderly people simply to find them accommodation. Third, it was suggested by representatives of the Board of Control that "communal homes should try to absorb one or two elderly people of this type" (NOPWC, 1954, p 32).

It would be easy to perceive such complaints about the treatment of the 'mentally infirm' as a humanitarian gesture from a variety of organisations. However, this may not be the case. Some of the duly authorised officers may have felt a loss of influence in the post-1948 arrangements; they wanted more control over the admissions policies of general hospitals and local authority homes. Combined with this was anxiety that mental hospital provision would lose status if associated with the containment of elderly people rather than the treatment of younger people. As one member of a hospital management committee expressed the problem:

> **The chronic aged sick are surely the biggest 'headache' confronting the mental health world. It appears that many of them occupy beds that might be more profitably occupied by younger patients who could be cured and returned to activity of some value to the national economy. (Maddison, 1954, p 983)**

What was the response of central government to this situation? In 1950, a circular was sent to hospital authorities urging that the 'mentally infirm', who would not benefit from specific treatment, should be sent to newly established long-stay annexes to which admission would be both from general and mental hospitals (Ministry of Health, 1950c). The memorandum also advocated the provision of short-stay psychiatric units in geriatric departments to allow both physical and mental assessments to take place. The extent to which new facilities were produced as a result of this circular is not known, although the evidence of the Boucher Report suggests very little in some areas. This report argued that of the 6,734 elderly patients in the mental hospitals serving the London area, 952 could equally well have been tended in general hospitals and a further 1,970 in welfare accommodation (Boucher Report, 1957, p 47). The report concluded that "there was no doubt that many aged persons were sent to mental hospitals who, though legally certifiable, could have been cared for elsewhere if the facilities had been available; a key problem was the reluctance of local authorities to accept such cases" (p 46). Such statements represent a significant shift of emphasis from the need to increase general hospital provision. Instead, the Boucher Report accepts that the majority of 'mentally infirm' elderly people can be directed to local authority residential care so long as their behaviour is not 'disturbed'.

This approach was supported by the Royal Commission on the Law relating to mental illness and mental deficiency, 1954-1957 (1957). Jones, in her history of the mental health service, does not mention the inappropriate certification of the elderly mentally ill as being a major factor in the setting up of the Commission (Jones, 1972, pp 289-312). However, the report of the Commission does discuss this issue. It claimed there was no evidence to show that old people admitted to mental hospitals were not in fact suffering from mental disturbance or deterioration which made them 'of unsound mind' within the meaning of the then Lunacy and Mental Treatment Acts (Royal Commission on the Law, 1957, p 112). This is perhaps surprising since an MP claimed that the evidence of Medical Officers of Health to the Commission showed that "80 percent of people over 65 years of age who are certified should never have been certified at all" (*Hansard*, House of Commons, vol 178, 29 November 1957, col 1494; speech by Norman Dodds). On the other hand, the Royal Commission felt that elderly patients were often forced to remain in mental hospitals when their treatment was over because they had nowhere else to go. The Commission argued that there was "a clear need for more residential accommodation of the type which should be provided by the local authorities, for persons suffering from a degree of mental infirmity which is manageable in such a home and which does not require care or treatment under specialist medical supervision" (Royal Commission on the Law, 1957, p 216).

The main findings of the Royal Commission were reflected in the 1959 Mental Health Act which tightened up conditions under which people could be compulsorily admitted into mental hospitals. *Circular 9/59* (Ministry of Health, 1959c) stressed that "there will be a need for hostels or residential homes for ... the elderly mentally infirm who do not need the services and resources of a hospital". Russell-Smith confirmed at the 1960 NOPWC Annual Conference that this Act meant that local authorities would have to take responsibility for greater numbers of the mentally infirm in their residential homes. However, this needed to be done in a way that ensured "the mentally normal in the Homes are not asked to bear an unfair burden"; there was a need for "more classification and grouping" (Russell-Smith, 1960, pp 43-4). Two small-scale surveys of local authority opinion by the NCCOP[11,12] suggested that local authorities were less convinced of their responsibilities in this area. Little thought had been given to the complexity of mental illness in old age or to the appropriate residential provision. The second report concluded that

> **... we envisage that local authorities will provide accommodation for a number of mentally confused aged in the Residential Homes for the physically infirm aged but that there will also be a need for special Homes, particularly for women, for those who would not fit easily into a more normal community or where the number of confused are too large for the residents of a normal home to tolerate'.**[13]

Nevertheless, local authorities did respond to this situation by building special residential homes for the elderly mentally infirm, and this tendency increased in the late 1960s. The number (66) opened in 1966-70 was more than double the number (32) for 1961-65 (Meacher, 1972, p 34).

By the mid-1950s, the 'infirm' were usually seen as a group which were a local authority responsibility, composed of both the 'physically infirm' and the 'mentally infirm'. Two questions remained unresolved, namely, how could local authorities be forced to accept appropriate cases, and how could disputes over borderline cases be settled?

The control of access to residential and hospital provision

Many argued that the split of responsibilities between regional hospital boards and local authorities was harmful to frail and sick elderly people. Often the suggestion was made that there ought to be a single authority with overall responsibility. As Hastings (MP for Barking) said in Parliament, "I do not think that we shall solve the problem of the aged and chronic sick until we have in every locality a single authority for all health functions and for welfare functions as well, so that the care of the old people whether they are well or ill, may be dealt with as a continuous process by a single authority" (*Hansard*, House of Commons, vol 312, 6 March 1953, col 741). The main alternative proposal was that a single officer should be created with the power to order admission to both hospitals and local authority homes. The proposed recreation of the old relieving officer led Wilkinson (Assistant Secretary, Ministry of Health) to remark acidly that "the old relieving officers are seemingly like poets – not really appreciated until after their death" (*Hospital and Social Service Journal*, 19 May 1950, p 557).

The AMC favoured the single authority solution. They believed hospitals should be returned to the local authorities and this case was frequently made out to the Ministry of Health and various government committees (*Municipal Review Supplement*, April 1954, p 92)[14]. Parker has summarised the argument in the following way:

> **The care of the chronic sick, they asserted, was one of the most notable failures of the Health Service. The difficulty of distinguishing between the sick and the healthy could only be solved by restoring hospital services to the local authorities so that the problem of co-ordination would be avoided. Such an arrangement would also mean that the hospital services would be run by elected rather than nominated bodies, a democratic principle very dear to the AMC. The Association also demanded**

> **that if local authorities did assume responsibility for the chronic sick they should receive an increased grant from the Exchequer as the accommodation they would provide would represent a saving of hospital beds. (Parker, 1965, pp 116-17)**

This message, however, was never received sympathetically by central government. The Guillebaud Committee, for example, concluded that "it is the 'inadequacy' of the services, and not the form of administrative organisation, which is the root cause of the problems relating to the care of the aged" (Guillebaud Report, 1956, p 215). This message seemed to be supported by the Boucher Report (1957, p 31). This claimed, as already indicated, that approximately 4,500 patients in chronic sick wards were no longer in need of hospital care and that the majority would be suitable for welfare homes, if only the appropriate staff and ground floor accommodation were available. The local authority associations themselves were divided over this issue. The CCA never argued for a return of hospitals to local authority control and as a result the AMC often felt compelled to dissociate itself from various memoranda prepared by the CCA which focused on the shortage of NHS facilities rather than the need for further administrative change (*CCA Gazette Supplement*, August 1958, p 180)[15].

The alternative argument of the need for a new post with the powers of the old relieving officer to order entry to institutions was justified on the grounds that "one of the most serious omissions from the present health service is the absence of a local officer charged with statutory responsibility for the care of the aged sick and having powers similar to those held by former relieving officers" (Reeve, 1953, p 393). This view was shared by many geriatricians, the AMC (*Municipal Review Supplement*, August 1954, p 202)[16], the NOPWC (1953, p 11) and by certain politicians (*Hansard*, House of Commons, vol 522, 14 December 1953, col 163; speech by David Llewellyn). Iain Macleod, when Minister of Health, suggested that the creation of such a post was far from unproblematic. Would such officers be employees of the local authority or the hospital authority? If of the local authority, would it be possible for them to direct that a hospital bed should be made available? Even more important, would they be lay people or medical officers (*Hansard*, House of Commons, vol 522, 14 December 1953, col 168)?

Most proponents of such a post – apart from those in the medical profession – failed to address this issue. Some counties argued that it should be a lay person employed by the local authority but this was never taken up by the CCA because of their belief that the real problem was a shortage of beds (*CCA Gazette Supplement*, 1951, p 293). More vocal was the medical profession in stressing that access to local authority residential homes should be through a geriatric unit. It has already been noted that this was a key feature of articles on healthcare for elderly people in the medical journals during the years 1945-48. Similar views were often expressed during the 1950s and early 1960s. Amulree, for example, argued in 1955 that:

> **It has hitherto been a vexed question whether these homes should be the responsibility of the National Health Service or of the welfare authority. In the absence of a joint-user agreement it seems probable that these homes should either be in the care of the regional hospital boards or that the medical staff of the hospital by whom the patients have been treated should be asked by the welfare authority to continue to supervise their health. This must not be regarded as a form of empire-building by the hospital staff, but a means of securing the most economical use of both welfare and hospital beds. (Amulree, 1953, p 574)**

In the early 1960s, Kay and his colleagues (1962) carried out detailed work in Newcastle on admissions to geriatric wards, welfare homes and mental hospitals. They found the criteria used for admission to be "haphazard" (Kay et al, 1962, p 187). This later led them to suggest that "since comprehensive assessment of the total situation before admission or placement is usually lacking it is possible that many patients are admitted to a unit which is not the most suitable one for their needs" (Kay et al, 1966, p 968). They argued that all services needed to be integrated through "comprehensive psychogeriatric assessment units" (p 969).

A variation on this theme was that medical officers of health and the staff of public health departments (that is, health visitors) should play the leading role in the assessment of community cases and the allocation of resources such as residential care. Irvine, for example, argued in 1950 that:

> **The transference of old people from a home to a hostel, from a hostel to hospital, and vice versa can be most readily effected when the decisions lie with medical men who understand the medical basis of the case. In Liverpool, Wigan, Preston and Reading and Kent, the health department is responsible for**

> **carrying out the authority's work under this Act. (Irvine, 1950, p 74)**

The Guillebaud Report did favour an increased emphasis on the role of the medical officer of health rather than the director of welfare services. It recommended that "all authorities who have not yet done so should review the working of their health and welfare services to see whether their efficiency might be improved, and the interests of patients better served, by combining their administration under one committee of the council, or under a joint sub-committee" because of the need "to effect a proper integration of the local authority services with the hospital and family practitioner services" (Guillebaud Report, 1956, pp 215-16).

Despite this, the overall attitude of government officials to the debate about the administration of hospital and residential care is not known. Were many of them sympathetic to the suggestion of more control of local authority services by geriatricians? Did they favour the abolition of separate welfare departments? Was there a struggle between the medical lobby and the local authority lobby within the Ministry of Health? Full answers to these questions could only be found in Ministry of Health file material that at the time of the research was not available for public inspection. What is known is that a complete medical takeover of access to residential homes was rejected. *Circular 14/57* on 'Local authority services for the chronic sick and infirm' stressed the need for a further increase in geriatric departments "both for assessment of cases and for active treatment" but went on to say:

> **It will be appreciated that the importance which has been attached in the preceding remarks to good liaison between hospitals and local authorities and to free interchange of cases does not in any way imply that all admissions to Part III accommodation should be in the geriatric units or medically controlled. Many, perhaps the majority of, admissions to care and attention accommodation will be governed by social reasons. A medical assessment should, however, be obtained where this seems to offer a possibility of effecting some improvement in an elderly person's condition. (Ministry of Health, 1957a)**

Circular 14/57, therefore, rejected the arguments of the medical lobby about how to control access to residential and hospital beds. Instead, the

Circular claimed local authorities and hospital authorities would be able to handle disputes in an objective way, so long as they were provided with sufficiently detailed guidelines about their respective responsibilities.

Official guidance on borderline cases

Throughout this chapter, reference has been made to the lack of agreed criteria for deciding the most appropriate placement of borderline cases between hospital and welfare authorities. The whole of the rest home argument can be seen as part of this boundary dispute, as can the early debate about the needs of the 'mentally infirm'. The guidelines that were published originated from the Boucher survey of services for the chronic sick and elderly. The survey teams were issued by Ministry officials with guidelines over the respective responsibilities of hospital and local authorities because "it was appreciated that different local interpretations could easily be made" (Boucher Report, 1957, p 6). These guidelines were later endorsed by the Guillebaud Committee (Guillebaud Report, 1956, pp 215-16) and then sent to local authorities through *Circular 14/57* (Ministry of Health, 1957a) and to hospital authorities through *Circular HM(57)86* (Ministry of Health, 1957b).

These circulars stated that welfare authorities were responsible not only for the 'active elderly person' in need of residential care but also for:

- care of the otherwise active resident in a welfare home during minor illness which may well involve a short period in bed;
- care of the infirm (including the senile) who may need help in dressing, toilet, etc, and may need to live on the ground floor because they cannot manage stairs, and may spend part of the day in bed (or longer periods in bad weather);
- care of those elderly persons in a welfare home who have to take to bed and are not expected to live more than a few weeks (or exceptionally months) and who would, if in their own homes, stay there because they cannot benefit from treatment or nursing care beyond help that can be given at home, and whose removal to hospital away from their familiar surroundings and attendance would be felt to be inhumane.

At the same time, it was not regarded as the responsibility of the welfare authority to give prolonged nursing care to the bedfast (except those in the last bullet above), nor as desirable that separate 'infirmary wards' should be created in large homes in which patients from other homes are concentrated.

Hospital authorities, on the other hand, were responsible for 'the acute sick and others needing active treatment'. They were also responsible for:

- care of the chronic bedfast who may need little or no medical treatment but do require prolonged nursing care over months or years;
- convalescent care of the elderly sick who have completed active treatment but who are not yet ready for discharge to their own homes or to welfare homes;
- care of senile confused or disturbed patients who are, owing to their mental condition, unfit to live a normal community life in a welfare home.

Hospital authorities did not have a responsibility to give "all medical or nursing care needed by an old person, however minor the illness or however short the stay in bed, nor to admit all those who need nursing care because they are entering on the last stage of their lives".

The Circular described the above as "a working guide". It admitted that no definition could hope to cover every set of circumstances that might occur but argued that local and hospital authorities do not in general have much difficulty in differentiating the types of case appropriate to each. In the odd difficult case, "the paramount consideration ... must be the 'interest' of the person requiring a service" although no guidance is given as to how this interest was to be assessed and interpreted.

Such a circular was riddled with problems of interpretation despite the optimistic tone. Could one always decide if a bedfast resident would die in three months or three years? How clear cut was the distinction between the senile and the senile confused? At what point did spending part of the day in bed justify a resident being labelled as bedfast and thus requiring admittance to a hospital? How could one know if removal to a hospital was inhumane? One suspects that the reality of the situation was that hospitals remained reluctant to accept patients from welfare homes while local authorities often retained their lack of enthusiasm for providing a nursing service for their sickest clients. Above all, there remained a demand from elderly people for places in residential homes and hospitals; pressure existed on both hospitals and local authorities to persuade the other to accept responsibility for as many elderly people as possible. The Circular could be used in arguments over specific cases but it did not by itself decide whether elderly people ended up in a welfare home or a geriatric unit. In other words, a bargaining process evolved between staff from hospitals and the personal social services which continues to the present day. One feature of such bargaining was that both sides had to make concessions. More specifically, what Davies calls "the swap" (Davies, 1979, pp 16-17) developed by which many hospitals refused to accept a referral from a residential home unless that home (or another in the local authority) would accept a patient from a geriatric unit of the hospital. Elderly people had few rights in this situation and it is likely that many continued to be moved around the various kinds of institutional care, according to the balance of power between the various professionals involved.

The guidelines provided by *Circular 14/57* remained in operation throughout the 1960s, although they were partially updated by *Circular 18/65* (Ministry of Health, 1965a) on 'The care of the elderly in hospitals and residential homes'. This circular was a byproduct of the attempt at 10-year planning in the early 1960s for hospital, and health and welfare services. The central argument put forward was that these exercises had underlined the need for joint planning between hospital authorities and local authorities:

> **The objective of joint planning is to ensure that, in the future, care is provided in each case by the right authority so far as it is possible to do so. This means joint planning of the amount and types of accommodation to be provided, and joint planning and execution of the arrangements for the ascertainment, diagnosis, admission, transfer or discharge of individual people according to their needs.**

Hospital authorities and local authorities were being asked to work together. To aid this process, the boundary lines between the two services were re-emphasised. With regard to local authorities this meant:

> **The elderly people whom (they) may need to admit or to retain in homes can broadly be described as those who are found, after careful assessment of their medical and social needs, to be unable to maintain themselves in their own homes, even with full support from outside, but who do not need continuous care by nursing staff. They include:**
>
> **i) people so incapacitated that they need help with dressing, toilet and meals but who are able to get about with a walking aid or with some help by wheelchair;**

> **ii) people using appliances that they can manage themselves or without nursing assistance;**
>
> **iii) people with temporary or continuing confusion of mind but who do not need psychiatric nursing care.**
>
> **They include also residents who fall ill, whether for short or long periods, whose needs are no greater than could be met in their own homes by relatives with the aid of the local health services. Where the illness is expected to be terminal, transfer to hospital should be avoided unless continuous medical or nursing care is necessary. Some incontinent residents (other than those with intractable incontinence and other disabilities) may also be manageable in a residential home.**

The local authority associations were not totally convinced that the new circular solved all their boundary dispute problems. The AMC described the circular as being of "some assistance" (*Municipal Review Supplement*, 1966, 'Care of elderly in hospitals and residential homes', Report No 3 of the Welfare Committee, January, p 24). Jordan, in an article in the *County Councils Gazette*, reviewed local authority expenditure on residential care for 1965-66 and concluded that one reason for staffing variations was that some residential homes were for residents in a more infirm condition than other homes were willing to accept (Jordan, 1967, p 179). *Circular 18/65* was still open to numerous interpretations. Members of the medical profession continued to argue that consistency could only be achieved if they controlled access to local authority homes. For example, Agate argued that "if it is accepted that the homes should be for people with manageable disabilities ... there must be a powerful case for the homes being under the overriding control of the geriatric physician for the area who would also assess the medical fitness of intending residents" (Agate, 1970, p 116).

This chapter has underlined the extent to which definitions of those who are sick and those who are in need of 'care and attention' have proved flexible over time. Increasingly the group defined as the 'infirm' have been seen as appropriate for local authority residential care. However, the question of the boundaries between such care and hospital provision continued to be problematic. A 1983 survey of residents from a variety of institutional settings concluded that "there is a great deal of overlap in dependency on nursing care between patients receiving long-term care in hospital geriatric units and residents in local authority homes" (Wade et al, 1983, p 222).

This finding led the authors to call for the creation of a new administrative body at local level, representing both health and social services, which would pioneer a new form of care which was capable of meeting a " broad spectrum of dependency" (p 224). However, as early as the mid-1960s, some commentators were already questioning the function of local authority residential care. Was it a positive form of state care or a repressive method of social control for those no longer productively active?

The quality of life in residential homes

Thomson (1983) has presented some detailed statistical work on residential care trends for elderly people for the period 1840 onwards. This demonstrated that the percentage of the elderly population in such care increased after 1948, as well as the actual numbers in such care. How is this to be interpreted? Does it represent a concession from the government to the needs of elderly people, or an unnecessary imposition of social isolation upon this group? So far in this chapter, the authors have considered various aspects of residential care for elderly people but made few judgements about its 'quality' or 'appropriateness'. This can no longer be avoided, and was the central theme of *The last refuge* by Peter Townsend.

This study of residential homes and institutions was based upon the following comprehensive material:

- statistical information concerning institutions and homes in all 146 counties and county boroughs of England and Wales;
- reports of visits to 173 of a random sample of 180 institutions and homes in all regions of England and Wales;
- simple statistical information concerning the sex, age, marital status, occupation, mobility, surviving children, contacts with visitors and length of stay of 8,517 residents of these 173 institutions (7,689 of whom were of pensionable age);
- questionnaires completed for 530 residents of pensionable age who had been admitted to these 173 institutions in the previous four months;
- reports on interviews with 65 chief welfare officers (or their deputies) of local authorities.

These data enabled Townsend to make detailed comments on the overall quality of life of elderly people in the three main types of local authority residential accommodation, namely former PAIs, old houses converted into residential units and new purpose-built homes.

His broader critique of institutions is considered in the next section. Before addressing this, it is appropriate to consider residential homes, using a narrower set of criteria, namely, the quality of buildings and the quality of staffing, and how this related to the policies of central government.

Very little guidance was given to local authorities on how to run their former PAIs. The 1958 Ministry of Health report, however, does give some indication of how conditions varied from one local authority to another:

> **Large dormitories and day-rooms have been broken up into units of more homely dimensions, walls have been plastered, floors relaid, ceilings lowered, bathrooms and lavatories modernised and ancient kitchens re-equipped. Some authorities have undertaken extensive work in replacing worn out heating and hot-water systems and installing passenger lifts to upper floors.... Nevertheless, there are still former institutions which have shown little change since 1948. Some of these buildings could not be effectively modernised without radical structural alterations. These may have been delayed because heavy demand prevented the authority from sparing accommodation even temporarily for the necessary works to be undertaken or because of restrictions on capital expenditure. In other cases, local authorities have been reluctant to incur expenditure on old premises which they hoped soon to relinquish. But a few authorities failed to do as much as they could for the comfort of residents in these buildings by such simple means as replacing worn out furniture and equipment and re-decorating in more cheerful colours. (Ministry of Health, 1959b, p 239)**

Many of the 39 former PAIs visited by Townsend seemed to fall into the final category described by the above report. Townsend felt that a third of his sample offered very inadequate facilities and another third were not much better. For example, 57% of the accommodation was in rooms with at least 10 beds (Townsend, 1964, p 32). Basic amenities such as handbasins, toilets and baths were not only insufficient but were often difficult to reach, badly distributed and of poor quality (p 34). As already indicated, the Ministry of Health had accepted by the early 1960s that "the vast majority of these institutions are such that, however adapted, they can never provide a proper home for the elderly" (Ministry of Health, 1963a, p 21) and it was calling upon local authorities to replace them all within the next 10 years.

The first postwar homes were mainly large houses converted from owner-occupation. At first, the Ministry of Health seemed to perceive this as an unproblematic (that is, cheap) means of establishing residential accommodation for elderly people outside former PAIs. However, the Ministry of Health's Annual Report for 1953 (Ministry of Health, 1945b, p 178) indicated some rethinking on this point, because growing difficulties in obtaining suitably sited buildings meant that expansion would have to depend to a large extent on the construction of new buildings. Other writers have suggested that the early converted properties were often not suitably sited and were often isolated from main residential and shopping areas. Kemp, for example, has complained of the large number of:

> **... conversions of large country and suburban houses in splendid grounds, offloaded on to the market by the erstwhile wealthy, left servantless and impoverished by the war. Though, in some areas, undoubtedly sumptuous, the one main fault with such properties was their isolation from the bustle of the world outside. Whilst ideal for a harassed broker seeking peace with his family after a long day at the stock exchange, such seclusion was not always the best life style for an elderly person, uprooted from familiar surroundings at the least adaptable time of life, and further, rendered inaccessible to the visitors, family and friends, who might have made this tolerable. (Kemp, 1973, p 496)**

Townsend's study of 48 converted properties suggested that problems did not end with isolation. He found many of them to have awkward stairways and passages, badly distributed toilets, a shortage of single bedrooms and a lack of lounge/dining room facilities (Townsend, 1964, p 64).

Physical standards in most former PAIs and in many converted properties left much to be desired. Could the same be said of newly built homes for old people? It should be remembered that the plans for each new home had to be submitted to the Ministry of Health for approval. Some of these early plans indicated a desire to retain dormitories and communal washrooms[17]. This led the Ministry of Health to form an Office Committee on 'Standards to be Observed in the Provision of Homes for Old People'. The work of the Office Committee also influenced Ministry of Health support or rejection of plans for adaptation and conversion. The aim of the Committee was to recommend suitable long-term standards for new buildings; it was then the responsibility of the appropriate division to apply these standards as closely as might be practicable in dealing with proposals for the adaptation of existing buildings. The Committee was not to be an executive body dealing with current cases but would have access to individual cases for the purpose of illustrating points of principle. A report on standards was produced by this Committee in May 1950. The report contained guidelines and suggestions; it did not contain rules. The argument against this had been made in an earlier draft:

> **... in attempting to recommend certain standards in the planning of Old People's Homes we should like to make it quite clear that we do not suggest that all Homes in the future should be planned to any rigid standards, nor that they should follow any type plan. The last thing that we should wish to see introduced in this country would be a typical Old People's Home to be repeated over and over again.**[18]

While a further draft was being prepared, recommended standards for premises to be adapted as old peoples homes were distributed to regional officers in April 1950[19]. These recommendations were confirmed by the May 1950 report of the Office Committee.

This final report admitted there had been "varying views on most of the problems enquired into and the Committee cannot claim that the experience so far available is sufficient to justify laying down final and complete standards for future adoption"[20]. For example, most authorities and voluntary organisations favoured small homes that have a high proportion of single bedrooms but "the predilection for single rooms and for small numbers is not always shared by the larger urban authorities". The report recommended that the new homes should cater for between 25 and 35 residents and be situated within easy reach of churches, shops, cinemas and good public transport. Such homes should not be more than two storeys and the internal layout should be simple without sudden changes of level, odd steps or unexpected corners, which might cause difficulties for old people who are uncertain on their feet or do not see very well. The homes should be suitable for use by wheelchairs, while fittings and furnishings should be varied and informal.

The report also laid down the following recommended minimum standards for the various rooms based on floor areas:

Single bed-sitting room	108 sq feet
Double bed-sitting room	180 sq feet
Bedrooms for more than two persons	80 sq feet per person

Dining room	15 sq feet per person
Total sitting room space	25 sq feet per person

With regard to bedrooms it stressed that "single rooms should be provided for the great majority of the residents" although some double bedrooms should be available for married couples. At the same time, rooms with three or four beds on the ground floor were seen as a good idea for the more 'infirm'. It stressed that "all single and double rooms should be designed and furnished as bed-sitting rooms" and should include built-in wardrobe, wash basin, two chairs, bedside table and chest of drawers. However, it was accepted that "old people often wish to bring some of their own furniture with them when they enter a Home and they should be encouraged to do so if they have suitable furniture".

The members of the Committee discovered that the Sub-Committee on 'House Building for Special Purposes' of the Central Housing Advisory Committee had also been considering standards of accommodation in hostels for old people; these hostels could be established under the 1949 Housing Act. The draft recommendations of this other committee were more generous in terms of floor space in bedsitting rooms (160 square feet compared with 108). In July 1950[21] a joint meeting was held together with representatives from the local authority associations and the LCC. The Ministry of Health representatives suggested that the question of cost needed to outweigh standards which might be theoretically desirable. The outcome of these negotiations was reflected in the supplement to the 1949 Housing Manual published in 1950 on behalf of the Ministry of Local Government and Planning:

> **After comparing the sizes of rooms in all the types of hostel we have considered and particularly those we have seen, we are of the opinion that 108 sq. ft. is the minimum consistent with a tolerable standard of comfort for the old person. We understand that this is the minimum recommended by the Ministry of Health for homes provided under the National Assistance Act and we endorse this recommendation. We feel, however, that old persons living in accommodation of the kind provided under the Housing Acts are likely to be more active and may wish to retain more of their own furniture. We suggest, therefore, in these cases 140 sq. ft. is a desirable standard and this is the standard shown in the specimen plans. (Ministry of Local Government and Planning, 1950, p 9)**

Despite the pressure for more generous standards from the Central Housing Advisory Committee, the Office Committee were meeting late in 1951, in response to the capital expenditure cuts required because of the rearmament programme, "to try and produce a larger home on more austerity lines at less cost than those erected to the approved standards"[22]. The ideas put forward included increasing the number of residents to between 30 and 50, to have 60% of beds in six-bedded rooms, and to reduce the size of single bed-sitting rooms to not less than 100 square feet.

During this period, numerous other organisations were encouraging an abandonment of the frequently stated policy of small homes for between 30 and 35 residents. The NCCOP argued that 60-bed residential units were more economical than smaller homes in its evidence to the Phillips Committee[23]. A similar argument was made by the AMC on the grounds that "residents in the homes now tend increasingly to require extra care and attention ... and the authorities find these needs can be more readily met in larger homes" (*Municipal Review Supplement*, 1954, p 201, Appendix C of Health Committee Report No 5). Others argued that the commitment to single rooms was illogical. E.C. Bligh (Chief Welfare Officer, LCC) argued that "the Ministry of Health was resolute in pressing local authorities to provide single rooms and even bed-sitting rooms for old people, but it was a fact that many old people had a horror of sleeping alone and it was a comfort to them to have others sleeping in the room with them" (quoted in *Hospital and Social Service Journal*, 27 April 1951, p 447). In the late 1950s, trade union representatives often called for larger homes on the grounds that this improved staff working conditions; it was easier to develop proper shift working and night cover for the more frail (see, for example, speech by L. Lewis at the Conference of Hospital and Welfare Administrators on 'The Elderly and the Chronic Sick', *Hospital and Social Service Journal*, 26 July 1957, p 785).

Circular 3/55 on 'Homes for the more infirm' indicated that such a shift in policy was to be carried out, using the following rationale:

> **The increased difficulty of looking after the old people now that an increasing proportion of those needing admission will be the very infirm, and, in particular, the higher ratio of staffing that will be needed, might be held to justify the building of larger homes, particularly in heavily populated areas.... After careful consideration of the various factors needing to be taken into account the Minister has come to the conclusion that in**

> **heavily populated areas where considerable numbers of old people have to be provided for and where suitable sites are difficult to find it may be reasonable to build homes of up to about 60 places. (Ministry of Health, 1955b)**

The circular also questioned whether infirm people needed or preferred single rooms. It was suggested that "residents who are likely to spend a good deal of their time in bed might prefer to be in double rooms, or in multi-bedded rooms where the very infirm could have more companionship and, from the staff point of view, could more easily be cared for". Appendix A of the Circular underlines this point by providing a sketch design of a 60-bed two-storey home accommodating 22 (4x4, 6x1) on the ground floor and 38 (5x4, 6x2, 6x1) on the first floor.

It would seem that several local authorities followed this advice. The Ministry of Health Annual Report for 1957 (Ministry of Health, 1958, p 136) referred to several of the new buildings opened during the year as homes designed specifically for the more 'infirm' type of resident on the lines suggested by *Circular 3/55*. The report for 1958, however, began to express doubts about the 60-bed home:

> **More thought still needs to be given to means of retaining a homely atmosphere within these larger buildings. The spacious entrance halls and wide staircases and corridors, which tend to appear in local authorities' plans for larger homes, are both unsuitable and extravagant, and it is doubtful whether the handsome main lounge which many welfare committees still consider essential for occasional concert parties and similar functions is, in fact, the best form of recreational space. (Ministry of Health, 1959b, p 241)**

Similar sentiments were expressed in the report for 1960 (Ministry of Health, 1961, p 112) which indicated that although some plans for 60-bed homes were approved during the year, many authorities were beginning to move away from the large residential home.

This further shift in departmental policy was confirmed by the 1962 *Building notes* from the Ministry of Health which were designed to simplify procedures between the Ministry and local authorities for approving various types of building project. *Building note no 2* was on residential accommodation for elderly people and, although the note dealt with homes for 30 to 60 places, it was stressed that "smaller homes, between 30 and 50 places, are generally preferable" (Ministry of Health, 1962a, p 1). The note also stressed a move back towards the previous policy on size of bedrooms:

> **The main need is for single and double rooms. Where multiple rooms are desired, the maximum should be four beds. About 96 to 110 sq. ft. is required for single rooms; 160 to 170 sq. ft. for doubles; and about 80 sq. ft. per person for four-bedded rooms. The arrangement should be to provide for not less than 40 to 50 per cent of the residents in single rooms, 30 to 40 per cent in double rooms, and not more than 10 to 12 per cent in four-bedded rooms. (Ministry of Health, 1962a, p 4)**

This *Building note* remained the main advice to local authorities through to the reorganisation of the personal social services.

The period 1948-62, therefore, saw considerable uncertainty about policy towards the design of purpose-built residential homes. Townsend expressed anger at "these vacillations on the part of the Ministry of Health about the design of residential homes" (Townsend, 1964, p 23) which he felt showed a lack of confidence in the general direction of postwar policy. A more generous interpretation would be that Ministry of Health officials reverted to the standards they believed in as soon as they were allowed by the Treasury and their political masters. At the same time, the discussion of residential care policy so far has illustrated the extent to which the Ministry of Health and the local authorities were concerned with costs and completion rates. Individual members of the Welfare Division might be concerned with the quality of life inside residential homes but the bulk of departmental discussion was finance-led.

This analysis also explains the lack of comment from the Ministry of Health or local authorities about appropriate training for the staff of residential homes. In Chapter Four, it was noted that this issue was not addressed in 1948 despite Bevan's comment that "the workhouse is to go" (*Hansard*, House of Commons, vol 443, 24 November 1947, col 1608). This aim was not seen as having implications for the retraining of staff brought up in the tradition of Poor Law service. Many of the staff in former PAIs interviewed for *The last refuge* were middle-aged and elderly persons who had given "a lifetime's service under the old Poor Law as well as the new administration" (Townsend, 1964, p 39). Townsend felt "it would be idle to pretend that many of them were imbued with the more progressive standards of personal care encouraged by the Ministry of Health, geriatricians, social workers and others since the war"; indeed, a minority of them "were unsuitable, by any standards, for the tasks they performed, men or women with authoritarian attitudes inherited from Poor Law days who provoked resentment and even terror among infirm people" (p 39).

Townsend emphasised the lack of retraining offered to such staff. Several senior staff in all these types of home did have nursing qualifications but there was little evidence of training or knowledge about the latest approaches to meeting the social needs of elderly people. Residential work with elderly people was seen as 'women's work' in which the appropriate qualities of warmth, gentleness and good housekeeping would flow naturally from the right type of applicant with the minimum of instruction. This can be illustrated by the early struggles of voluntary organisations to gain support from central and local government for training initiatives in this field.

In March 1949, the Secretary of the NOPWC wrote to the Deputy Secretary, Ministry of Health about "the promotion of a scheme of training for Matrons and Assistant Matrons in Old People's Homes"[24]. In the long term, NOPWC hoped to develop a one-year course but at first they wished to start a one-week residential course at the London School of Economics for 45 people from 11-18 September 1949. The Deputy Secretary was initially enthusiastic and suggested that a senior officer from his Welfare Division sat on the training sub-committee of NOPWC. In May 1949, the Ministry of Health issued *Circular 50/49* (Ministry of Health, 1949a) which stressed that residential homes were to expand and that this created a need for "training not only those who are to be appointed to new Homes but also those already employed in the existing establishments". The September course of the NOPWC was outlined and the following subject areas listed:

- the psychological problems of old people
- modern methods of rehabilitation
- the place of the home in the community
- the importance of the individual
- food values, with special reference to old people
- general problems of catering
- occupations and recreation for old people
- special problems of old age
- household management with special reference to the importance of record keeping, staff management and hygiene in homes

- statutory and voluntary provision for the aged.

The circular encouraged local authorities to send their staff on this course. It indicated that a long-term review of training requirements was being carried out by the Ministry and the NOPWC.

Almost from the beginning, the officials at the Ministry of Health had "reservations about the need for a one year course"[25]. The NOPWC were encouraged to develop a six-month course involving three months' theoretical work and three months' practical. The first course was planned for September 1950. Grants or bursaries were to be provided by local education authorities and from the NCCOP. *Circular 25/50* (Ministry of Health, 1950d) from the Ministry of Health outlined the diploma course but this circular found little favour with the local authority associations. The Secretary of the AMC claimed "arrangements embodied in the circular are somewhat nebulous" especially over whether local authorities would have to find the salary of an employee who went on the course. He also queried whether the NOPWC was "sufficiently representative of local authorities if it is to become a recognised body for training purposes"[26].

Both the AMC and the LCC produced papers on their own attitude to training. Ministry of Health officials summarised the AMC position in the following way:

> **They hold the view that it is essential that officers of local authorities who are primarily concerned in this matter should be allowed to work out detailed training arrangements before any schemes other than experimental schemes are put into force on a national basis.... They understood that the Ministry agree that the present training courses being carried out by the National Old People's Welfare Committee and the National Corporation for the Care of Old People would be entirely without prejudice to the future pattern of training arrangements, and that no implications whatever flow from the holding of these courses.**[27]

The Welfare Department of the LCC was even more blunt. Its paper argued that the most important qualifications for a matron of a small home are not dietetics or geriatrics but a flair for homeworking, sympathy with old people and above all, commonsense and administrative ability[28]. The LCC clearly saw most residential care jobs as women's work, and not especially skilled at that.

These papers were discussed at a conference held on 30 June 1950 in which a deputation from the AMC, CCA, and LCC met senior officials from the Ministry of Health. The Under Secretary informed the meeting that "Circular 50/49 had unintentionally overstated the Ministry's position, vis-à-vis the National Old People's Welfare Committee in regard to long-term planning of training". At the meeting, "it was further agreed that there did not appear to be a need for a long (six month) course"[29] for residential staff. The AMC and LCC representatives stressed their desire to carry out their own training. Ministry of Health officials claimed that there was a need for a national training body with local authority representatives to replace the old Poor Law Examination Board.

Nevertheless, the diploma course did get off the ground with the help of bursaries from the NCCOP for workers from the voluntary sector. More refresher courses were also held. For example, six short refresher courses were run from September 1950 to September 1951 (NCCOP, 1951) while the diploma continued, although further shortened to four months. In the following year male candidates were excluded from the course because of difficulties of placing them with local authorities (Ministry of Health, 1953, p 120). The hostility of the local authority associations, or at least the AMC and LCC, also remained at a more general level. In 1952 the Care of Elderly Persons Sub-Committee of the AMC produced a report on the *Training of matrons, assistant matrons and wardens of old people's homes.* Although the report claimed this was "a field in which local authority action might well be taken", it went on to state that "it would not seem that at the present time there is any need for a lengthy course, and it is suggested that the period of training should be of not more than two weeks' duration and should be suitable both as a refresher course ... and as a course for those who have been newly appointed" (*CCA Gazette Supplement*, February 1953, p 20)[30]. The ideal matron or warden was seen as a mature person with a pleasant outlook on life and plenty of tact and gentleness. Experience in nursing was seen as a great advantage but not essential. The two-week course would cover the following three main areas:

- general: housekeeping, including the purchasing and storage of food in bulk; some knowledge of bulk cooking but bearing in mind the special requirements of old people;
- special needs of old people;
- Minor ailments of old people[30].

In November 1952 a joint meeting of representatives from the CCA, AMC and LCC met to consider the AMC report on training. This meeting provoked considerable aggression from the LCC representatives about the four-month NOPWC course which they described as "unnecessarily long"[31]. Representatives from the AMC "considered that the initiative in providing both training and refresher courses ought to come from the local authorities themselves". Defence for the NOPWC courses did, however, come from the CCA representatives who said "they had no reason to suppose that county councils were otherwise than well satisfied with the courses being run by the National Old People's Welfare Committee and they would not wish to see any steps taken to disturb the existing arrangements in the absence of any evidence that they were inadequate or not working satisfactorily".

Such attitudes meant it was difficult for the NOPWC to finance their diploma and refresher courses. However, in 1954 a grant from the King George VI Foundation made it possible for the NOPWC to continue these courses, and to extend the scheme to include courses for voluntary workers helping the much larger number of elderly people living in their own homes. This scheme became known as the King George VI Social Service Scheme and a further 10-year grant was made in 1958. The four-month diploma course and the refresher courses continued as before. The 1961 handbook of the NOPWC suggested the following types of applicant were attracted to the four-month course:

> **The majority of the applicants selected to take these courses are between the ages of thirty and fifty and they come from a wide variety of backgrounds. They have included widows, women who have lived at home looking after relatives, housekeepers, business women and clerical workers, teachers and nurses, as well as those already working as assistants in homes who seek promotion within the service. (NOPWC, 1961a, p 145)**

The NOPWC saw the job as a demanding one, requiring a wide combination of personal qualities and practical skills. The essential qualifications were seen as "a genuine respect and liking for elderly people, an imaginative approach to their needs and an ability to make and sustain sound personal relationships with people of all ages" (NOPWC, 1961a, p 144). The NOPWC and the local authority associations agreed that residential care was women's work; they disagreed over the level of expertise required to carry it out. However, the NOPWC was able to influence only a small number of staff. By December 1958 only 200 trainees had been through the scheme (Ministry of Health, 1959b, p 243).

The late 1950s and early 1960s saw no change in this situation. The Younghusband Report (1959) on the recruitment and training of social workers reserved only a single paragraph for the training of residential staff, and fieldwork staff were seen as a much higher priority. The impact of *The last refuge* upon such complacency is not known. However, the Ministry of Health did begin to express concern at the inability of local authorities to obtain sufficient residential staff because of poor working conditions. The 1961 annual report of the Ministry of Health stated:

> **The care of the very infirm makes heavy demands on staff at all levels, and recruitment, especially of assistant matrons and resident assistants, continues to present difficulties in almost every part of the country. The considerations which appear most to affect recruitment are the standard of accommodation for staff and the status accorded to the work. It is important to provide suitable staff accommodation of a proper standard, and essential that staff should have adequate opportunities for rest and privacy ... this peculiarly taxing type of work. Training and Refresher courses for matrons and assistant matrons have continued to be held by the National Old People's Welfare Council though these no more than touch the fringe of need. (Ministry of Health, 1962b, p 92)**

The NCSS decided to finance a survey committee into how staff shortages in all forms of residential care could be overcome. This was chaired by Professor Lady Williams and the final report was not published until 1967. *Caring for people: Staffing residential homes* surveyed the staff of nearly 2,000 homes in the public, voluntary and private sector and found that over 80% of all full-time care staff were without any formal qualifications for their work (Williams Report, 1967, p 45). They also found that over 80% of resident care staff were women and nearly two thirds were married women.

The report envisaged an increase in demand for residential homes especially from older people. It was felt that this demand could only be met if new sources of recruitment were found such as older women, more men and married couples. In particular, the report argued that "bringing up a family is the kind of experience that can make an excellent foundation for the training that is necessary for residential work" (Williams Report, 1967, p 148). Considerable thought was given as to what the nature of that training might be, and the main recommendation was that "the accepted pattern of training for those who wish to take up residential work as a career should be a two-year course providing a common context of study for all students, with special sections enabling the student to concentrate on his main fields of interest" (p 179). It was also agreed that for some older and experienced students, a one-year course of a specialized nature should be set up, in the first instance for an experimental period of five years. The development of in-service training was also seen as essential. The core element of such training would be to instil "knowledge of complex human personalities and relationships" which would give "the ability to learn and comprehend something of the working of the mind and the emotions and the ways in which people's behaviour and ideas have been fashioned by their lives, their families and their social background" (p 32).

As a result of the report, the Ministry of Health asked the Council for Training in Social Work (CTSW) to set up one-and two-year diploma courses for residential staff. However, the first of the two-year courses was abandoned because of lack of applicants (Younghusband, 1978a, p 183). By 1971 there were eight full-time one-year courses for senior staff and in-service training was also being developed by CTSW (Younghusband, 1978a, p 184). The development of these courses was, of course, interrupted by the implementation of the main proposals of the Seebohm Report (1968) (see Chapter Seven).

The last refuge: the response of central government

Staffing and buildings are only pointers to the possible quality of life offered in residential homes; they say little about the actual experiences of elderly residents. And yet *The last refuge* is often remembered as a bitter attack upon the failure of the state to end the use of PAIs after 1948; the problem was not residential care but the use of inadequate buildings and poorly trained staff. However, that is not the central theme of *The last refuge* which is rather the presentation of evidence that all existing forms of residential care fail to offer a living environment that meets the needs of elderly people. The residents suffer from a loss of occupation, they feel isolated from family, friends and community, they fail to make new relationships, they experience a loss of privacy and identity and there is a collapse of powers of self-determination. Townsend concludes that the long-stay institution fails to give residents "the advantages of living in a 'normal' community" (Townsend, 1964, p 190) and should be abandoned as an instrument of social policy.

What were the alternatives? Townsend argued that many residents were placed in residential homes because they lacked adequate income and housing rather than because they were frail. Despite the trends discussed in the previous sections, Townsend found that "between a half and two-thirds are comparatively active and are physically and mentally capable of managing most or all personal and household tasks with little or no help" (Townsend, 1964, p 193). With regard to the group defined as the 'infirm', Townsend proposed two main policies. The first of these was for an expansion of sheltered accommodation so that all housing authorities would provide at least 50 dwellings per 1,000 population aged 65 and over in 'sheltered' schemes within a period of 10 years. This would be a considerable undertaking since:

> **By 1958 there were only 134 schemes with 2,938 dwellings in county council areas of England and Wales, although another 64 schemes with 1,376 dwellings were planned. There were another 84 schemes comprising 1,254 dwellings in county boroughs. As many as 27 county councils and 32 county boroughs had no schemes in operation. (Townsend, 1964, p 200)**

Townsend claimed such housing should largely replace residential homes as then understood and administered.

Second, he argued that a family help service should be established to develop systematic visiting schemes, to administer sheltered housing schemes and to organise the provision of domiciliary services such as home help, meals, laundry and night attendance. The overall principle should be that "when the individual can no longer do some necessary personal or household task for himself, and his family cannot do it for him, then it should be the duty of the home and welfare services to help, and to go on offering (and giving) help so long as he is able to live there" (Townsend, 1964, p 202). This required a rapid expansion of the domiciliary services. Finally, those who were sick should receive treatment from the NHS. The division between the 'sick' in hospital and the 'infirm' in residential homes was artificial and so the diminished number of residential homes "should be administered by hospital management committees, under the general direction of regional hospital boards" (p 207). The emphasis should again be on returning elderly people to their own homes as soon as possible rather than offering a long-term home.

The last refuge was not an isolated attack upon the limitations of institutional life. This period saw a whole series of books and articles about different kinds of institutions from a variety of perspectives. However, many of them agreed that institutions 'cut' people off from normal society and normal social relationships, and that this has a deleterious impact upon their personality and behaviour. Barton, for example, claimed to have discovered a disease called "institutional neurosis" which is "characterised by apathy, lack of initiative, loss of interest, especially in things of an impersonal nature, submissiveness, apparent inability to make plans for the future, lack of individuality, and sometimes a characteristic posture and gait" (Barton, 1959, p 53). In other words, mental hospital patients often develop a secondary illness as a result of their loss of normal social relationships. A sociological as opposed to medical approach was offered by Goffman who looked at mental hospitals and mental patients in the USA. He felt such hospitals were total institutions "defined as a place of residence and work where a large number of like-situated individuals, cut off from the wider society for an appreciable period of time, together lead an enclosed, formally administered round of life" (Goffman, 1968, p 11). Goffman also discussed homes for those felt to be "both incapable and harmless" (p 16) such as frail elderly people, and these were also seen as total institutions. All total institutions operated in the following way:

> **A basic social arrangement in modern society is that the individual tends to sleep, play and work in different places, with different co-participants, under different authorities, and without an overall rational plan. The central feature of total institutions can be described as a breakdown of the barriers ordinarily separating these three spheres of life. First, all aspects of life are conducted in the same place and under the same single authority. Second, each phase of the member's daily activity is carried on in the immediate company of a large batch of others, all of whom are treated alike and required to do the same thing together. Third, all phases of the day's activities are tightly scheduled, with one activity leading at a prearranged time to the next, the whole sequence of activities being imposed from above by a system of explicit formal rulings and a body of officials. Finally, the various enforced activities are brought together into a single rational plan purportedly designed to fulfil the official aims of the institution. (Goffman, 1968, p 17)**

Again, the same theme is present. Institutions such as residential homes are 'cut off' from normal society and are an artificial way to live. Batch living is the opposite to family life. If institutions are 'cut off' from the rest of society, then residents and patients may be very much at the mercy of staff. In Britain, the dangers of this were exposed by a group called Aid for the Elderly in Government Institutions (AEGIS) which claimed in the mid-1960s that there was widespread abuse of mental and geriatric patients by hospital staff. Their book, *Sans everything: A case to answer,* (Robb, 1967) received massive publicity and was a major factor in the establishment of an NHS hospital advisory service in 1969 (*The Hospital*, 1969, 'NHS Hospital Advisory Service', June, pp 205-6).

Finally, in the early 1970s, *Taken for a ride* by Michael Meacher was published. This was a study of special homes for elderly people with dementia. He claimed these protect "small ordinary homes from the disturbances of disapproved or even repugnant behaviour and enable these homes to preserve their more select and exclusive image by offering an alternative repository for the confused elderly" (Meacher, 1972, p 475). Unfortunately the implications of such separatist policies for residents and staff were profound:

> **For staff what is signified is that there is something 'wrong' or abnormal about the residents: for why else should they be there, and how else is dissociation justified? Any quirk of behaviour is then naturally interpreted as derivative from the single underlying cause of admission, mental infirmity. Consequently a series of practices are adopted by administrative and care staff – such as dumping without explanation ('taking for a ride'), infantilizing procedures, heavy sedation, physical restrictions like the use of geriatric chairs, ritualised questions and similar devices – the cumulative impact of which may generate the need for defensive psychological manoeuvres on the part of the residents. To the extent that the latter employ a strategy of compensation or dissociation or retreat negatively into paranoia or withdrawal or even assume the ploys of panicky tactical defensiveness, they expose themselves to the label of impression and provoke the rationalisation that their condition is organic rather than reactive. (Meacher, 1972, p 476)**

An alternative approach was required. A comprehensive system of domiciliary psychogeriatric assessment should be available and the focus should be on enabling elderly people to remain in their own homes through a major expansion of day care and domiciliary services. Overall, the task was "to preserve the family structure intact as the natural care agency, and secondly to maintain and encourage work or other positive family commitments as long as possible" (Meacher, 1972, p 308). Family care was natural; residential care was not.

There is no evidence of any general support from central and local government officials for this generalised critique of institutions although the rest of this chapter and the next two will discuss how a complex reassessment of state provision did take place in the late 1960s. Indeed, many officials[32] felt anger at *The last refuge* which they saw as a biased account of residential life that failed to acknowledge the post-1948 achievements (for an indication of discontent from local authority officials, see Beglin, 1965, pp 199-205). There were problems with residential care and there was a need to expand domiciliary services but the overall situation was improving. Central government continued to argue that residential care could deal with the social and medical needs of older people more appropriately on a long-term basis than hospitals. This was the central thrust of both *Circular 14/57* and *Circular 18/65*. The 10-year plans for both hospitals and health and welfare social services reflected this theme. The 1962 hospital plan envisaged a reduction in beds 'reserved' for geriatric cases (Ministry of Health, 1962c, p 5); the 1963 10-year plans for health and welfare services encouraged a major expansion of residential care (Ministry of Health, 1963a, pp 13-14). In terms of the proposed capital programme, just over half of the money was to be devoted to residential homes for elderly people (£117m out of a capital building programme total of £223m) (Ministry of Health, 1963a, p 367). Local authorities were asked to revise their plans in each of the following two years (Ministry of Health, 1964a; 1966a). These plans and their revisions replaced the return by local authorities of their building programmes for the ensuing two financial years. In other words, it was "intended to use the revised plan as the future building programme ... and to plan the allocation of loan sanctions accordingly" (Ministry of Health, 1963b). The stated policy behind the capital programme for residential accommodation was to replace all unsatisfactory premises, whether former PAIs (Ministry of Health, 1965b) or converted dwellings, and to bring the provision of places in homes for elderly people by all 146 local authorities up to the national average in 10 years' time, derived from the plans returned to the Ministry by the individual authorities. Yet many felt the changed mechanism did not represent a coherent attempt to link provision to need:

> **Although the Government have published a document which purports to be a national plan for the development of health and welfare services over the next 10 years, it is extremely difficult to regard it as a plan at all ... there is no evidence of the Government having given any leadership at all to local authorities to assist them in working out their proposals.(National Labour Women's Advisory Committee, 1964, p 10)**

In other words, there were no objective criteria employed, arbitrary standards were devised from meaningless averages and doubts were expressed about the feasibility of the policy:

> **The norm involved a perfect circle. It was, in fact, simply an average of local authorities' own records. But local authorities used to take it as an initial figure which was presumably based on intensive study. (Bosanquet, 1978, p 110)**

The periodic economic crises of the Labour governments from 1964-70 did lead to restrictions in public expenditure and cutbacks on capital projects. Table 6 indicates, however, that loan sanction for residential homes remained a central feature of expenditure decisions. At first, the procedure for loans had been linked into submissions of revisions of the 10-year plans (Ministry of Health, 1968a, p 117; DHSS, 1969a, p 124). However, the 10-year plan revisions were quietly discarded because of the uncertainties created through the pressure on public expenditure. Instead, in May 1969, the Ministry of Health, through *Circular 10/67* (Ministry of Health, 1967)[33], had asked local health and welfare authorities to submit three-year rolling capital programmes. The Department of Health and Social Security (DHSS) conducted a census of residential accommodation on 30 April 1970 "to provide an adequate statistical picture of the problems which local authorities face in providing residential accommodation" (DHSS, 1969c). On 30 April 1970, there were 2,126 local authority homes for elderly and physically handicapped people with 96,763 places, and 1,035 voluntary homes with 32,486 places. About half of the 322,486 places in voluntary homes were sponsored by local authorities (DHSS, 1975, pp 1-5, 7).

The residential care sector, therefore, continued to expand. Was there an even greater expansion of services that might enable elderly people to remain in their own homes? Attempts were made to reduce the stigma associated with national assistance but the new system of supplementary pensions failed to transform the financial position of pensioner claimants. Thomson believes there is a direct causal link between the level of cash pensions and rates of residential care. He claims that "maintenance of the elderly in institutions was and remains a counterpart to maintenance of the old by cash pensions, and variations in institutional experiences over a century and more can be shown to have a functional relationship with the availability and value of pensions" (Thomson, 1983, p 64). Using a variety of measures including Family Expenditure Surveys, he concludes that the retirement pension has remained 'fixed' in value at about 40% of the income of the average non-aged working-class adult but that "the total 'package' of incomes which the elderly enjoy, drawn from pensions, benefits, employment, occupational superannuations, investments, rents and the like has had its value eroded" (Thomson, 1983, p 64).

Table 6: Loan sanctions (1963-69)

	Total of loan sanctions recommended for local health and welfare capital building schemes	Total of loan sanctions recommended for residential accommodation under the 1948 National Assistance Act
Year	£m	£m
1965-66	16.5	9.4
1966-67	23.2	12.5
1967-68	26.1	14.0
1968-69	27.5	14.2

Note: the low figure for 1965-66 (£16.5m compared with £22.2m for 1964-65) reflects the government decision in mid-1965 to defer building starts for six months. The figures exclude the cost of capital works financed by means other than loan sanctions.

Source: Ministry of Health (1968a, p 119); DHSS (1969a, p 124)

At first glance, the situation with regard to housing appears much brighter. Butler et al indicate how in the mid-1960s, local authority housing departments began to be aware of an imbalance in the housing stock towards three-bedroomed family units. The chosen remedy was to increase small unit developments and between 1966 and 1971 279,761 small units were built, which was 27.3% of the total. However, they point out that the distribution of such units remained patchy; 386 housing authorities still had fewer than five one-bedroomed units per 100 people over the age of 65, 318 had only between 5-10 units, while only 270 had more than 10 units per 100 people over 65 (Butler et al, 1979, p 8). A small percentage only of such housing would have been in sheltered housing schemes that included a warden. Design guidance was offered to local authorities on such schemes during the 1950s and 1960s (see, for example, Ministry of Housing and Local Government, 1958; 1962), but it was not until *Circular 82/69* (Ministry of Housing and Local Government, 1969) that the Ministry of Housing and Local Government made any real attempt to clarify the role of such housing. This circular established the concept of 'Category 1' and 'Category 2' schemes. Category 1 schemes, generally bungalows, were to be "self-contained dwellings to accommodate one or more old people of the active kind". The tenants should be "couples who are able to maintain a greater degree of independence who can manage rather more housework and who may want a small garden". The more costly Category 2 schemes would consist of flats and have a wider range of additional services such as a common room, laundry, public telephone and so on. These should be for "less active old people, often living alone, who need smaller and labour saving accommodation". By this stage, another boundary dispute was beginning to emerge. How did the residents of sheltered accommodation differ from those of residential homes? Townsend might answer "very little", other than that they had retained their independence and were still part of the community. Others were soon to have doubts. Some were to claim, according to Butler and his colleagues, that "such housing is encouraging the segregation of the elderly from the rest of the population, stigmatises them and creates what has been described as geriatric ghettoes" (Butler et al, 1979, p 15; for a critique of sheltered housing, see Gray, 1977, pp 20-1).

However, this debate had not really started during the period prior to the establishment of social services departments in local authorities. More relevant is to stress that awareness of the housing needs of elderly people remained limited. A greater emphasis upon sheltered schemes was beginning to emerge but this affected only a minority of elderly people. Many more of them lived in privately rented and owner-occupied properties. Many of these properties were in need of improvement and repair. It was not until the early 1980s that any thought was given to specific difficulties of elderly people in such accommodation (see, for example, Wheeler, 1982, pp 299-330).

The period from 1964-70 saw no great expansion of domiciliary services such as home help, meals on wheels, laundry and chiropody services. These continued to develop slowly, despite rhetoric about the need to keep elderly people in their own homes and despite awareness of the growing costs of residential care. Bosanquet has argued that in 1948 residential homes represented a reasonable response to the major dilemma presented by PAIs and yet by the late 1960s "homes have come to loom larger and larger as things that are good in themselves rather than as practical solutions to a pressing difficulty" (Bosanquet, 1978, p 109). Both the last section of this chapter and Chapter Six attempt to explore some of the reasons for the continued reliance on institutions, despite the criticisms of *The last refuge* and associated works.

Demographic trends and service provision for elderly people

Perhaps the most striking feature of debates about residential care for elderly people after the publication of *The last refuge* was the complacency. It was argued that former PAIs needed to be closed down, and the quality of staffing improved. Residential homes were cheaper than hospitals and elderly residents enjoyed living in them. The Chief Welfare Officer at the Ministry of Health claimed in 1964 that:

> **... the true centre of the picture so far as geriatric services are concerned, really has shifted, or is rapidly shifting, to care in the community supported by domiciliary services, and the important thing is to remember that residential homes are in fact a vital and most important part of community service. (Aves, 1964, p 12)**

This positive view of residential life was also to be found in Harris' 1968 Government Social Survey on *Social welfare for the elderly*. She claimed that most residents were quite content to be living in a home so that "the gloomy picture of old people's homes being inhabited by masses of unhappy, discontented residents is not supported by any evidence from this inquiry" (Harris, 1968, p 50). It has already been noted that the Williams Committee on *Caring for people* tried to estimate the training needs of residential staff in both children's and old people's homes. With regard to the latter, the argument was made that demand would increase because:

> **Looking at TV is more enjoyable when one can discuss the programme with others: a game of cards is possible without the need to invite others in for the purpose and there are all sorts of additions to social life that help one to pass the time agreeably. The purpose-built homes for old people now being built are usually delightfully planned and well equipped; if they further develop to give their residents help in living an interesting and sociable life it could easily happen that a much larger proportion than at present would choose to live in them rather than maintain their separate homes. (Williams Report, 1967, p 114)**

In other words, residential homes were homely places where the lonely and isolated could be brought to end their lives in companionship and friendship.

But such an analysis provides no explanation of the reasons for such complacency. Why did it take until the 1970s and 1980s for central government to become concerned about the high cost of residential care as well as hospital care? Why was *The last refuge* not used to emphasise the need for reduced provision of this kind rather than the expansion that actually occurred? Townsend believes it is important to study the self-interested behaviour of those people who work in public services. Have trade unions and profession groups blocked 'reform'(Townsend, 1981)? The self-interest of those in central government also needs to be considered. Civil servants at the Ministry of Health had fought to obtain an extensive building programme for residential homes, despite numerous difficulties. It would take an enormous shift in the policy climate to force them to reassess such fundamental priorities. *The last refuge* could be used to reinforce their building programme resource demands (that is, to close former PAIs) rather than to challenge the central assumptions of their overall welfare policy towards elderly people.

The first half of this chapter argued that the thinking of government officials towards welfare services was finance led. *The last refuge* was about quality and content rather than overall costs. Townsend emphasised that his proposals were not a cheap alternative, especially because of his desire to expand pensions and sheltered accommodation. He did not focus on the financial waste of institutional care other than insofar as these resources could be used to offset the cost of other reforms. Many senior officials in central and local government responded to *The last refuge* by claiming that residential care remained the most economic provision for the most impaired. In a 1965 article, Beglin, the Director of Welfare Services for

Bradford, argued that "domiciliary support services could not expand sufficiently to give adequate support to such people, without being so costly in manpower and finance as to be prohibitive" (Beglin, 1965, p 204). The same point was made in 1967 by Speed, the County Welfare Officer for Devon. He listed all the services required by infirm elderly people who lived in their own homes and concluded:

> **I think it is easy to see that the cost of maintaining an old person in the community can be in the region of £10 per week. There may, therefore, be a point at which we must say that the community cannot afford in terms of manpower to provide a home help for more than so many hours per week. This would be because home helps are in limited supply, and because an employee in a residential home would be able to provide a similar service to a number of old people at the same time. (Speed, 1967)**

In other words, a belief in the utility of residential care may have retarded the development of domiciliary services.

Another less obvious factor in the lack of response to *The last refuge* concerns the limited interest in demographic trends during this period. The authors of this book have been struck by the reduced interest from medical journals, social work journals and parliamentary debates in the social and medical care of elderly people during the mid-1960s in comparison with the mid-1950s and how this relates to fluctuating interest in the so-called 'burden of dependency' created by such people. Concern about demographic trends was widespread in the late 1940s and early 1950s. Riley has called this concern "pronatalism" which she defines as "despondency and alarm over the low birthrate, both past and as anticipated by demographers, which took the 'solution' to be the encouraging of women to have more children" (Riley, 1981, p 60). A typical writer of the period was Eva Hubback in *The population of Britain*. She warned that "though we cannot predict an exact time-scale, as long as the average family is two or less, the population must ultimately fade out unless falling numbers are made good by immigration"(Hubback, 1947, p 99). She saw the key issues as being how to strengthen the wish for more children among the great majority of potential parents and secondly how to facilitate the carrying out of this wish. This leads her to argue for a major attempt to educate people about the need for population expansion and secondly for a series of social reforms such as family allowances, tax relief schemes and nurseries.

Two years later such sentiments received strong official support. The 1949 Royal Commission on Population warned that:

> **If the future brings a further reduction in average family size – not necessarily a very large one – the decline of annual births will become rapid, with serious consequential effects – supposing no immigration – on the trend of population. Well before the year 2000 the numbers of children and of young adults would be falling rapidly; by that date the population of working age and the total population would be entering a similar decline. (Royal Commission on Population, 1949, p 99)**

The Royal Commission went on to argue that a failure of a society to reproduce itself indicated something wrong in its attitude to life, yet at the same time there was acceptance that many women were seeing a real conflict between having more children and living a tolerable life. The theme of "taking the strain out of motherhood and housework" was again pushed to the fore:

> **The general aim should be to reduce the work and worry of mothers of young children. To this end these family services should be developed so that help can be made available, through home helps, sitters-in, day nurseries, nursery schools and other means, for the care of children and the running of the household in normal circumstances. (Royal Commission on Population, 1949, p 187)**

It was hoped that such policies would encourage a high birthrate, especially among "the better educated and more intelligent" (Royal Commission on Population, 1949, p 156).

A subsidiary theme to the 'pronatalist' debate was the assertion that the population of elderly people was rising and that their financial rights would be considerable under the new pension arrangements. Beveridge himself had warned that "it is dangerous to be in any way lavish to old age, until adequate provision has been assured for all other vital needs" (Beveridge Report, 1942, para 236). The Nuffield survey (Rowntree, 1980) that did so much to expose the poor conditions of many elderly people both in the community and in institutional care still made repeated warnings about not giving way to the political demands of pensioners at the expense of the young and those at work. The general theme was that elderly people were a burden on the rest of society. State expenditure was seen as a "hopeful investment" (Hubback, 1947, p 134) for the young, but not for elderly people. The Royal Commission laid considerable emphasis upon this theme. It argued that "the number of old people (over 65) will grow steadily over the next 30 years, the increase amounting to at least 2-3 millions and very probably much more" (Royal Commission on Population, 1949, p 99). It was felt that the general public would be startled if they realised the full cost of pension legislation for this growing group especially since "the old consume without producing which differentiates them from the active population and makes of them a factor reducing the average standard of living of the community" (Royal Commission on Population, 1949, p 113).

Some authors felt that the warnings of the Royal Commission were not taken seriously enough. Vaughan-Morgan, Maude and Thompson (1952), in a 1952 pamphlet published by the Conservative Political Centre, lamented that the report of the Royal Commission had never been debated in Parliament and consequently, there was a failure to appreciate the need for a population policy. They went so far as to claim that in 25 years time, every man and woman at work would be devoting more than 12 hours a week to producing goods and services for consumption by old people who had retired from work. Milder versions of these views were often to be found in gerontological, social work[34] and medical publications[35]. Sanderson (Assistant Secretary, Nuffield Foundation) claimed that "while it was common to speak of old people as having 'earned' their retirement, those who retired could only be supported from current production" (Sanderson, 1949, p 24). Sheldon (1955, pp 15-26), in his presidential address to the Third Congress of the International Association of Gerontology, warned that demographic trends created "a problem destined to grow on a frightening scale". Indeed, he felt "the tide is on the flood, and any search for a general social philosophy of old age must take account of the possible levels that may be reached by the spring tide that for this country is predicted to arrive in about twenty years' time" (Sheldon, 1955, p 16).

How did central government respond to this situation? The Phillips Committee was appointed in July 1953 "to review the economic and financial problems involved in providing for old age, having regard to the prospective increase in the numbers of the aged" (Phillips Report, 1954, p 1). Its report stressed the high cost of pensions which it saw as involving the transfer to elderly people of incomes currently derived from the exertions of others; contributions would not cover pension costs and the deficit would have "to be met out of general taxation, and, to some degree, out of the savings of the tax-payer, so that it will actively impede the very process of capital accumulation on which, implicitly, it rests" (Phillips Report, 1954, p 34). The report recommended that this should be reflected in future decisions about pension rates. In some respects, therefore, the report reaffirmed negative attitudes to old age. At the same time, it played down the importance of demographic changes by exposing what Titmuss angrily called "the noisy barrage of faulty statistics" (Titmuss, 1955, p 47). The Phillips Report argued that Beveridge and the Royal Commission on Population had overestimated the growth of the elderly population by assuming too high a reduction in mortality rates in old age. The trends expected by the Phillips Report were "neither new, sudden, nor (taking young and old together) particularly large" (Phillips Report, 1954, p 11). Titmuss argued that the Phillips Report proved "the present alarm is unjustified" (Titmuss, 1963, p 56); the 'burden' of pensions would be much less than predicted in the 1940s.

The demographic debate of this period created a climate of concern about the 'burden of dependency' caused by elderly people upon the rest of the population. This concern focused usually upon the cost of pensions but the 'flood' of dependency was also seen as having implications for health and welfare services, especially in relation to bed blockages in the NHS. Pension and benefit levels remained an issue in the 1960s but this was no longer debated with a background of concern about demographic trends. Reference might be made to how smaller families, greater geographical mobility and the increased numbers of women in full-time work had reduced the pool of potential 'family' carers, but this was seen as requiring an expansion of residential care rather than a thorough reassessment of state intervention in the lives of sick and frail elderly people. *The last refuge* could not make such people a priority concern with politicians and civil servants who were far more concerned with issues such as race and juvenile crime in the inner city. Concern about service provision for elderly people would only be fully awakened when demographers again began to stress a major growth in the number of elderly people and to question whether this could be 'afforded' by the rest of the population.

The above analysis is offered as a reflection on the failure of *The last refuge* and associated works to lead to the abandonment of residential homes as the main form of welfare provision for elderly people. Does this mean that there was general agreement with the Nuffield survey of 1947 that the independence of elderly people should not be encouraged? This issue and its relationship to domiciliary services and 'family' care is the central theme of the next chapter.

Notes

[1] DHSS 94031/1/74, *Residential Accommodation: General. Discharge of chronic sick cases from hospital.* See, for example, letter from Bournemouth and East Dorset Group Hospital, 9 August 1950.

[2] DHSS 94031/1/60, *Medical society for the care of the elderly.*

[3] DHSS 94031/1/74, letter from Carruthers (Principal) to SW Metropolitan Regional Hospital Board, 8 September 1950.

[4] The Ministry of Health's 1952 Annual Report referred to the reimposition early in the year of control over the distribution of steel, entailing a severe curtailment in the quantity available for new construction (Ministry of Health, 1953, p 118). The last of the building controls, as opposed to continued restrictions on capital investment, was removed on 10 November 1954 (Ministry of Health 1955a, p 133).

[5] DHSS 94031/1/48, *Provision of residential accommodation for the aged.* Letter from Bevan to Messer, 24 June 1949.

[6] DHSS 94020/1/112 Part A, *National Assistance. Welfare services: Capital investment programmes.* Memorandum from T. Williams to Principal Regional Officers, 20 April 1951.

[7] NCCOP Archives: Advisory Council – Book One. Minutes of 51st Meeting, 5 June 1951.

[8] NCCOP Archives: Advisory Council – Book One. Letter from Thigh (LCC) to Simson (Secretary, NCCOP), 26 June 1950.

[9] NCCOP Archives: Advisory Council – Book One. Comment by Dr Godber (Ministry of Health) during discussions on the Oxford Rest Home, 16 March 1950.

[10] NCCOP Archives: Governor's Minutes – Book Three. Evidence submitted to the Phillips Committee, 27 April 1954.

[11] NCCOP Archives: Governors' Minutes – 9th Book. Minutes of 87th Meeting, 13 February 1962. See report by Secretary on 'The mentally infirm aged'.

[12] NCCOP Archives: Governors' Minutes – 9th Book. Minutes of 93rd Meeting, 30 July 1963. See report on 'Accommodation for the mentally infirm aged' by the 'ad hoc' committee of Dr G. Townsend, Dr A. Exton-Smith, Lady Norman, Dr F. Post and Dr T. Wilson.

[13] Ibid; p 11.

[14] The memorandum of evidence to the Guillebaud Committee stressed that "the difficulties arising from the present separation of functions can most satisfactorily be solved by the restoration to local authorities of the hospital service".

[15] The Children and Welfare Committee of the CCA noted that the AMC did not need to negotiate with the Ministry of Health on the report of the working party on the 'Care of the Elderly Sick' because of the recommendation to the Phillips Committee and the Guillebaud Committee that hospitals should be administered by local authorities.

[16] A memorandum to the Phillips Committee stated that "the problems of the chronic sick and very infirm point to the need for a single officer with overall responsibility".

[17] DHSS 94031/1/4, *National Assistance Act 1948: Standards to be applied to residential accommodation provided under the National Assistance Act 1948.*

[18] DHSS 94031/1/31A, *National Assistance Act 1948. Standards to be observed in the provision of homes for old people Proceedings of the Office Committee.* See Report on 'Observations of visits' by M.Tebbitt (Architect) and G.Aves (Chief Welfare Officer), 7 April 1949.

[19] DHSS 94020/1/106, *National Assistance Act: Buildings.* See Division 12 Memo No1/50 on 'Acquisition and adaptation of premises for residential accommodation', 5 April 1950.

[20] DHSS 94031/1/31A. See report of the Office Committee on 'Standards to be observed in the provision of new homes for old people', 12 May 1950.

[21] Ibid; meeting to consider standards of accommodation for old people under the National Assistance Act, 6 July 1950.

[22] DHSS 74031/1/31/1B, *Residential accommodation, General: National Assistance Act 1948. Alternative standards of accommodation in homes for old people: Proceedings of Office Committee.*

[23] NCCOP Archives: Governors' Minutes – Book Three. 45th meeting of Governors, 27 April 1954. This meeting considered 'Evidence submitted to Phillips Committee'.

[24] DHSS 94020/1/93A, *National Assistance Act 1948: Training for work with old people, 1949-50.* Letter from Dorothea Ramsey (NOPWC) to Sir John Wrigley (Ministry of Health), 18 March 1949.

[25] DHSS 94020/1/93A, memorandum from Chief Welfare Officer, dated 24 March 1949.

[26] DHSS 94020/1/93A, letter from Secretary of the AMC, dated 8 February 1950.

[27] Ibid; comments from Ministry of Health official on AMC paper 'Training for welfare staff', 30 June 1950.

[28] Ibid; abstracted from *LCC Welfare Department: Notes for conference,* undated.

[29] Ibid; minutes of meeting about training for residential staff between Ministry of Health officials and representatives from AMC, CCA and LCC, 30 June 1950.

[30] *CCA Gazette Supplement*, February 1953, p 20. Memorandum by Care of Elderly Persons Sub-Committee of the AMC on Training of Matrons, Assistant Matrons and Wardens of Old People's Homes.

[31] Ibid; p 19. Minutes of Meeting on 11 November 1952 between CCA, AMC and LCC to discuss AMC memorandum on training.

[32] For example, this view was expressed to us during interviews with Dame Geraldine Aves (formerly Chief Welfare Officer, Ministry of Health) and Elizabeth Hope-Murray (formerly Deputy Chief Welfare Officer, Ministry of Health).

[33] The same request was made in May 1968 and in addition it was announced that revisions of the 10-year plans would not be called for "having regard to the difficulties authorities may have in formulating revised plans in present circumstances" (Ministry of Health 1968b). In June 1969 there was no mention of development plans in the circular asking for the three-year returns on capital projects (DHSS 1969b).

[34] See, for example, report on the 1955 Welfare Conference organised by the AMC, CCA and LCC in *Hospital and Social Service Journal,* 4 March 1955, pp 205-6. The speech by Dr H. Paul (Medical Officer of Health, Smethwick) placed an especially high emphasis upon elderly people as a burden upon the rest of the community.

[35] See, for example, Roberts (1949). Roberts spoke of how "national prosperity" was diminished by measures which promote the survival of the unfit without making them fit and by those which merely prolong invalidism at a level incompatible with functional efficiency.

SIX

Avoiding institutional care: the changing role of the state, the family and voluntary organisations

Introduction

The legislative framework for service development for older people laid down by the 1946 National Health Service Act and the 1948 National Assistance Act placed the emphasis on institutional provision. And yet the first section of this chapter underlines how there was agreement by the early 1950s that elderly people should remain in their own homes for as long as possible. Despite this, there was no dramatic shift of resources from hospitals and residential homes to domiciliary services, housing and income maintenance schemes.

This chapter focuses narrowly on arguments about those domiciliary services that were eventually to be located in social services departments. What kind of arguments were made in their favour and how did perceptions vary about their function? What was seen as the role of voluntary organisations in service provision? How did these arguments relate to perceptions about the responsibilities of families to their elderly relatives?

Staying at home and care by the 'family': the arguments

There was a broad consensus throughout the 1950s and 1960s that elderly people should remain in their own homes for as long as possible for their own happiness and also to reduce financial pressure on the state. The first of these arguments was strongly put by Townsend:

> **Home was the old armchair by the hearth, the creaky bedstead, the polished lino with its faded pattern, the sideboard with its picture gallery, and the lavatory with its broken latch reached through the rain. It embodied a thousand memories and held**

> **promise of a thousand contentments. It was an extension of personality. (Townsend, 1963, p 38)**

The 'financial pressure' case was put forward by Sheldon at the 1954 International Association of Gerontology Conference. He stressed the burden of old age dependency on the rest of the community in terms of hospital and residential care provision. This created a need to encourage and support "their general vigour under natural surroundings and their craving to maintain independence up to and even beyond the best possible moment"; this would reduce "the demands on permanent accommodation" (Sheldon, 1955, pp 15-26).

The Ministry of Health shared such sentiments. The 1953 Annual Report spoke of the "universal recognition of the urgency of the task of enabling old people to go on living in their own homes as long as possible" (Ministry of Health, 1954b, p 187), while the 1954 report said that "the importance of enabling old people to go on living in their own homes where they most wish to be, and of delaying admission to residential care for as long as possible is now generally recognised" (Ministry of Health, 1955a, p 138). The 1958 report spoke of "the emphasis laid in the last few years on measures to enable elderly persons to remain in their own homes for as long as possible" (Ministry of Health, 1959b, p 252). The 1960 report made an even stronger statement when it claimed that

> **... the general objective of both health and welfare services, working in co-operation, is to maintain the elderly in the community and to accept admission to hospital or residential care as the right course only where an old person himself accepts the necessity for this and when he has reached a point where the community services are no longer sufficient. (Ministry of Health, 1961, p 122)**

Such views were echoed by members of all three main political parties. Throughout the 1950s and 1960s, parliamentary debates about services for elderly people were full of rhetoric about the need to keep such people in their own homes. For example, in a 1953 debate, Llewellyn claimed that "the House will agree that, ideally, we should try to keep people as long as possible in their own homes" (*Hansard*, House of Commons, vol 522, 14 December 1953, col 163), while Thompson stressed in 1958 that "more emphasis ... (should) be placed on the care of old people for as long as possible in their own family and in their own homes" since "that is what elderly people themselves want" (*Hansard*, House of Commons, vol 582, 12 February 1958, col 535). Political pamphlets and research reports tended to follow a similar line. Vaughan-Morgan, Maude and Thompson, in their 1952 pamphlet for the Conservative Political Centre, agreed that "we should devote all our energies to enabling old people to continue living in their own homes" (Vaughan-Morgan et al, 1952, p 19). This was justified in the following way:

> **There they are surrounded by the things and people they know and love. There they are required to help themselves in a hundred ways, all calculated to stimulate their physical and mental processes and so maintain their interest in life. At home, insignificant and unimportant possessions and habits, in which the old increasingly find solace, assume positions of great prominence. (Vaughan-Morgan et al, 1952, pp 19-20)**

In the mid-1960s, the National Labour Women's Advisory Committee was talking of "the widely accepted view that the first priority of the Welfare State should be to make provision in such a way that old people are enabled to live an independent existence within the community for as long as possible" (National Labour Women's Advisory Committee, 1965, p 3).

Local authority associations, professional bodies and voluntary organisations also expressed similar views. For example, the 1953 report of the NOPWC emphasised that "it has long been realised by the National Committee that everyone wishes to live in his or her own house if possible" (NOPWC, 1953a). And yet, of course, this consensus is illusory; there has always been conflict and disagreement about how to define and understand 'if possible' and 'for as long as possible'. This conflict is at the core of the debate about how to define the respective roles of the state, the voluntary sector and the family towards the care of frail and sick elderly people.

Indeed, it is impossible to understand attitudes to the provision of domiciliary services by local authorities and voluntary organisations without a consideration of assumptions about the 'natural' obligations of the 'family' in the care of elderly relatives. Much of this debate talks about the 'family' and whether the welfare changes of the 1940s had undermined the willingness of the 'family' to take on such obligations. Protagonists in this debate have usually assumed that women have a responsibility to stay at home and look after dependent members. This is usually taken to mean children but there were also strong views about the care of frail and sick elderly people, especially in the light of worry about demographic trends (see previous chapter).

Just after the war, there was a demand for women workers in certain key industries where there was a labour shortage, but such opportunities retained a strong element of 'for the duration only', and little attempt was made to develop good childcare facilities for women in these industries (Riley, 1981). The main emphasis of this period, however, was upon the role of women in motherhood. Even the literature on 'dual career' families stressed that childcare was the primary responsibility of women (see also, for instance, Brittain, 1953). Myrdal and Klein, for example, in *Women's two roles: Home and work* stated that:

> **We could have gone further in our calculation and suggested that married women could give an average of 15, or even of only 10 years to their children instead of 20. The correspondingly greater increase in the labour force and, as a result, in the total production of goods and the supply of services would be tremendous, and would make possible a considerable rise in the standard of living. If we did not make this suggestion it is because it seems neither practicable nor desirable that mothers of very young children should go out to work. (Myrdal and Klein, 1956, p 188)**

Myrdal and Klein put considerable stress on the need to improve standards of living and to use consumer durables to ease the strain of housework and motherhood. More recently, Wilson has also emphasised the importance of this theme during the 1950s:

> **The revolution in the production of small-scale consumer durable goods affected women first and foremost in creating or expanding opportunities for their employment and in – supposedly – easing their lot in the home. Somehow the installation of Hoovers, refrigerators, electric mixers, and washing machines was held to give housewives equality. Quite apart from the fact that only a minority of women had access to these aids, while many still laboured at home without even hot water, there was an awful complacency about this myth. (Wilson, 1980, p 12)**

The work of Wilson is an example of 1980s feminist writing that has done so much to challenge previous conceptions about women's role and the family. However, as Bond has pointed out, "most of the discussion of woman's role in the literature has focused upon her functions in relation to the present and future work-force, and has made little reference to her role with regard to the retired work-force" (Bond, 1982, p 12). This is despite the fact that the early 1950s saw considerable discussion about the need to enforce women's role (often called the 'family') in the care of frail and sick elderly people. Concern about this issue was expressed by politicians, local authority officers, members of the medical profession, social workers and staff of voluntary organisations.

The medical profession and surveys of hospital provision offer the most forceful examples of such attitudes. The key concern was bed turnover; one senior administrative medical officer claimed "the bottleneck will grow", if "their relatives cannot or will not receive them" (Hughes, 1951, p 38). McEwan and Laverty, in their 1949 survey of hospital provision in Bradford, were convinced that many old people were not wanted by their children. There was often a shortage of space in their homes, and there was concern about implications for the family budget and many women were at work in the textile industry. The key problem, however, was 'the Spirit of the Age' which undermined individualism and family responsibility through an overreliance on the state. The authors warned that "if once it were to become fashionable to transfer the care of the elderly from the family to the state without loss of 'face' and without a guilty conscience, a very big hospital and socio-economic problem would confront the community" (McEwan and Laverty, 1949, p 107). Thompson was associated with surveys of hospital provision for sick elderly people in the Birmingham area and he argued:

> **It is ... possible that slackening of the moral fibre of the family and a demand for material comfort and amenity out-weighs the charms of mutual affection.... The power of the group-maintaining instincts will suffer if the provision of a home, the training of children, and the care of its disabled members are no longer the ambition of a family but the duty of a local or central authority. (Thompson, 1949, p 250)**

Nearly 10 years later, Rudd, a consultant physician from a Southampton geriatric unit, was using equally extreme language:

> **The feeling that the State ought to solve every inconvenient**

> **domestic situation is merely another factor in producing a snowball expansion on demands in the National Health (and Welfare) Service. Close observation on domestic strains makes one thing very clear. This is that where an old person has a family who have a sound feeling of moral responsibility, serious problems do not arise, however much difficulty may be met. (Rudd, 1958, pp 348-9)**

Other leading geriatricians of the 1950s such as Brooke (1950) and Warren (1951) expressed similar if less extreme views. The primary responsibility for the care of sick and frail elderly people lay with 'the family' and this had not been changed by the welfare reforms of the 1940s. Articles in *The Almoner* (see, for example, Macdonald, 1950, pp 227-9) suggested that those medical social workers attached to geriatric units in the 1950s shared many of these views, but were also aware of the difficulties of forcing reluctant families to provide a home for elderly parents. For example, a sub-committee of the Geriatric Almoners' Group argued in 1951 that "even when, by all the laws of justice, a family should be made to accept the responsibility of looking after an old parent, the almoner has always the uneasy fear that if this is done, they will so vent their resentment upon the patient that the step taken will defeat its own ends" (Sub-Committee of the Geriatric Almoners' Group, 1951, pp 252-4).

Such views were often supported by politicians during the 1950s. Vaughan-Morgan, Maude and Thompson in their 1952 pamphlet (p 28) claimed that there was clear evidence of a decline in the willing acceptance of family responsibilities, a point often supported by other politicians from the same party during this period. This point was being made as late as 1958 by Sir Keith Joseph (*Hansard*, House of Commons, vol 582, 12 February 1958, col 534). Labour politicians seemed to have been much less convinced of family irresponsibility. Kenneth Robinson in 1953, for example, stressed "we should also think of the young mother with two or three small children to look after who may find it physically impossible to look after a sick and elderly mother and father as well" (*Hansard*, House of Commons, vol 512, 6 March 1953, col 718). However, this did not mean necessarily that the existence of these responsibilities was being challenged; only the feasibility of them being carried out in certain types of situation. Such attitudes were exposed in the National Labour Women's Advisory Committee survey some 11 years later. This document is usually presented as progressive for its time but it argued with regard to the home help service that:

> **... those local authorities who choose to assist those less in need by less frequent and shorter visits must ask themselves whether they are providing a service which, in some cases, could just as well be supplied by private help or the help of neighbours and relatives, and whether they are providing too universal a service at the expense of those in greatest need. (National Labour Women's Advisory Committee, 1965, p 7)**

Both officers and councillors from local authorities were prone to express strong sentiments on this issue. Bligh (1951), Chief Welfare Officer for the LCC, criticised the weakening of 'filial piety' as reflected by the abolition in 1948 of Section 14 of the Poor Law Act, that is, children no longer had a legal responsibility to relieve and maintain their poor old parents. The AMC, in evidence to the Phillips Committee, spoke of "the reluctance of many families to care for their aged relatives" (*Municipal Review Supplement*, June 1954, p 108) especially after they had entered hospital, and this placed pressure on local authority residential accommodation. In 1959, the Chief Welfare Officer for Manchester was lamenting the "changed attitude towards aged dependants" (*Hospital and Social Service Journal*, 9 January 1959, p 36) while a colleague was warning that "it would be an administrative nightmare if there was a decline in family responsibility" (*Hospital and Social Service Journal*, 9 May 1950, p 495; speech by Dr G. Wynne Griffith, Royal Society of Health Annual Congress).

Some voluntary organisations were perhaps more reluctant to pass judgements about the 'weakness' of the family in post-Beveridge Britain. Indeed, the annual reports of the NOPWC tended to argue that the family did care about its elderly members, and it needed support from services that could best be provided by voluntary organisations. As early as 1955, it was stressing "there is no lessening of family responsibility" (NOPWC, 1955, p 7), although the assumption that such responsibility was appropriate was still taken for granted. It was still assumed that the 'family' should care wherever possible. However, the NCCOP took a different view. It was not so sure that the 'family' was still caring and whether the impact of voluntary organisations upon this situation was always positive:

> **Beyond doubt, there is an increasing tendency to regard this provision of help and care as a burden and to throw it, with so many other burdens, upon the State. Family life and family responsibilities have, in the past, been among the finest features of our national heritage.**

> **It would be a thousand pities if voluntary committees and organisations should help, albeit unconsciously, to break down this great tradition by undertaking the entire responsibility for old people whose relatives can make some contribution towards their care. (NCCOP, 1950, p 26)**

Throughout all these references to family responsibility, two questions are being posed. Does the 'family' still accept its responsibilities towards elderly parents? Do domiciliary services and provision from voluntary organisations support or undermine the 'family' in this respect? As Sheldon put it, "we must do everything possible to assist the family in the care of its aged dependants without at the same time relieving it of the necessity for still taking an interest in the matter" (Sheldon, 1950, p 319). Empirical evidence about these issues during the 1950s and early 1960s is examined in the next section.

Staying at home and care by the 'family': the evidence

The first major study was Sheldon's *The social medicine of old age* in 1948. The fieldwork was, of course, carried out prior to the implementation of the welfare state 'reforms' and involved interviews with a sample of nearly 600 elderly people from Wolverhampton. Sheldon stressed that "contact with old people in their own homes immediately brings to light the fact that the family is of fundamental importance" (Sheldon, 1948, p 140). The key role in the performance of domestic chores and the management of illness was carried out by wives and daughters. He found that "whereas the wives do most of the nursing of the men, the strain when the mother is ill is yet to fall on the daughter, who may have to stay at home as much to run the household as to nurse her mother" (p 164). Sheldon felt the burden upon such women needed to be shared with the rest of the community and this required the establishment of a national domestic help service (p 166).

Small-scale later studies confirmed these findings. Families did care but the bulk of this caring was carried out by wives, daughters and daughters-in-law. The importance of this was stressed by Exton-Smith (1952) in his survey of patients discharged from St Pancras Hospital and by Isaacs and Thompson (1960) in their review of holiday admissions to a geriatric unit. The 1958 NCSS survey of 100 people over 70 years of age found that, "in all, the impression of family ties was one of unity and strength, not of irresponsibility and weakness" (NCSS, 1954, p 25). Chalke and

Benjamin, in their 1953 survey of pensioners from Lewisham and Camberwell, found that some four fifths of women and nearly two thirds of men received visits from near relatives and they concluded that "the alleged negligent 'spirit of the age' is in reality a factor of minor importance" (Chalke and Benjamin, 1953, p 589). Thirteen years later, Lowther and Williamson used evidence from their survey of 1,500 patients discharged from a geriatric unit in Edinburgh to show that relatives would accept the home care of elderly parents so that the "belief in the decline in filial care of the elderly is unfounded and an as yet unproven modern myth" (Lowther and Williamson, 1966, p 1460).

The most powerful challenge to this myth, however, is associated with the work of Peter Townsend. His influential book, *The family life of old people*, was first published in 1957 and this detailed the family system of care that existed in the East End of London during the mid-1950s. The records of local GPs were used to provide a sample of 261 people of pensionable age; 203 of them were eventually interviewed and 139 of the 203 were women. A central theme of the book was the extent to which elderly people provided family services as well as received them, and that this created an intimate bond between the three generations. Children shopped for elderly parents while the parents provided meals or looked after grandchildren. The care of grandchildren was a key task and involved "fetching them from school, giving them meals, looking after them while their parents were at work, or sitting in during the evening" (Townsend, 1963, p 62). However, these tasks were much more commonly performed by grandmothers than grandfathers. In return, elderly people received considerable help from their families in terms of both regular domestic chores and nursing during illness. Townsend points out how:

> **As women got older and more infirm their relatives took over first the shopping, then the heavy cleaning and washing, and only in the last resort the cooking and the payment of rent and other regular outgoings.... More than half those helping with home tasks were daughters, and most of the remainder were daughters-in-law, sisters, and nieces. (Townsend, 1963, p 61)**

A similar situation was found during periods of illness. Half the women and half the men had been confined to bed through illness at some stage in the previous two years. During such periods, the main care for men was provided first by wives and then daughters. On the other hand, "daughters were the chief source of help for fifty-eight per cent of women, other relatives (mainly sisters, daughters-in-law and nieces) for twenty-six per cent, husbands for ten per cent and neighbours or friends for the remainder" (Townsend, 1963, p 66).

Townsend balanced his stress upon the reciprocal nature of these relationships by arguing the need to develop services both to support this system of care and also to help those who were outside it. Prolonged illness and impairment of an elderly parent did impose severe strain upon daughters and daughters-in-law who had taken on the primary tending role. Second, some elderly people were isolated from this system of care because they lacked children, because their children did not live in the locality or because they had only sons. Both groups, that is, the over-strained daughters and isolated elderly people, needed support from a major expansion of publicly-provided domiciliary services, such as home care and district nursing.

Townsend developed these themes not only through his survey of institutional residents in *The last refuge* (1964, pp 191-240) but also through his major contributions to the cross-national survey of elderly people over 65 which was carried out in the United States, Denmark and Britain. This latter study provided a national picture of family care in this country to supplement his original case study approach and the results were written up in both *The aged in the welfare state* (Townsend and Wedderburn, 1965) and *Old people in three industrial societies* (Shanas et al, 1968). Research evidence from over 4,000 interviews stressed that illness and impairment among elderly people was more widespread among those living in their own homes than those in institutions.

However, those in their own homes tended to have more extensive family resources than those in institutional care. Such relatives, and especially female relatives, provided an enormous amount of domestic and nursing care which far outstripped anything provided by the state or voluntary organisations. The extent of this is underlined in Tables 7 and 8 taken from *The aged in the welfare state.*

Table 7: Percentage of persons ill in bed last year who received different kinds of help from different sources, Britain (1962)

	Persons ill in bed last year		
Source of help	Receiving help with housework	Receiving help with shopping	Receiving help with meals
Spouse	30.5	30.3	35.6
Child in household	22.2	22.2	21.6
Child outside household	13.2	15.1	12.9
Relative in household	6.7	7.2	7.1
Relative outside household	4.1	4.9	3.9
Other in household	2.2	2.1	2.2
Friend or neighbour	3.2	9.7	5.9
Social services	4.8	1.8	1.4
Private domestic help	4.8	1.7	1.6
Other help outside	0.9	1.4	0.9
None	7.3	3.5	7.0
Total	100.0	100.0	100.0
Number	1,159	1,160	1,161

Note: nearly 3,000 persons not ill in bed in previous year excluded. Information not available for 18, 17 and 16 persons respectively.

Source: Townsend and Wedderburn (1965, p 36)

Table 8: Percentage of persons having difficulty in doing heavy housework, who received help with housework from different sources, Britain (1962)

	Persons having difficulty with heavy housework		
Source of help	Men	Women	Men and women
	%	%	%
Spouse	37	11	19
Child in household	20	26	24
Child outside household	8	12	10
Relative in household	4	6	5
Relative outside household	2	3	3
Others in household	3	2	2
Friends and neighbours	1	3	3
Social services	8	9	8
Private domestic help	10	12	11
Others outside	3	7	6
None	7	16	13
Total	103	107	104
Number of persons	625	1,296	1,921
Number of replies	651	1,366	2,017

Source: Townsend and Wedderburn (1965, p 40)

The minority of elderly people who did receive services from the state and voluntary organisations tended to be similar to those in institutional care; they lacked family resources. Such findings led Townsend to conclude:

> **... the health and welfare services for the aged, as presently developing, are a necessary concomitant of social organisation, and therefore, possibly of economic growth. The services do not undermine self-help, because they are concentrated overwhelmingly among those who have neither the capacities**

nor the resources to undertake the relevant functions alone. Nor, broadly, do the services conflict with the interests of the family as a social institution, because either they tend to reach people who lack a family or whose family resources are slender, or they provide specialised services the family is not equipped or qualified to undertake. (Shanas et al, 1968, p 129)

Rather than being restricted from a fear of undermining the family, domiciliary services needed to be expanded rapidly to support families and help the isolated.

Townsend had comprehensively answered the two crucial questions. The family did care, and this care was not undermined by the provision of support services. However, this research and the other studies reviewed had rarely questioned the disparity between female and male care for elderly relatives. Sheldon had spoken of "sweated labour" (1960, p 1225) but this was to be eased by domiciliary services, and the lack of sweat on male brows was not questioned. It was also usually assumed that the family ought to care, and a failure or refusal to provide physical services such as cleaning, shopping, or nursing, was seen as implying a lack of emotional care. If a woman loved her mother, it was expected that she would carry out these household tasks rather than expect another agency to do it for her, unless she was rich and could afford private domestic help. In the words of Meacher, the 'family structure' was seen as "the natural care agency" (Meacher, 1972, p 508). And yet Townsend was aware that such definitions of roles and responsibilities were socially defined rather than just 'natural'.

... the answer to the practical question 'does this individual need help?' may depend on a number of hidden assumptions: that the service has to be restricted on grounds of cost or limited manpower to a particular number of people, that the family should normally be expected or obliged to provide care, that with few exceptions individuals should be obliged even in old age, to be self-reliant in at least some respects. These are not just individual value assumptions. More often they are the value assumptions of society or at least of certain sections of the population. (Townsend and Wedderburn, 1965, p 45)

Who should run domiciliary services?

Whatever their limitations in relation to assumptions about the 'natural' role of women, these early sociological and medical surveys of elderly people and their families did begin to shift the attitudes of politicians and government officials about the need for an expansion of domiciliary services. Voluntary organisations were encouraged to develop such services as visiting schemes and luncheon clubs (see, for example, Ministry of Health, 1962d; 1962e). The legal right of local health authorities to provide chiropody services under the 1946 Health Service Act was confirmed by *Circular 11/59* (Ministry of Health, 1959d, Section 28). The 1962 amendment to the 1948 National Assistance Act gave local authorities the power to develop their own meals on wheels services. The 1968 Health Services and Public Health Act and the 1970 Chronically Sick and Disabled Act both considerably increased the power of local authorities to provide domiciliary support services.

The 1968 Act gave local authorities a general responsibility to promote the welfare of the elderly and made the home help service a mandatory duty rather than a permissive power. Kenneth Robinson (Minister of Health) stressed that the power to promote the welfare of elderly people would include practical forms of help such as aids and adaptations, "preventive and advisory forms of service" such as housing wardens, and a general visiting service (*Hansard*, House of Commons, vol 754, 7 December, cols 1679-803). The 1970 Act arose from a private member's bill and greatly extended the responsibilities of local authorities towards chronically sick and disabled people, the largest number of whom are elderly. Among its numerous provisions was not only a confirmation of the importance of aids and adaptations but also the right for this group to apply for the installation of a telephone by the local authority.

Such lists of legislative developments and exhortation by circular can give the impression of unimpeded incremental progress towards a more 'liberal' policy of social welfare provision for elderly people. However, there is a major difference between legislative intent and service development; it has already been shown how service provision remained dominated by residential care throughout the 1960s and early 1970s. There was also a continued debate about the respective roles of the family, the state and voluntary organisations. Who should have the responsibility for running domiciliary services – central government, local authorities or voluntary organisations? To what extent should such services be expanded? These themes run through the rest of this chapter.

One possibility considered in the 1940s and early 1950s was that the main responsibility for the development of welfare services for elderly people who lived in their own homes should lie with the National Assistance Board (NAB). As already seen, the 1940 Old Age and Widows Pension Act had given the Board a duty not only to assess elderly people for supplementary pensions but also to "promote the welfare of elderly people". During the 1940s, there was much discussion within the Assistance Board about how seriously to take this instruction: did it mean more than providing cash? Chapter Three showed that this 'duty' was used by certain officials to justify helping to form the OPWC and, also, to encourage the growth of voluntary hostels during wartime. In the mid-1940s, it was the policy of the Assistance Board that elderly people could be visited for welfare reasons as well as for the assessment of benefit, while some staff were calling for the establishment of a "definite welfare section"[1]. However, increasingly, Assistance Board staff were encouraged to send lists of those in need of social visits to voluntary organisations, such as the Red Cross[2]. Staff shortages within the Assistance Board meant that social visits had to be reduced, although Clarke argued that there was also a desire to distance the Board from "the old style parochial philanthropy – good works and kind words; they abhor the thought of meddling" (Clarke, 1948, p 150).

Despite this, authors such as Samson stated that it should be the duty of social security staff to watch over the general welfare of elderly people; such officers "should be specially selected and trained in the needs and psychology of old people" (Samson, 1944, p 58). Chapter Four indicated that this view was supported by the Rucker Committee on the Break-up of the Poor Law. Local authorities should be allowed to provide specialised domiciliary services only for certain narrowly defined groups of the handicapped. This definition should not be drawn too wide to avoid including all old and infirm people. Such a system would be 'extravagant' and in any case:

> **In our view, the overall duty of providing general welfare services – for the old, the infirm, the subnormal and others – should rest with the Assistance Board and the Ministry of National Insurance. The powers of the Assistance Board in this regard would be, in effect, a continuance of the Poor Law duty to care for all in need of assistance. Thus, in the new pattern of social services, there will be, outside the field of local government, means of providing a general domiciliary welfare service for all who are likely to need help of this kind.[3]**

Under these circumstances, it is strange that Section 2 of the 1948 National Assistance Act merely stated that "the Board are to exercise their functions in such manner as shall best promote the welfare of persons affected by the exercise thereof". No mention was made of the active promotion of the welfare of elderly people, and that part of the 1940 Act was repealed. The new terminology did seem to reduce the chances of the NAB taking on a general welfare function towards elderly people. This proved to be the case.

This became clear when the AMC first began to pressurise for increased legislative powers to develop domiciliary services for elderly people. In October 1950, the AMC had formed a Care of Elderly Persons Sub-Committee and this raised the issue of boundaries between local authorities and the NAB. It pointed out that Section 2 could be taken to mean:

> **... the Assistance Board is responsible for the welfare of aged persons living in their own homes if they are in receipt of national assistance but we ourselves are not inclined to adopt this interpretation. We merely quote it as an example of the doubt which exists in relation to the respective spheres of influence of the Board and of the local authorities. (*Municipal Review Supplement*, 1951, 'Coperation between local authorities and the National Assistance Board', April, p 82)**

This committee argued that the AMC should call for local authorities to have a general power to promote the welfare of elderly people, unless it could be shown that the NAB already had such a power. A meeting was eventually held between representatives of the AMC, the CCA, the Ministry of Health and the NAB (*Municipal Review Supplement*, October, 1952, p 209). The Ministry said there was no need for legislative change and that voluntary organisations could provide the necessary services. This was supported by the CCA. The NAB reported that they were in touch with only 1,300,000 of the 6,000,000 people of pensionable age. NAB officers did draw the attention of pensioners to the various services available, if it appeared these were required. However, an NAB representative stressed:

> **... that services such as helping with shopping or home visiting were jobs for neither central nor local government officials; this sort of thing was better left to voluntary organisations. The Board's officers make a practice of getting in touch with these voluntary organisations where their services are needed.**

The NAB had no intention of carrying out the responsibilities suggested by the Rucker Committee.

This remained the situation throughout the 1950s and early 1960s. On the election of a Labour Government in 1964, discussions took place about the future of the NAB. The 1966 Ministry of Social Security Act combined the NAB and the Ministry of Pensions and National Insurance in a new Ministry. National Assistance was renamed Supplementary Benefit in the hope of improving take-up and reducing stigma. During the debate about the future of the NAB, Douglas Houghton, who was Coordinator of Social Services in the Labour government, raised the possibility that NAB social security officials should play a much fuller role in the assessment of the welfare needs of elderly people (Cooper, 1983, p 76). Nothing came of this suggestion. Stevenson felt that "there is little doubt that the rank and file of officials saw the merger with the Ministry of Pensions and National Insurance as an indication of a diminution of interest in 'welfare'" (Stevenson, 1973, p 31). Despite this, pressure for a more 'welfare' perspective was exerted by certain members of the newly formed Supplementary Benefits Commission. Olive Stevenson was appointed the first Social Work Adviser to the Commission and she encouraged the development of employment review officers and special welfare officers. The latter group did visit a large number of elderly claimants (17% of referrals from May to July 1969) but the bulk of referrals concerned the long-term sick and fatherless families. Special welfare officers spent most of their time dealing with what were considered to be examples of financial mismanagement (Stevenson, 1973, pp 154-5).

The growth of home nursing and the home help service

The overall responsibility for domiciliary welfare services was not to be taken over by the NAB/Supplementary Benefits Commission. What other alternatives existed? Local health authorities had the power under the 1946 National Health Service Act to provide home nursing and home help services. How did these services develop during the period? A central aspect of their development was the health/welfare division at the local authority level and this is dealt with at length in the next chapter. In this section, the focus is on service provision issues, and how the debate about them reflected attitudes towards people remaining in the community for 'as long as possible'.

At first glance, the home nursing service did expand during the 1950s and work with elderly people took up a greater proportion of its time. (Figures supplied in this paragraph are abstracted from the Ministry of Health, 1963a, p 17.) For example, in 1961, about 431,000 (49%) of those attended by home nurses were elderly people, compared with 379,000 (32%) in 1953. The number of nurses had also expanded. At the end of 1961 there were 7,658 home nurses (whole-time equivalent) or 0.17 per 1,000 population compared to 6,829, or 0.15 per 1,000 in 1953. Such figures seemed to satisfy the Ministry of Health. The 1961 Annual Report claimed that "it is clear that the service is being carefully and effectively deployed, with increasing emphasis on the needs of the elderly" (Ministry of Health, 1962b).

The National Labour Women's Advisory Committee survey, on the other hand, felt that this was a totally inappropriate response to those needs. The survey pointed out that there was a general increase in the number of cases helped by home nurses between 1949 and 1953 but that from 1954 onwards there had been a decline until by 1962 fewer cases were being helped than in 1949. The total number of visits had also increased between 1949 and 1957 but had declined subsequently. This meant that although elderly people formed an increased part of the home nurse caseload and although patients were receiving a more intensive service it could be argued:

> **... that a significantly smaller proportion of the elderly has now been helped by this service than in 1949 and that the development of this service has been totally inadequate to deal with the demand. The growing number of the elderly in the population, the growing emphasis upon home nursing care as an alternative to hospitalisation and upon aftercare and preventative domiciliary nursing, make the relative and absolute decline of this service a matter for grave concern. (National Labour Women's Advisory Committee, 1965, p 11)**

The survey committee felt projections in the 10-year health and welfare plans were totally inadequate and would fail to reverse this trend. These plans hoped that by 1972, 9,790 home nurses (whole time equivalent) would be in post which would provide 0.19 nurses per 1,000 of the population (Ministry of Health, 1963a, p 17).

How did the service develop in the late 1960s? Table 9 indicates that an unspectacular increase did take place but one that certainly did not represent a major shift of policy emphasis towards domiciliary rather than hospital or residential care.

Table 9: Home nursing, England (1968-71)

Number of staff and whole-time equivalents				
30 September	1968	1969	1970	1971
Number of home nurses	10,108	10,186	10,388	10,871
Whole-time equivalents	8,163	8,300	8,609	9,069
Number of patients visited				
30 September	1968	1969	1970	1971
Patients aged 65 or over at the time of first visit	465,779	522,580	530,464	570,611
All patients (including those 65 or over)	837,001	933,719	955,098	1,020,792

Source: DHSS (1971b, p 202; 1972, p 211)

Was the growth of the home help service any more impressive? The 10-year plans indicated that in 1961 (Ministry of Health, 1963a, p 18), home helps assisted about 250,000 households, or 75% of the total, because a member of the family was elderly or 'chronically ill', and this work probably took up more than 75% of their time. The proportion, as well as the numbers, had grown since 1953, when about 115,000 households, or 57% of the total, were assisted for these reasons. Townsend and Wedderburn felt that the results of their survey of elderly people showed the home help service to be totally inadequate. They claimed that many in need were not receiving the service (see Table 10); that those in receipt often needed a more intensive service; and that the extent of variation of provision between local authorities was a national disgrace (Townsend and Wedderburn, 1965, pp 45-9).

Table 10: Summary of numbers in the elderly population requiring the home help service, Britain (1962)

	Estimated number aged 65+
Total elderly population in private households	5,825,000
Home help	
Feeling a need for help with housework	332,000
Not feeling such need, but having difficulty with housework and having no one to help	268,000

Source: Townsend and Wedderburn (1965, p 69)

Such views were supported by the National Labour Women's Advisory Committee survey. They described the development of the home help service as being "superficially spectacular" but in reality, "patchy, unplanned and characterised by regional variation and confusion as to scope and standards" (National Labour Women's Advisory Committee, 1965, p 10).

Table 11: The home help service, England

Number of staff (whole-time equivalents in brackets)

30 September	1968	1969	1970
Organisers			
Whole-time	867	878	924
Part-time	129	137	143
	(49)	(52)	(59)
Total	996	1,015	1,067
	(916)	(930)	(983)
Home helps			
Whole-time	2,846	2,605	2,574
Part-time	60,514	60,571	61,170
	(26,982)	(26,902)	(27,071)
Total	63,360	63,176	63,744
	(29,828)	(29,507)	(29,645)

Total staff	64,356	64,191	64,811
	(30,744)	(30,437)	(30,628)
Number of cases in which service was given			
30 September	1968	1969	1970
Maternity	18,757	15,828	13,485
Old age (65+)	334,096	354,959	373,321
Chronic sickness and tuberculosis	29,865	30,221	30,563
Mentally disordered	1,784	1,797	1,913
Other	25,016	25,044	23,926
Total	409,518	427,849	443,208

Source: DHSS (1971b, p 203)

The 10-year plans of local authorities had envisaged an increase to 37,083 whole-time equivalent home help staff or 0.73 per thousand population by 1972 (Ministry of Health, 1963a, p 18). Table 11 indicates that little progress was made towards this figure. However, the Ministry of Health had itself commissioned research which questioned the adequacy of such incremental growth. In 1967, the Government Social Survey had carried out a detailed investigation of the home help service on behalf of the Ministry in order to investigate the way in which the home help service was operating, and to attempt to form an estimate of the extent, if any, to which the service was failing to meet adequately the needs of the community. The research involved sending a questionnaire to all local authorities in England and Wales responsible for the home help service together with detailed interviews of samples of home helps, organisers, recipients and housewives. The report concluded that "in order to satisfy the unmet need of present recipients and to provide home help for those who are eligible by present standards but are not currently receiving it the size of the home help service would need to be increased to between two and three times its present size" (Hunt, 1970, p 25).

In other words, throughout the 1950s and 1960s the expressed demand for the home help service had been greater than the ability or willingness of local authorities to supply the service. Research has also indicated a mass of further unreported or unexpressed need for the service. Such pressures required either more resources or an imposition of rationing mechanisms. How was the failure to expand the home help service more quickly explained and justified? What rationing criteria were implemented, and what values about the role of the family did these expose?

Harris, in her 1968 research on social welfare services for the Government Social Survey, indicated that the legislation gave local authorities considerable scope to define priority and need in relation to the home help service. The 1946 National Health Service Act stated that local authorities should "provide domestic help for households where such help is required" and mentioned 'the aged' as one of the groups which might qualify. Local authorities were given little guidance on how to interpret such ambiguous words. As Harris pointed out, this allowed "generous Authorities to act generously" and "frugal Authorities to provide less liberally" (Harris, 1968, p 2). The implementing Circular (Ministry of Health, 1947b) for this part of the 1946 Act gave no detailed guidance on this issue but merely argued that:

> **... the discharge of the Local Health Authorities' duties under other sections in Part III of the Act, particularly those relating to the care of mothers and young children, domiciliary midwifery, home nursing and the care and after care of persons suffering from illness or of mental defectives will be seriously hampered without an adequate and efficient domestic help service.**

No mention was made about the particular needs of frail and sick elderly people, and it could be implied that these were not seen as a high priority.

Chapter Three showed that some senior officials at the Ministry of Health were concerned that the home help service could become an expensive general service for elderly people rather than one that emphasised the specific needs of maternity cases and the sick. Despite this, the home help service did increasingly become orientated towards the needs of elderly people rather than other client groups. The ambiguity of the wording of the 1946 Circular was not used to exclude all elderly people from the service. The reasons for the reorientation of the service towards the so-called 'aged and chronic sick' are not known for certain (this is the expression used in the early Ministry of Health annual reports – see, for example, Ministry of Health, 1955a, p 95). One possibility is that demand for the service reflected the shortage of hospital beds and residential home places in the 1950s (see Chapter Five).

The Phillips, Guillebaud and Boucher Reports all stressed the value of the home help service as an economy measure that reduced pressure on institutional care. This argument appeared to be accepted by the Ministry of Health despite its earlier reservations. *Circular 14/57* spoke of "a great increase in the proportion of the time devoted by the home help service to the care of the aged, as the value of the contribution which this service can make to help them to continue to live in their homes has been increasingly recognised" (Ministry of Health, 1957a).

However, we have already seen that the 1950s and early 1960s were characterised by the debate about whether or not domiciliary services such as the home help service undermined the willingness of families to care for their elderly parents. This was mirrored in another aspect of the priority/need debate, namely should the service be an intensive or an extensive one? Ostensibly, this debate was about whether large numbers of elderly people should be helped with a minimal service or whether the service should be restricted to those 'in greatest need' who required a very intensive service. Behind this debate, however, lay certain assumptions and anxieties about 'need' and how it should be met. Were priority cases for the home help service defined in terms of the characteristics of the client, or was it also appropriate to consider the level of potential support from families? Should those with nearby relatives be excluded from the service, or at least made a low priority?

Most commentators have agreed that family support is a factor that should be taken into account during client assessment, but few have claimed that the availability of 'family' support should completely exclude the elderly person from consideration for the service. Nepean-Gubbins, an LCC home help organiser, spoke of the need to consider both the medical condition of the patient and the availability of family support. People with 'families out at work all day' would receive more home help hours than where this was not the case (Nepean-Gubbins, 1958). Amulree made a similar point in claiming that "many families whose younger members have to go out to work would be more willing and better able to shoulder their filial responsibility if home helps were available" (Amulree, 1952, p 32). However, others felt priority should be placed elsewhere. Boucher, Senior Medical Officer at the Ministry of Health, stressed that:

> **It is not possible with our present resources to spread our attention among all the old people in a district; it is important to concentrate our efforts on those likely to make most demands, including the very frail and those old people living alone or relying entirely on the support of one hard-pressed relative or neighbour. (Boucher, 1958, p 8)**

In other words, the home help service should go to the very sick and very frail, especially where there were no family resources or where those family resources were slight. Wright and Roberts, in a 1958 article for *The Lancet*, were even more blunt. They claimed the home help service had drifted into being a monopoly of the 'aged infirm' who now considered they had an automatic right to the service. They asked:

> **How far are we justified in diluting the time given to those who need it badly so that those whose need is less may share in a service to which they consider themselves entitled?.... The service can certainly no longer be haphazard in its organisation, nor can it hope to fulfil the needs of old people unless intelligent care and thought is given to each case and its work is supplemented by enlisting every possible source of help from relatives, friends, neighbours and voluntary organisations. (Wright and Roberts, 1958, pp 235-6)**

The authors did not specify what mechanisms should be used to enlist such support, and what should be the response if the family refused to offer such help.

After 1948, the Ministry of Health did not produce a circular specifically on the home help service until 1965 (Ministry of Health, 1963c) and even then, the issue of an intensive versus extensive service was not addressed, let alone how the service should relate to the availability of care from relatives. *Circular 25/65* merely indicated that the home help organiser was 'essential' and should be skilled in the assessment of need. The Circular also indicated that the Institute of Home Help Organisers was trying to develop its own courses to teach members such skills. Central government silence on this issue was not ended until the early 1970s. *Circular 53/71* (DHSS, 1971a) implemented Section 13 of the Health Services and Public Health Act. This stressed that Section 13 referred to households, not individuals, so that "authorities who until now have felt unable, for example, to assist relatives caring single-handed for elderly people may now find advantage in the reconsideration of how to accommodate this need". However, even this was a less than comprehensive statement of the various issues involved; it was also a statement that would struggle to survive in a harsher economic climate.

What is known about the attitude of local authorities to these issues? The local authority associations never showed any inclination to debate the function of the home help service and how priorities should be set within it. These were perhaps seen as professional rather than political concerns, although they were more than willing to debate the respective roles of residential and hospital care. The Harris and Hunt surveys do give some indication of local authority practice during the latter part of the 1960s. Harris looked at eight local authorities in England and Wales and three from Scotland. Where children were living with a sick or frail elderly parent, she found that:

> **In all areas a home help would be allocated if the son or daughter was working, but in four places the help would be limited to those rooms used exclusively by the old person. In one of these areas, the help is withdrawn on those occasions when the working son or husband is on holiday, and in another it is expressly stated that no able-bodied person may benefit from the home help's services. (Harris, 1968, p 17)**

One authority took the view that if a daughter who had to work found it too much for her both to look after her mother and continue working, it was appropriate to offer the daughter a job as a home help to her mother, so that she at least had a small income. Another authority took the view that if the child who was working was a son, the home help would keep the whole house clean, but if it was a daughter, then the service should be restricted to the old person's rooms. Hunt provided less detailed information on this issue but did find that:

> **... in assessing the amount of help to be given, a majority of organisers said they took at least some account of relatives living nearby (although many qualified this by saying that the circumstances of the relatives would be taken into consideration and no organiser would refuse a home help simply because relatives lived nearby). (Hunt, 1970, p 23)**

The research by Townsend (Shanas et al, 1968, p 129), of course, confirmed that the home help service tended to go to those with no family or those with only slender family resources.

The authors of this book would argue that most local authority and central government officials and politicians assumed that families should physically care for their frail elderly parents and that the bulk of this work would be carried out by women rather than men. Such self-evident truths were not seen as requiring explicit statements. If such views were shared by the elderly population and their children, then they would have been likely to have had a significant impact on expressed demand. Women would take on what they saw as their responsibilities and would not expect help from local authority domiciliary services.

However, it should be recalled that other rationing mechanisms were also available at this time. In terms of those people accepted as clients, many of their needs may have been met by home helps outside normal working hours. This was often mentioned with pride. Nepean-Gubbins claimed a good home help does the following type of task for her clients:

1 bakes food for them when cooking for her own family;
2 takes a day's leave to act as guide to a blind person on an outing;
3 goes back in her own time to put the aged person to bed;
4 takes them into their own home for Christmas or on a Sunday;
5 does their washing in her own home;
6 washes the old lady's hair and attends to other matters of personal hygiene. (Nepean-Gubbins, 1958)

The frequency of this kind of task performed on an unpaid basis by home helps was confirmed by Harris (1968, p 66) and Hunt (1970, p 18). As Bond pointed out, "the service, as well as the clients, often benefit from this unpaid caring in that it enables scarce resources to be stretched even further than would otherwise be possible" (Bond, 1982, p 27). Bond further argued that this situation was accepted and at times encouraged throughout the years since 1948 because "the home help service is predicated upon part-time dual role women workers who act as substitute housewives and surrogate daughters doing women's work in a woman's world" (p 6). She pointed out how many home helps had both a full-time unpaid and unsupervised job as housewife and mother, as well as a part-time poorly paid but doubly supervised (by client and organiser) job at work. In their paid work, they were expected to meet both the physical and emotional needs of a group of highly dependent people; this could be achieved only by drifting into an acceptance that this requires them to carry out unpaid work in this part of their lives as well.

Another rationing mechanism has been the power to charge for the services. This can be used to discourage demand. Section 29 of the National Health Service Act stated that:

> **... a local health authority may, with the approval of the Minister,**

> **recover from persons availing themselves of the domestic help so provided such charges (if any) as the authority consider reasonable, having regard to the means of those persons.**

The implementing Circular gave local authorities considerable discretion by giving them freedom "to determine in each individual case whether any, and if so what, charge – within the limits of the standard charge specified in the tariff – would be reasonable, having regard to the means of the person concerned" (Ministry of Health, 1947b).

The proportion of the gross cost of the home help service raised by such costs has never been large and has been declining since the late 1950s. The reason for this decline was the growth of elderly clients as a proportion of the overall home help caseload. The majority of these elderly clients were on low incomes and many were in receipt of financial help from national assistance/supplementary benefit. This created conflict between the local authority associations and the NAB/Ministry of Social Security since the former felt the latter should make a contribution to the local authority when claimants received a service. (For useful discussions of this, see Judge and Matthews, 1980, pp 60-3; Parker, 1965, pp 94-5. More detailed information can be found in *CCA Gazette*, January 1961, p 71; March 1961, p 105; *Municipal Review Supplement*, November 1960, p 259.) However, the Ministry of Health always took the view that such cases should receive a free service and that any attempt to impose minimum charges in such cases could be 'ultra vires'. *Circular 25/65* was very critical of local authority pricing policy in general and claimed "some of the present arrangements for charges deter people in genuine and even urgent need of the service from taking full advantage of it" (Ministry of Health, 1965c).

An alternative approach would have been for the local authorities to have expanded their home help service on a much larger scale. This would have reduced the need to deter people by the paying mechanism or any other rationing device. Four reasons are put forward to explain why the service did not expand along the lines envisaged by Townsend and others. The first of these is linked to the previous charging issue. The local authority associations complained vehemently about the minimum charges issue, because they felt they were not receiving sufficient resources from central government to expand welfare services for elderly people; this debate became especially heated after the publication of the 10-year plans. As seen in the previous chapter, local authorities felt they were being asked to take on the former responsibilities of hospital authorities. The 1963 Annual Report of the AMC expressed this attitude by stressing how:

> **... representatives of this Association, the County Councils Association and the London County Council in October met the Ministers of Health and Housing and Local Government to urge upon them the need for increased grant to take account of the expanding services of local authorities in these fields, particularly in relation to some services (eg home helps) where local health authorities were more and more undertaking functions hitherto undertaken by the hospital authorities. (*Municipal Review Supplement*, October 1963, p 191)**

This may have created a climate in which it was difficult to obtain support from local authority politicians for an expansion of the service.

A second possible reason for the failure to expand the home help service may have been difficulty in obtaining home help staff. In the 1960s there were a number of references to such shortages as an explanation for the slow growth of the service. *Circular 25/65* was based on information supplied by 20 health authorities and this claimed that "difficulties in recruiting may have hindered some authorities in providing an adequate service" (Ministry of Health, 1965c). In the 1960s there were numerous job opportunities for women who wanted to obtain part-time work. Despite this, no major attempt was made to improve the working conditions of home help staff in order to make the job more attractive. Instead, attempts were made to improve the image of the service. The early advocates of the service had spoken of the need for a uniformed service that was distinguishable from normal domestic service (see Chapter Three). There were other alternatives. Short in-house training courses could be developed for the home help as a means of bolstering morale and improving recruitment (see, for example, Wright, 1964, pp 7-8; Parker, 1968, pp 85-7). Hunt found that new home help recruits still looked upon themselves as domestics and the welfare aspect was seen as secondary to their new job (Hunt, 1970, p 11). *Circular 53/71* took up this point and argued:

> **The status of service is a most important factor in attracting recruits. Potential recruits may often be deterred by the image of a limited domestic service and good background publicity can play a great part in establishing the service as a wide-ranging and versatile means of enabling individuals or families to remain in their own homes and of providing much-needed practical help in difficult situations. Local press and radio features are likely to be suitable media for what must be essentially local**

campaigns for very localised work. (DHSS, 1971a)

Many local authorities were sceptical about this 'go out and get them' approach being advocated by the DHSS. Sumner and Smith, in their 1965 fieldwork in 24 local authorities, reported in *Planning local authority services for the elderly,* found that many authorities failed to use employment exchanges or to advertise (1969, p 227); they concluded that there "was some evidence of lack of knowledge of techniques for recruiting and selecting staff" (p 244).

A third possible explanation for the lack of growth in the home help service was stressed in the previous chapter. There remained a belief that at certain levels of illness, frailty and impairment it became more economic to encourage the client to enter a residential home or hospital. This was seen in terms of both money and staff. This debate is not rehearsed again. The final explanation for slow growth concerns the feasibility of developing home help care at night-times and at weekends. The need for this has often been emphasised by central government. As early as 1957, the Ministry of Health was claiming that "as the experience of progressive authorities has shown, the value of this service can be still further enhanced if it is imaginatively planned, with due regard, for example, to the times at which the old person most needs assistance (maybe evening attendance)" (Ministry of Health, 1957a). Such views were supported by Sainsbury's research on elderly people in Fulham receiving a home help; district nursing; or meals on wheels (Sainsbury, 1964, pp 11-12). She found that a quarter of the home help group recipients needed help with household tasks during weekends while half those in the district nursing group needed the kind of attention at weekends that could best be provided by a general care service. However, the research by Sumner and Smith stressed some of the blockages to such developments that existed because of the attitudes of local authority health and welfare staff. They found that:

... some officers were not concerned to try to expand the present services, because they considered that too much was being asked of the domiciliary services. This applied especially in the case of the need for the services at night and weekends. (Sumner and Smith, 1969, p 179)

In other words, cover at nights and weekends should be provided by relatives, and if that was not possible then institutional care was the only alternative.

Voluntary organisations and domiciliary services

The 1946 National Health Service Act gave local authorities the power to develop certain domiciliary services for elderly people. Further service provision duties were not required by the 1948 National Assistance Act which merely gave local authorities powers to make grants to those voluntary organisations involved in the provision of meals services and recreation facilities. Local authorities had no power directly to provide laundry schemes, meals services, lunch clubs, recreation clubs, visiting schemes or skilled counselling help. Early circulars from the Ministry of Health emphasised the importance of voluntary organisations in the provision of this kind of service.

Circular 51/49 (Ministry of Health, 1949b) stated that Section 136 of the 1948 Local Government Act could be used by local authorities to make general grants to voluntary organisations involved in developing general welfare services for old people. *Circular 11/50* (Ministry of Health, 1950a) (see Chapter Four), on the welfare of old people, stressed the urgent need for voluntary organisations to develop services of a personal kind which were not covered by statutory provision "and which indeed can probably best be provided by voluntary workers actuated by a spirit of good neighbourliness". The Circular went on to list the services in question, such as regular visiting for the lonely and isolated, help with shopping, letter writing, mending and so on. The Circular ended by urging local authorities to do "everything in their power to encourage further voluntary effort to meet the needs of old people".

The Ministry of Health appeared well pleased in the early years with these arrangements. The 1952 Annual Report of the Ministry of Health claimed cooperation between local authorities and voluntary organisations was "firmly established in most parts of the country". There was "growing recognition of the important part that voluntary effort can play in supplementing the statutory services by providing services for the welfare of old people living in their own homes" (Ministry of Health, 1953, p 120).

What volume and scope of domiciliary services were actually provided by these voluntary organisations? No attempt is made to detail all the activities of the main organisations, but some idea of the level of activity is given by looking at how services had been developed and supported by the NOPWC, WRVS, BRCS and NCCOP up to the early 1960s. The second half of this section then looks at some of the obstacles and difficulties faced by these organisations during this period.

The NOPWC claimed to be a national focal point for information and advice on all aspects of the care of elderly people, and it brought together in consultation some 50 national voluntary societies and 6 government departments as well as representatives of OPWCs throughout the UK, and individuals with special experience. By 1960, there were 1,603 local OPWCs, together with 62 regional and county committees (NOPWC, 1960a, p 4). Local OPWCs were meant to be the coordinating body for local services. It was believed that by bringing together local organisations – both statutory and voluntary – which provide such services, the needs of elderly people could be kept under review and developments or new activities planned. Such committees varied enormously in the extent to which they achieved such coordination, and in the extent to which they became service providers. The 1960 Annual Report of the NOPWC does give some useful case studies of the scope of such service provision. These examples are likely to be biased towards active committees but they do give some flavour of the work. Marylebone OPWC, for example, was involved in the following activities:

> **The Borough Council's main grant has been increased from £975 to £1,075 plus £250 to pay for assisted holidays for old people. The Meals-on-Wheels service delivered 6,101 meals in 1959. The Association is responsible for the service and the WVS distribute the meals. The two parts of the Borough have a twice weekly service, the fifth day being reserved for more urgent cases but it has not been possible to serve any person daily. During 1959 information was supplied to the Welfare Committee of the LCC for a report on the costs of local meals services. 619 home chiropody treatments were given and the fee charged was 2/- a time. Regularity of visiting has made it possible to lengthen the intervals between visits, the average time now being nine weeks. The Association felt indisputably that the home treatment had helped to keep many old people moving around in their own homes, with great advantage to themselves and a reduction of calls on hospital services.**
>
> **The friendly unofficial visiting of lonely old people, which was the first work undertaken by the Association, continues to be of real value. The monthly meeting with the Borough Health Inspector and the Secretary provides not only opportunities for learning about conditions met during visiting, but about**

> **many kindnesses shown to old folk by churches and other groups. It is a great advantage to have six churches represented on the Visitors' Committee. One church has a hundred members engaged in visiting.**
>
> **Home decoration was an innovation made possible through the kindness of students connected with a Methodist Church who gave spare time to decorate rooms for eight pensioners. The Association provided paint and other equipment and paid expenses of a chimney sweep and tea for the workers. (NOPWC, 1960a, p 34)**

One of the services mentioned in the Marylebone report was the visiting scheme. In 1964, John Moss, when chairman of NOPWC, had stated that "the primary function of an old people's welfare committee is to provide personal service of which perhaps visiting is the most important" (NOPWC, 1964, p 2). *Circular 11/50* (Ministry of Health, 1950a) had spoken of the need for regular visiting of the lonely and isolated. NOPWC discussions about the causes of loneliness and the role of visiting schemes in its alleviation never suggested that this was a problem only for those with little or no family support. And yet it is hard to avoid the impression that central government and voluntary organisations saw their priority as helping not only the elderly bereaved but also those with few family resources. If Bond was correct to describe home helps as surrogate daughters (Bond, 1982, p 29), then perhaps voluntary visitors were meant to perform the same role on a free basis. The 1957 review of the causes of loneliness by NOPWC spoke of how one cause was usually assumed to be "separation from relatives by distance or death, or even, as time progresses, fewer relatives as a result of the trend towards smaller families" (NOPWC, 1957, p 33). The 1960 Annual Report looked at the organisation of visiting schemes and stressed that "the special responsibility of an old people's welfare committee in relation to visiting is to provide a service for those who have no visitors and emphasis should be laid on finding this type of elderly person and determining their degree of need" (NOPWC, 1950, p 45). The intention is clearly to target the service towards those who lack family support, although there is also obviously a concern about those cut off from neighbours, friends and all outside activities.

The WVS in 1962 had both a Food Department and an Old People's Welfare Department. The former was responsible for 846 meals on wheels schemes that delivered 3,461,099 meals in that year. The latter department was responsible for 22 residential clubs, 3 nursing homes and trolley shops in 188 welfare homes. In terms of domiciliary services, the WVS provided 88 all-day clubs, 2,011 Darby and Joan clubs, 374 chiropody clinics (WVS run), and 97 chiropody clinics (WVS assisted)[4]. These services were organised through local offices and as early as 1955 "old people's welfare specialists"[5] had been appointed to the staff of regional and to most of the county and county borough offices. Their task was "to ensure that there is an efficient organisation throughout the country to develop domiciliary care for old people in all its branches".

It has proved harder to obtain an accurate picture of the activities of the BRCS[6]. However, the organisation had 22 residential homes for the non-sick in 1962 and six homes for the 'aged sick' (BRCS, 1962, p 51). The organisation was responsible for numerous visiting schemes to hospitals and residential homes and such visiting often continued after people had left these institutions. By early 1955, 36 BRCS foot clinics were in operation (1955, p 26) and most of these continued to operate in the early 1960s. In 1962, BRCS ran 443 old people's clubs and 208 meals on wheels schemes.

Chapter Three described how the NCCOP was established to investigate the many problems connected with old age, and to make grants to voluntary organisations to enable them to test out ways of improving the situation. The Corporation soon became convinced that it was crucial to evaluate the levels of support that could be offered by domiciliary services to people in their own homes. Could this reduce the pressure on hospital and residential care and if so at what cost? The 1953 report of the NCCOP stated that:

> **The Governors in their last report expressed the opinion that there was a need for voluntary committees to turn their attention from the provision of Homes to the provision of domiciliary services as a means of enabling old people to remain in their own homes. It is their firm conviction that, in general, this is a field in which voluntary agencies can do most useful pioneering work and that the task of providing new communal Homes is now one for the local authorities save in exceptional circumstances. (NCCOP, 1953, p 6)**

This policy shift was likely to have a major effect on only one of the three main voluntary organisations. The WVS had guaranteed funding from central and local government. The BRCS had a grant application rejected by the NCCOP as early as 1948 because of their unwillingness "to give much detail of the way in which their large reserves were being spent"[7]. On the other hand, local OPWCs and councils of social service did receive numerous grants for administration and to develop services such as chiropody and laundry from NCCOP.

However, NCCOP expenditure on grants in the early 1960s remained heavily skewed to residential care. Voluntary organisations proved to be rather reluctant 'pioneers' of domiciliary services. The NCCOP often expressed annoyance (NCCOP, 1962, pp 7-8) at the continued interest of voluntary organisations in residential schemes rather than in experimenting with domiciliary services. By this time, there was growing evidence of unrest, especially from local government, about the achievements of voluntary organisations in domiciliary service provision. Slack looked at the operation of London OPWCs during the late 1950s and concluded:

> **The picture that has been presented has shown that there has been substantial growth over the past seventeen years in the services that have been provided to assist old people in London. Much remains, however, that is incomplete and some services were noticeable only by their absence. The impetus of the war and the first post-war years, which led to the rapid developments of the earlier years, slowed down and although this allowed for some consolidation there has been dissatisfaction about the present position and the time is ripe for further expansion. (Slack, 1960, pp 32-3)**

The limitations of the 1948 National Assistance Act meant such expansion was dependent upon the voluntary organisations. Slack claimed this had created "a wind of discontent" (Slack, 1960, p 22) from the local authorities which could only be overcome by amending Section 29 of the 1948 Act so that local authorities could provide the same services for elderly people as they could for the physically impaired.

One difficulty faced by the voluntary organisations was that of finance. Voluntary organisations had three main alternatives. They could raise their own funds; they could approach a charitable trust such as the NCCOP; or they could seek finance from central and local government. All of these alternatives raised difficulties. Fundraising required projects that would attract public sympathy. It may be that some voluntary organisations felt that a residential home possessed these qualities rather than a visiting scheme or chiropody service. Money available from the NCCOP began to decline in the mid-1950s as the original charitable funds were used up and the organisation became more concerned with its information/research dissemination role[8]. The availability of grants from local government often depended on location and reputation. Slack noted how there was often a reorganisation or reconstitution of many of the original OPWCs in London during the mid-1950s, frequently linking them more closely with or even tying them to the borough council or council offices. Slack goes on to explain that:

> **These constitutional changes, in part of a very fundamental nature, indicate that the work of some of the original old people's welfare committees made little impact on or failed to satisfy the demands of borough councils or their senior officers; and that grant aid was often conditional upon closer control by the borough council. (Slack, 1960, p 27)**

Various suggestions were made to overcome these problems. Finer (1955, p 8), for example, proposed that £3m or £4m should be given to a government-appointed committee that would have a similar constitution to the University Grants Committee and which would assess applications from voluntary bodies who wished to experiment with new services or provide on a voluntary basis services in supplementation to the existing statutory ones. This proposal was never taken up by central government, which instead continued to extol the virtues of voluntary organisations (see, for example, Ministry of Health, 1962d; 1962f), and to ask local authorities to be sympathetic to grant requests (Ministry of Health, 1964b).

The difficulty of raising finance was particularly acute in relation to meeting the administrative needs of voluntary organisations. It was increasingly recognised that domiciliary services could be organised and delivered only if there were paid administrative staff working for the voluntary organisations. However, this was hard to justify in fundraising appeals (Roberts, 1970, p 79)[9] and often received little sympathy from local authorities. Slack (1960, pp 70-83) argued that the shortage of paid organisers was a weakness of London OPWCs and this argument was accepted by the NOPWC (1961b, pp 45-7). The NOPWC approached the NCCOP about this problem and received a sympathetic response. In February 1962, the NCCOP agreed to set aside £10,000 at the rate of £2,000 a year for five years which would be used to help meet staff and administrative costs of OPWCs in selected areas. The three aims of these schemes would be to encourage local authorities to fund organisers, to encourage other trusts to offer funds, and to persuade local OPWCs of the need for paid organisers[10].

The problem of administration was not felt so acutely by the BRCS and the WVS, and yet the administrative requirements of, for example, the meals service were considerable. It is interesting that the WVS rapidly withdrew from the organisation of most home help schemes in the early 1950s. In 1949 they had full responsibility as agents of the local authority for 144 schemes[11] but by 1950 this had been dramatically reduced to 20 schemes[12], while the 1966 Annual Report announced that one of the remaining three schemes had been taken over by the local authority[13]. The main reason behind this trend was probably a local authority belief that the home help service should be directly run by local government. Municipal boroughs were the first to take over the service from the WVS. It could also have been that the WVS lacked the administrative capacity to organise and administer these schemes on the required scale. The WVS certainly found difficulties in the cost and complexity of administering meals on wheels schemes.

A WVS survey of 27 of their meals schemes in 1955 found that many "had poor equipment and served poor quality food" and an example was given of one large county borough which was "quite content to dole out from the van tepid milk pudding from an uncovered and uninsulated baking tin"[14]. The main task was seen as being to improve the quality of training offered to meals organisers so that they appreciated both the need for high nutritional content in the food and the welfare element of the service, that is, keeping an eye on those 'at risk'. The second requirement was to get what was called the 'tools for the job'. The high cost of kitchens and transport was a major difficulty for the WVS. Some local authorities felt that the 1948 National Assistance Act allowed them to meet such expenses while others claimed it allowed them only to meet food and delivery costs. In 1961 the National Survey by Amelia Harris of the meals on wheels service in England, Scotland and Wales was published. This underlined the regional variation of the service, the failure to provide a service during school holidays and the extent to which most recipients received a meal on only one or two days per week. Her conclusion was that the organisation of the service should be taken away from the voluntary bodies:

> **A possible way of meeting the full demand would be for Local Authorities to take responsibility for administering the scheme, arranging for the supply of a meal suitable for old people,**

> **supplying drivers and transport, and garaging and maintaining vans.... The voluntary organisations could then devote their resources to delivering and serving the meals, maintaining the personal interest and social contact. (Harris, 1961, p 83)**

The response of the voluntary organisations, local government and central government to such suggestions is examined in the next section of this chapter. At this stage it is important to stress that voluntary organisations were increasingly seen as struggling to administer domiciliary services.

Another key problem faced by voluntary organisations was a shortage of volunteers. Slack (1960, pp 132-3) pointed out how the early postwar enthusiasm for such work began to peter out and OPWCs found it increasingly difficult to recruit volunteers. Harris (1961, p 80) reported that nearly 40% of meals schemes had difficulty in maintaining the existing service due to lack of volunteers. Not only this but volunteers were easier to find in wealthier areas, so that meals provision had become skewed in favour of these areas and against those with a lower economic status. Local authority staff often believed that the overall shortage of volunteers meant that domiciliary service expansion could not be achieved by the voluntary organisations. Sumner and Smith, for example, found that:

> **A major reason in some areas was that voluntary organisations suffered from the same problems of labour shortages as the local authority services themselves. Half of the case study authorities referred to lack of voluntary manpower for the meals-on-wheels service, and a quarter to shortage of manpower for voluntary visiting. (Sumner and Smith, 1969, p 324)**

Voluntary organisations were short of finance, were struggling to cope with the administrative demands upon them and suffered from a shortage of volunteers.

They also had a tendency to 'squabble' among themselves which was hardly conducive to any coordination of their respective activities. In theory, OPWCs should have played the lead role in such a coordination, but this often failed to occur for at least three reasons. First, many local authorities were reluctant to cooperate since they saw it as their responsibility to carry out such coordination (Slack, 1960, pp 28-56). Second, many OPWCs lacked a capacity or willingness to address coordination issues. Slack was very critical of those committees which were content to concentrate upon summer outings and Christmas parties rather than the coordination of a coherent plan of domiciliary provision (Slack, 1960, pp 87-111). NOPWC proved willing to accept this criticism (NOPWC, 1961b, pp 5, 44)[15]. Attempts were made by NOPWC to emphasise the importance of the coordination role as opposed to general social activities[16], but in London at least this does not appear to have solved the problem. Slack reinvestigated OPWCs after the reorganisation of local government in London. She found that OPWCs now formed "bewildering administrative patterns" (Slack, 1970, p 7). Many committees still followed the old boundaries; they often lacked representatives from key organisations; and many made little if any attempt to coordinate local voluntary services[17].

The third blockage to effective coordination faced by voluntary organisations was the extent of hostility towards each other, especially in terms of the relationship between the WVS and the NOPWC. This hostility had existed since the 1940s. It surfaced over discussions about the impact of food rationing upon elderly people (see Chapter Three). WVS viewed the desire expressed by NOPWC to develop their own meals services as a clear attempt to persuade the Ministry of Health of the need to "get the Local Authorities asked to form Old People's Welfare Committees"[18]. In June 1948, Lady Reading complained to the Deputy Secretary at the Ministry of Health that "the creation of Old People's Welfare Committees locally has led to a great deal of rather hazy thinking regarding financial liability"[19]. When the Ministry of Health encouraged local authorities to make contributions to voluntary organisations under the 1948 Local Government Act, WVS staff complained to several officials at the Ministry of Health that this meant "more unnecessary money from the rates"[20]. Local OPWCs were clearly seen as a threat to the central role of the WVS in service provision for elderly people. *Circular 11/50* (Ministry of Health, 1950a) reinforced such attitudes because it stressed the coordination role of OPWCs but made no specific mention of the WVS. Lady Reading demanded that a further circular be issued by the Ministry of Health along the following lines to correct this situation:

> **Following Circular 11/50 the Minister would like to draw the attention of local authorities to the position of large voluntary bodies, such as the WVS, the Red Cross, St John's Ambulance and others that have already undertaken a large proportion of the welfare work for old people. These voluntary organisations have the personnel to undertake further work and it is hoped that local authorities will encourage this by working closely**

> **with these bodies and helping them by grants under Section 21 of the National Assistance Act when necessary.**[21]

The request for a circular along these lines was refused[22]. However, the underlying tensions continued to influence relations between the two organisations at both national and local level. All WVS members were informed from central office that they were responsible to their headquarters staff so that "if they became a member of another operational body in the form of an Old People's Welfare Committee, confusion results, since they are then responsible to and receive guidance from, two different bodies for the same work"[23]. WVS members could, therefore, attend such meetings to give information about what they were doing but they could not be full members. WVS Darby and Joan clubs were also informed that they could not affiliate to OPWCs. This remained the policy throughout the 1950s although a reconsideration of policy did take place in the early 1960s.

A 1960 WVS Circular confirmed that WVS clubs should cooperate with other bodies but that this must never involve affiliation or the payment of a fee. It was also stated that:

> **... when members accept nomination to these Committees they should keep in mind that their responsibility for work undertaken is to the WVS and if the local Committee's policy on any particular issue appears to conflict with WVS Headquarters' instructions, the WVS representative on the Committee should abstain from voting on that issue and ask for advice from the Regional Office through the usual channels.**[24]

At the same time, the Circular was conciliatory in tone by stressing that "if WVS co-operates fully" with local OPWCs in their task of coordination, and at the same time maintains its own identity and realises the responsibility it has to its own service, then the work for old people will go forward smoothly. The reasons for this change in tone appear two-fold. The WVS was under pressure from members unhappy at the restrictions on them in relation to OPWCs[25]. At the same time, WVS was also concerned at the growing criticism of the work of voluntary organisations in domiciliary service provision; much of this criticism focused round the inadequacies of meals on wheels services throughout the country (Harris, 1961).

Central government throughout the 1950s continued to believe many domiciliary services should be provided by voluntary organisations, although towards the end of this period it began to show concern at the lack of growth of these services and the failure to coordinate statutory and voluntary provision. The desire to reduce residential and hospital care costs was beginning to make domiciliary services more important in the eyes of central government.

The County Councils Association took a similar position. One of its representatives had argued in a 1952 meeting at the Ministry of Health that "the main effort in the field of welfare of old people being on their own should be left to voluntary organisations" (*CCA Municipal Review Supplement*, October 1952, p 209)[26]. Their 1954 evidence to the Phillips Committee had claimed:

> **... that a partial solution of the problem which will arise from the anticipated increase in the aged population can be found in the encouragement and development of voluntary service and that much good can come from an extensive but wise use by local authorities of their statutory powers to make contributions to voluntary organisations. (*CCA Gazette Supplement*, June 1954, p 113)**

However, by the early 1960s, the CCA had been persuaded of the need to amend the 1948 National Assistance Act to allow local authorities to provide a direct meals service where voluntary organisations were unable to develop such facilities (*CCA Gazette Supplement*, January 1960, p 5).

The AMC, however, were far more critical of voluntary organisations and the existing legislation. They believed chiropody services, laundry schemes, meals services and visiting schemes needed to be provided directly by local authorities in many instances. Their evidence to the Phillips Committee claimed that the:

> **... experience of the past four years has shown ... that, whilst voluntary organisations can make a valuable contribution, there is, nevertheless, the need for greater freedom for local authorities and, where necessary, wider powers to provide directly the various domiciliary services which are needed to deal with the increasing number of old people living in their own homes. (*Municipal Review Supplement*, August 1954, p 189)**

Such views were often supported by local authority staff from both welfare and health departments.

Chapter Four described how the Association of Directors of Welfare Services called for extended powers under the 1948 Act from the very beginning and how *Circular 11/50* (Ministry of Health, 1950a) represented an attempt by the Ministry of Health to deflect this discontent. The Association, however, continued to press for such change. *The Hospital and Social Service Journal* claimed that the dominant issue at its 1961 AGM was "the care of the elderly in their own homes and the extension of statutory powers to enable Welfare Departments to give the maximum assistance to cases" (*Hospital and Social Service Journal*, 16 June 1961, p 698). Slack indicated how medical officers of health in London shared these feelings of frustration with existing legislation (Slack, 1960, pp 20, 22). In 1959, an editorial in *The Medical Officer* called for "a systematised development of the meals on wheels service" (*The Medical Officer*, 14 August 1959, p 7) and stressed that this could be achieved only through its development as a public service.

The 'reform' of the meals on wheels service

Central government gradually came to accept the need for local authorities to play a greater role relative to voluntary organisations in the provision of domiciliary services, although it was not until 1962 that the 1948 National Assistance Act was amended so that local authorities could directly provide meals on wheels services. On 22 January 1957, Lord Amulree led a debate in the House of Lords on the needs of frail elderly people. He criticised Section 31 of the 1948 Act for not giving local authorities the power to provide a direct meals service in areas where voluntary agencies were unable to do so. The Earl of Home replied for the government and stressed that "this aspect of the legal powers of local authorities to provide meals directly, and the consequent need to rely entirely upon voluntary associations is one to which I think further attention ought to be given, and I will recommend that to my right honourable friend" (that is, the Minister of Health) (*Hansard*, House of Lords, vol 201, 22 January 1957, col 34). On 6 February 1957, Frank McLeavy, Labour MP for Bradford East, introduced a private member's bill to the House of Commons which would "amend section thirty-one of the National Assistance Act, 1948, and to empower local authorities to provide meals, domiciliary and other facilities for old people" (*Hansard*, House of Commons, vol 564, 6 February 1957, col 452). McLeavy stressed his appreciation of the "splendid work" of the voluntary agencies but went on to argue that "there is nothing like a network of services operating throughout the country" (col 452). Such a network would enable the elderly to remain in their own homes which "is cheaper to do ... than to provide either hospital beds or residential homes" (col 453).

At first glance the bill appeared uncontroversial. Several local authorities such as Preston (Parker, 1965, p 127) and Rochdale (Brown, 1972, p 143) already had powers to provide a direct meals service through local acts. There was widespread criticism of the weakness of general local authority powers in this respect. Nevertheless, it was five years before Section 31 of the 1948 Act was amended. The reasons for this delay were not primarily lack of interest from central government or obstruction from the voluntary organisations, but rather the reluctance of the local authority associations to take on further statutory responsibilities without increased financial support from central government. Both the NOPWC and the WVS decided to support the bill. The NOPWC expressed concern to the Minister of Health that "the Bill may lead to local authorities ... seeking to control the work of voluntary organisations"[27]. The real need was to encourage local authorities to be more generous with grant aid so that "the existing voluntary services among old people could be expanded where necessary at comparatively small cost to local authorities". At the same time, the NOPWC accepted that it would be helpful to give local authorities powers to provide mobile meals services where necessary. The WVS were more positive. As already explained, their own internal research had pointed to deficiencies in the service and the need to persuade local authorities to offer grant for more than just the food and delivery costs of the service, that is, transport and kitchen equipment. The WVS, therefore, argued:

> **The one important factor is that the service should be extended to meet to the full the need of old and sick people. To achieve this, the resources of the Local Authorities would be of infinite value.... At the same time it is clear that in the years to come old people are going to need more care than the state can provide, and it is hoped that if the Bill becomes Law, Local Authorities will run their schemes in co-operation with voluntary bodies.**[28]

The WVS argued that this was important because the use of volunteers was cheaper than paid labour and they had the time to offer a more personal service.

The second reading of the bill was moved by Ronald Williams (MP for

Wigan) because of the illness of McLeavy. It soon became apparent that the bill had run into certain problems which were explained by the Minister of Health, Dennis Vosper. The CCA were opposed to the bill as long as the proposed services would have to be paid for out of the general rates. However, exchequer funds could only be supplied through a money resolution which would have to be placed before Parliament by the government. Vosper made it clear that there was no hope of this happening for at least two reasons. First, the bill was confusingly worded (*Hansard*, House of Commons, vol 569, 10 May 1957, col 1414), and second, "the whole future of local government is at the moment under consideration" (col 1416). It did not make sense to increase the responsibilities of local authorities until this matter had been resolved. The bill never reached its third reading.

Despite this, central government appears to have been convinced of the need to extend local authority powers in relation to meals services. The 1959 Annual Report of the Ministry of Health stated that:

> **The provision of meals is a service which is growing slowly, and, with the exception of a very few areas, still only touches the fringe of the need. The proposed legislation on services for old people, announced by the Minister in the House of Commons on 10th November, includes a power for local authorities themselves to provide meals. (Ministry of Health, 1960, p 143)**

The WVS were enthusiastic about this proposal despite the increase of local authority powers. Lady Reading felt that it would mean the loss of the service in some London boroughs but "on the whole it will mean a great expansion"[29] for the WVS. She wrote to Walker-Smith, Minister of Health, and argued:

> **... although we are the largest operators we are very conscious that there is a tremendous need to expand this service which we believe plays so large a part in enabling frail old people to continue to live in their own homes, with great benefit to themselves, and consequent saving in capital and nursing costs of residential units. We feel that the proposed legislation will give an impetus to many Local Authorities, and that in making direct provision the majority of these will ask for our help which we shall most gladly give as we always welcome**

> **opportunities to continue our wartime practices of working direct to Local Authorities.**[30]

The sticking point, however, remained the local authorities. They continued to show enthusiasm for such legislative change, but insisted that it should be accompanied by increased central government financial support (*Municipal Review Supplement*, April 1961, p 77) and that there should be no restrictions on their right to impose charges (*CCA Gazette Supplement*, January 1950, p 5).

Any doubts about the sketchiness of existing meals provision were removed by Amelia Harris' 1961 survey of *Meals on wheels for old people* which was financed by the NCCOP as a result of the interest generated by the 1957 private member's bill. There was a desire to obtain a picture of the extent and intensity of present provision; to assess the administrative needs of the service; and to clarify the objectives of the service, that is, was nutrition or social contact more important? Harris uncovered 453 voluntary schemes of which 77% were run by the WVS, 11% by OPWCs and 4% by the Red Cross (Harris, 1961, p 3). These schemes covered 20,595 recipients of which 40% received one meal a week; recipients in the North East and Wales were especially likely to be dependent upon this very limited service. Harris found that "of the 453 schemes, 162 close completely for part of the year" (Harris, 1961, p 12), either because they were dependent on school meals, or helpers were on holiday. As already explained, 40% of schemes were having difficulty in maintaining the present service due to lack of personnel. Delivery staff had only the briefest of contacts with clients, and so Harris felt that the service should concentrate upon the nutritional quality of the food.

The Chairman of the NCCOP was in no doubt about the conclusion to be drawn from the information collected by Harris; he argued that:

> **... the scale on which this service should be provided to meet all needs is beyond the scope of voluntary finance and their resources of manpower: and it is clear that the time has come when local authorities, in spite of the ever increasing demand on them, should become responsible for this important service. (Gibbs, 1961)**

A shortened version of the report was sent to all MPs[31].

The WVS were angered by the critical tone of the report and upset at the subsequent press coverage[32]. Harris, for example, had pointed out that the schemes for which WVS had sole responsibility served almost half their recipients with only one meal a week. Lady Reading wrote to *The Times*[33] and stressed that WVS meals provision had expanded since the fieldwork was carried out in 1958. This could be further expanded if local authorities could be empowered "to build, equip and lend kitchens to voluntary organisations as well as to supply equipment and transport". Harris had also wanted to turn volunteers into "a messenger service" and had undervalued the individual welfare as opposed to nutritional aspects of the service.

The impact of this report upon the Ministry of Health is not known. However, when a new private member's bill on direct meals provision was presented to Parliament in 1962 for its third reading, it received "the full support of the Government". Indeed, Geoffrey Johnson-Smith (MP for Holborn and St Pancras South) opened the third reading by explaining that:

> **There is no secret about it that there has been a change in the Government's attitude towards this piece of legislation, because they have made it possible for expenditure under the Bill to rank for rate deficiency grant in England and Wales and for exchequer equalisation grant in Scotland. Authorities which qualify for these grants are, in the main, the poorer authorities, and it is in the areas of those authorities that the social responsibility for looking after the needs of elderly people is so acute. (*Hansard*, House of Commons, vol 657, 6 April 1962, col 821)**

The previous objections of the local authority associations were thus overcome.

During the debate, numerous speakers listed their own views about the virtues of meals on wheels provision for elderly people. Little mention was made of the need for nutrition, although there was consensus that such a service would "reduce the needs of old people to use the homes provided by local authorities" (*Hansard*, House of Commons, vol 657, 6 April 1962, col 826). Instead, much of the talk focused on the burden of cooking experienced by the elderly who live on their own. Johnson-Smith called it "a dreadfully dreary job" (*Hansard*, House of Commons, vol 657, 6 April 1962, col 823) while another MP spoke of how "old folk will not be bothered to cook a meal if they are on their own" (col 832).

A second theme was that the delivery of a meal brought social contact for the isolated. Alan Glyn (Clapham) claimed that "it brings to the homes of old people not only a meal, which they may be unable to cook for themselves, but also friendliness" (*Hansard*, House of Commons, vol 657, 6 April 1962, col 836); Johnson-Smith felt that "we shall be bringing them into contact with life and showing them that they are not neglected" (col 824). The third main theme was that regular contact with the isolated elderly through a meals service would enable a check to be kept on their health and social needs.

All three themes were summed up by Edith Pitt (Parliamentary Secretary to the Minister of Health) when she stated that what "is so important ... is that not only may a hot meal be provided for people who might not otherwise take the trouble or be able to provide it for themselves but that someone will call upon them who is interested and who will put them in touch with other branches of the social services if there is need" (*Hansard*, House of Commons, vol 657, 6 April 1962, col 845).

The new amendment had two subsections. The second empowered local authorities to provide a direct meals service or to use a voluntary organisation as its agent. The first encouraged local authorities to be more generous and imaginative in their grant aid to voluntary organisations for the provision of this service. Any doubt as to the legality of meeting financial costs beyond those of food and delivery were removed since local authorities could now assist voluntary organisations to provide meals or recreation for old people, by making contributions to the cost of the service; providing, by gift or loan or otherwise, furniture, vehicles or equipment; permitting them to use premises belonging to the local authority; and making available the services of local authority staff connected with the premises or vehicles which the organisation is permitted to use. This subsection reflected the aspirations and influence of the WVS and this was equally true of the implementing circular which argued:

> **The meals on wheels service is one specially suited to voluntary organisations.... The Minister is confident that local authorities will do all they can, with their additional powers, to help the voluntary organisations to give the utmost service of this kind. Authorities will now be able to help voluntary organisations by making available premises, vehicles, furniture and equipment, in addition to financial contributions or to use a voluntary organisation as their agent for providing this service. (Ministry of Health, 1962e)**

Local authorities were being encouraged to move from just giving grants to voluntary agencies to providing all the facilities necessary for the maintenance of a meals service. The WVS believed that this would lead to an expansion of their influence. However, the 1962 Act and the implementing circular were ambiguous about who should be seen as running the meals service. The long-term trend was that local authorities took over meal preparation and client assessment, even when the voluntary agency remained responsible for the delivery of meals. The respective roles of voluntary organisations and local authorities were changing; local authorities increasingly saw themselves as being in overall charge of the meals on wheels service.

What both groups continued to lack, however, was any clear statement from central government about the objectives of the service and how this should relate to 'family care' and eligibility criteria. The Ministry of Health was content to assert that this service offered "the support needed to enable many who are frail or handicapped to continue to live at home" (Ministry of Health, 1962e).

The 1968 Annual Report (DHSS, 1969a, p 25) of the Ministry of Health indicated that the decade since Harris carried out her fieldwork had seen a considerable expansion of meals provision. The total number of meals served at home or in clubs and other centres was recorded at over 18 million. Of these about 7 million were provided entirely or mainly by local authorities, about 7.3 million by voluntary organisations and the rest under joint schemes. The total number of meals served to people in their own homes was 12,615,035.

Local authorities provided information for two sample weeks in May and November about the number of people served with meals at home and the number of days on which meals were served. The average weekly total number of meals served in the two weeks was 260,565 while the average number of people served was 101,813. The largest number of people (56,107) were served on two days only, while the number served on one day only was about 12,500.

The national pattern was that many urban authorities especially in London were providing a direct meals service, while others were developing specific agency arrangements which limited the role of the voluntary organisation to delivery (Slack, 1970, p 70). The volume of meals delivered had expanded, but little progress had been made in making the service more intensive (that is, meals to be available on more days per week) despite exhortations from the annual reports of the Ministry of Health (1966a, p 30)[34] and the WRVS[35].

Local authorities and the promotion of the welfare of elderly people

After the 1962 Amendment Act, local authorities remained quite limited in their powers in relation to elderly people. They still had no legal right to offer counselling services, to develop visiting schemes or to establish 'at risk' registers. Their responsibility to provide aids and adaptations was not clearly defined. Many services remained a permissive power rather than a mandatory duty. There was no general remit to develop preventive services along the lines of the 1963 Children and Young Persons Act which stated that "it shall be the duty of every local authority to make available such advice, guidance and assistance as may promote the welfare of children by diminishing the need to receive children into or keep them in care".

Many individuals and groups continued to argue that this situation should be changed. The proposals for a family help service by Townsend in *The last refuge* (1964, p 205) included two legislative suggestions. Section 29 of the 1948 National Assistance Act empowered local authorities to take action to promote the welfare of persons who were blind, deaf or dumb and others "who are substantially and permanently handicapped by illness, injury, or congenital deformity or such other disabilities as may be described by the Minister". Townsend suggested that this could be interpreted broadly to include elderly people. If this was felt to be impossible, then the legislation should be amended. Christie argued that this amendment required only "one stroke of the pen" so as to add 'the aged' to those groups covered by Section 29. This was seen as essential since "only by making the Welfare Authorities statutorily responsible can they and the voluntary organisations work together with the maximum effectiveness for the maximum numbers" (Christie, 1964, p 213). Ruck, in *London government and the welfare services* argued that voluntary organisations were more concerned with offering entertainments for the 'hale and hearty' rather than domiciliary services for 'the frail or solitary' (Ruck, 1963, p 35). He agreed with Townsend and Christie on the need to amend Section 29 and so place primary responsibility for service development on local authorities.

Such views were echoed in *Our old people: Next steps in social policy,* a pamphlet published by *Socialist Commentary*:

> **Our second recommendation is therefore that the statutory duty to help old people should be extended by making mandatory many services which are now permissive. This could**

be achieved by adding the words 'infirmities associated with old age' to Section 29 of the Act. (Morris et al, 1966, p ix)

This pamphlet was produced by a group of politicians, academics and professionals who were to have a considerable influence upon future events. Both Kenneth Robinson (Minister of Health 1964-68) and Douglas Houghton (Coordinator of Social Services, 1964-66) were early members until their appointment to the Labour Cabinet in October 1964. The group also included two members of the Seebohm Committee in J.N. Morris and Robin Huws Jones. The Association of Directors of Welfare Services were continuing to make similar legislative demands and at their 1965 AGM it was Douglas Houghton who responded on behalf of a Labour government. He promised that a body of official advisers had been appointed to look into the scope of Section 29 and that "we are reviewing new services for the elderly and handicapped with a view to deciding whether any expansion can be undertaken by local authorities" (*The British Hospital and Social Service Journal*, 14 May 1965, p 882).

It took another three years for the 1968 Health Services and Public Health Act to be passed. As already indicated, this provided local authorities with new permissive powers in relation to domiciliary services, It gave them a general responsibility to promote the welfare of elderly people, and it made the home help service a mandatory duty. These clauses, however, were not implemented until April 1971 with the establishment of social services departments. When there seemed to be so much evidence about the need for such change and the direction it should take, why did it take so long for the legislation to be framed and then implemented? April 1971 was six years after Houghton's reassuring noises to the Association of Directors of Welfare Services, and despite the fact that two key cabinet ministers had helped in the early research for *Our old people* (see Morris et al, 1966).

The main factor was discussed in the conclusion to the previous chapter. Health and welfare services for elderly people were very low on the political agenda. A debate on 'the care of the elderly' was held in the House of Commons in July 1967 as a response to the allegations about geriatric and psycho-geriatric hospitals in *Sans everything* (Robb, 1967) and the importance of domiciliary services was stressed by several speakers. However, one MP complained about "the sparseness of our numbers" (*Hansard*, House of Commons, vol 750, 11 July 1967, col 456; speech by Gregor Mackenzie) which Dr Shirley Summerskill responded to by claiming that "one of the reasons why we do not see a huge turn-out of hon. members is that the subject has no glamour" (col 485).

There was no shortage of 'glamour' subjects to attract attention. Poverty, race and urban decay were all social priorities for a Labour government even if such priorities were seen as dependent upon economic growth. Such concerns were not a straightforward response to the 'rediscovery of poverty' associated with such academic research as *The poor and the poorest* by Abel-Smith and Townsend (1965). It was also a response to a feared social unrest generated from such diverse influences as Enoch Powell with his "rivers of blood" speech on race, and Shelter with their exposure of housing conditions in the inner cities.

Elderly people were not completely neglected. Leading pressure groups and academics interested in gerontological issues concentrated upon trying to persuade the Labour government of the need for radical pension and financial benefit reform for elderly people (see, for example, Hall et al, 1975, pp 410-67). *The Poor and the poorest* (Abel-Smith and Townsend, 1965) had confirmed the extent of poverty in old age. The consequent social security reforms were just a minor part of the large programme of policy and organisational restructuring associated with that period. This included the creation of new super departments at the national level (DHSS, DoE), while the reorganisation of the NHS and local government were also under consideration. More relevant to the 1968 Health Services and Public Health Act, the Seebohm Committee were producing proposals for restructuring the personal social services. It was decided that the relevant sections of the 1968 Act could not be implemented until these more general issues of social service organisation had been resolved.

The need for more and better domiciliary services was, therefore, extremely low on the political agenda. There was some concern at the high costs of hospital and residential care, but less acceptance of the more fundamental critiques of institutional care offered by Townsend and others. Keeping elderly people 'in the community' was not a big issue.

It was argued in Chapter Five that the one factor that might have changed this would have been a wider appreciation of the implications of future demographic trends. Some information and predictions were available, but these were not widely debated by professional groups and politicians[36] as had occurred in the early 1950s. Kelsall, in his 1967 book on *Population* (pp 59-63) argued that the over-65 population would decrease as a percentage of the overall population even though their actual numbers would increase. This was seen as a 'problem' because the elderly might lobby for high pensions that would place an unfair burden on those in society involved in active production.

However, Kelsall pointed out that many elderly people could be encouraged to remain in work. Economic growth was still seen as easily achievable and ensuring full employment. Kelsall gave no consideration to the growing numbers of so-called 'old old' who could not possibly be available for work. This was much more clearly appreciated by the authors of *Our old people*. Table 12 outlines their population projections. Their analysis of the implications of these projections raised issues more in tune with subsequent events than Kelsall. They claimed:

> **The 5½ million old people (ie those aged 65+) in England and Wales in 1961 formed 12 per cent of the total population; this is likely to rise to about 13 per cent in 1981; the 'old olds', the over 75s, who are likely to need more help will rise by 40 per cent. Another salient fact is that, even on a conservative estimate, about a quarter of old people are 'alone' – without spouse or children. (Morris et al, 1966, p v)**

This pamphlet, however, was unusual for the period in its attempt to reawaken issues in social policies for elderly people through an emphasis upon demographic trends. The Seebohm Report did make a similar point by stressing that the over-75 population was expected to rise by another 35% between 1971 and 1991 (Seebohm Report, 1968, p 91). Services for elderly people were described as "underdeveloped, limited and patchy" (Seebohm Report, 1968, p 90) and local authority powers needed to be increased through the legislative changes proposed by the Health Services and Public Health Bill. At the same time, the Seebohm Report gave little indication that services for elderly people were one of the major issues facing the personal social services. Much more focus was given to the overall health/welfare division, services for children, and the need to tackle urban unrest in inner cities through a focus on community need rather than individual families.

Table 12: Population (in thousands) of England and Wales in 1961 and projected to the end of the century

Age (years)	1961	(Census)	1981		2001	
	Males	Females	Males	Females	Males	Females
45-64	5,663	6,172	5,762	5,802	6,604	6,443
			2%*	-6%*	17%*	4%*
65-74	1,419	2,102	2,021	2,624	2,070	2,384
			42%*	25%*	46%*	13%*
75+	684	1,292	954	1,800	1,213	2,071
			39%*	39%*	77%*	60%*
Total aged 65+ Male and Female						
		5,497		7,399		7,738

Note: These figures show the percentage increase over the 1961 figures.

Source: Morris et al (1966, p v)

Previous discussions on the attitudes of local authority associations to domiciliary services suggested that the AMC would have been pressing for early implementation of the 1968 Act since it gave local authorities the legislative powers they had always asked for. Instead, they were bitterly opposed to Clause 13 which made the home help service a mandatory duty rather than a permissive power. The AMC argued that the "clause was an attack upon the freedom of democratically elected local authorities" (*Municipal Review Supplement*, March 1968, p 131). In any case, the "home help services are in fact provided according to the needs and requirements in the area of each authority and the purpose of creating a statutory duty under these circumstances is not evident". The AMC believed the real problems were an inability to recruit suitable staff and a lack of finance. There was less pressure upon central government to implement the 1968 Act than might have been expected. There was no firm consensus about the extent to which local authorities should take over primary responsibility from voluntary organisations for all domiciliary service provision. The end result was that these clauses of the 1968 Act were not implemented until April 1971.

'Family' care and domiciliary services

As already suggested, it is possible to perceive the years between 1948 and 1971 as a period of incremental progress for domiciliary services for elderly people. Commentators from a range of perspectives have suggested this. Brown, for example, as early as 1965, claimed:

> **... the concept of welfare of old people has widened into one of full community care, and local authorities are increasingly concerned to promote the welfare of all old people rather than simply cater for the minority with the actual or potential need for admission to homes. (Brown, 1965, p 92)**

The original service had been a residual one, focusing on the provision of institutional care for those with no or little family. Increasingly, a preventive service was developed that used domiciliary services to help a wider range of elderly people to remain in their homes. Tunstall argued that to achieve successful prevention, required local authorities to advertise the availability of domiciliary services and to consult on a regular basis every elderly person about their social needs (Tunstall, 1963, pp 17-18).

The Seebohm Report did not go that far. It favoured some form of register, but stressed that this should contain only those most 'at risk'. Overall, the report argued that "much of the failure of the existing social services can be attributed to their inability to discover those with physical, mental and other difficulties before they have deteriorated to such an extent that preventative action is only marginally possible" (Seebohm Report, 1968, p 91). Meacher may have criticised the "conservatism" (Meacher, 1970, p 93) of the Seebohm Report in relation to its proposals for elderly people, but the thrust of his arguments was the same. The key task was "the development of effective techniques of primary and secondary prevention" which required a policy of seeking out demand rather than waiting for people to opt in. This could only be achieved through regular visiting of all persons of retirement age, together with special priority for members of known 'risk' groups, and the implementation of a more effective system of coordination and psychogeriatric assessment (p 80).

Much of this chapter has been about the slowness of the movement towards such a policy and some of the complex reasons for this. However, there was widespread agreement that personal social services for elderly people were moving – if only slowly – in this direction. The overall task was to establish a broad-based preventive service that reduced the need to admit elderly people into residential and hospital care. The argument was over the respective roles of the state and voluntary organisations in service provision under such a policy, and the point at which illness, frailty and impairment could no longer be coped with outside an institutional setting.

The definition of those 'at risk' had widened and it was no longer considered to be those without family support. Instead the task was to support the carers. This was stated not only by academics such as Meacher (1970) and Townsend (1968, p 129), but also asserted by the Seebohm Report:

> **In particular, of course, services for old people in their own homes will not be adequately developed unless greater attention is paid to supporting their families who in turn support them. The problems of old people living alone have attracted much attention, but many of those who are most dependent live with younger relatives who often are themselves getting on in years. (Seebohm Report, 1968, p 96)**

The DHSS supported such views. *Circular 53/71* (DHSS, 1971a) on the home help service stressed the importance of not restricting the service to those without 'family' care.

However, at another level, little had changed. It was still assumed the 'family' ought to care and the naturalness and fairness of this arrangement was rarely challenged. This led to warnings that the task of domiciliary services was to support the 'family', and not to replace it. For example, one of the justifications used by the AMC for their opposition to a mandatory home help service was that relatives might look upon it as a right and refuse to cooperate in carrying out household and nursing tasks in the client's home (*Municipal Review Supplement*, March 1968, p 131). The NCCOP had similar doubts about the 1968 Act:

> **These services were never intended to work alone; they were intended as a support for those prepared to help themselves and their families and only to take over where there are no families and no friends. (NCCOP, 1969, p 39)**

In the late 1960s, the argument was about how to offer support to the 'family' without taking over from it. This rhetoric was not to survive the growing fiscal pressures upon the state and the rising numbers of dependent elderly people. By 1976, Moroney was warning:

> **If the elderly person is living with relatives, especially children, the service is withheld on the assumption that the family will provide needed care. In other situations, it would appear that even when family members cannot or will not provide care, the service is refused on the basis that they should do so. In practice, then, some authorities are still guided by the principle of family responsibility as enunciated in 43rd Eliz. (Moroney, 1976, p 56)**

Moroney was pointing out that the process of incremental change described in this chapter has had little influence upon attitudes to family responsibility. However, the underlying assumptions of Moroney are the same as those of Meacher and Townsend. The task should be to support the 'family' in its role of primary care giver. This does not include a challenge to assumptions about the naturalness of this type of care.

To do this is seen as inviting chaos; society would be swamped under a tide of demands from dependent elderly people. Moroney indeed argued that this tide could be stemmed only if families were offered more help (Moroney, 1976, p 58). As Stacey and Price stated:

> **Notions of the 'proper place' and 'proper behaviour' are deeply ingrained and emotionally loaded, such that acute discomfort is felt when the norms are violated. For to the actors concerned, the norms have come to appear as 'natural', as part of an externally given order without which there could only be chaos. (Stacey and Price, 1981, p 8)**

This explains what Wilson has called "the stunning silence" (Wilson, 1982, p 46) about the effect of welfare policies on women during the 1950s, 1960s and 1970s. Women accepted that it was their duty to look after sick and frail elderly parents and in-laws, and this view was shared by central government, local government and voluntary organisations. From 1948-71 this attitude was never challenged. The debate was about how best to ensure such responsibilities were carried out.

Notes

[1] PRO AST 7/664, *Welfare and the visitation of old people*. See minutes of Regional Officers' Conference, 17 February 1944.

[2] Ibid; arrangements with Voluntary Organisations for Visiting Lonely Pensioners, undated.

[3] PRO CAB 134/698. A copy of the Rucker Report on the Break-Up of the Poor Law is attached to the Minutes of the Seventh Meeting of the Social Services Committee, 12 July 1946.

[4] WRVS Archives. See Box file: *WVS/WRVS Headquarters Annual Reports, 1954-62* for 1962 Report.

[5] Ibid; 1955 Annual Report.

[6] The annual reports of the BRCS contain little factual information. Certain key policy files, especially those on meals on wheels, have been shredded.

[7] NCCOP Archives: Governor's Minutes – Book 1. See minutes of meeting between NCCOP and BRCS representatives, 8 July 1948.

[8] NCCOP Archives: Governor's Minutes – Book 6. Minutes of 68th Meeting, 11 March 1958: "The Corporation can no longer afford to make grants to known and tried types of scheme and it is submitted that its funds should now be used to encourage new thought and new practical schemes".

[9] Her history of NOPWC claims "administration is not an appealing object for fund-raising".

[10] NCCOP Archives: Governor's Minutes - 9th Book. Minutes of 87th Meeting, 13 February 1962.

[11] WRVS Archives: Box file: *WVS/WRVS Headquarters: Annual Reports 1948-53*. See 1949 Annual Report for section on the Health Department.

[12] Ibid; Annual Report for 1950.

[13] WRVS Archives: *WVS/WRVS Headquarters Annual Reports for 1963-68*. See annual report for 1966.

[14] WRVS Archives: File F.61, *Meals on wheels, 1946-56*. See report on 'The survey and expansion of the WVS meals-on-wheels service', 9 March 1956.

[15] Her criticisms probably influenced the contents of NOPWC (1962).

[16] This theme consistently appeared in the NOPWC annual reports. See, for example, NOPWC, 1965, p 2 which remarked how some OPWCs provided the focal point for services "but in some others those primary functions of an old people's welfare committee – co-ordination of services and their mobilisation for every individual in need of them – are still neglected in favour of easier and narrow tasks".

[17] During the late 1960s and early 1970s, NOPWC continued attempts to clarify the functions of OPWCs. See Age Concern Archives: Box File 30: on *The future function of OPWC committees.*

[18] WRVS Archives. File OP5: *Old people's welfare policy, 1946*-50. See memorandum from Young to Reading, 1 March 1968.

[19] Ibid; letter from Reading to Hawton, 25 June 1948.

[20] Ibid; this information is contained in a memorandum from Young to Reading, 13 April 1949.

[21] WRVS Archives: File OP5: *Old people's welfare policy, 1946-50.* Letter from Reading to Wrigley, 2 February 1950.

[22] Ibid; letter from Wrigley to Reading, 20 February 1950.

[23] WRVS Archives: Box File A1/38 WVS: *Outline of policy and terms of reference, 1942-51.* See 1948 memorandum on 'WVS and Old People's Welfare Committees'.

[24] Age Concern Archives: Box File C47/29/WRVS: *Women's Royal Voluntary Service, 1948-60.* This contains a copy of a memorandum on 'Relations of WVS with Old People's Welfare Committees', 15 March 1960.

[25] Ibid; see letter from Massey (WRVS) to John Moss, 13 April 1960.

[26] See minutes of meeting between the local authority associations, the Ministry of Health and the NAB.

[27] WRVS Archives: File F.61: *Meals on wheels and old people's welfare, 1957-59.* This contains a copy of a memorandum from NOPWC to Minister of Health on Draft National Assistance Act 1948 (Amendment) Bill, 24 May 1957.

[28] Ibid; memorandum on 'The future of the meals-on-wheels service', 21 April 1953.

[29] WRVS Archives: File F.61: *Meals-on-wheels and old people's welfare, 1957-59.* Memorandum dated 13 November 1959.

[30] Ibid; letter from Reading to Walker-Smith, 2 December 1959.

[31] NCCOP Archives: Governor's Minutes – Book 7. Minutes of 77th Meeting, 12 January 1960.

[32] WRVS Archives: File F.61: *Meals on wheels policy, 1958-72. The Times* covered the survey on 17 January 1961.

[33] Ibid; letter printed on 20 January 1961.

[34] "There is still room for a considerable expansion of meals services, not only to reach large numbers of old people, but also to increase the number of days a week meals are served (Ministry of Health, 1966a, p 30)."

[35] WRVS Archives: Box File: *WVS/WRVS Headquarters Annual Reports, 1963-69.* See 1969 report which stated "it is very regrettable that the number of people receiving one meal only has increased when it was hoped the figure would have been nil by the end of 1969".

[36] For the period 1963-71 neither the professional journals (*The Medical Officer, Lancet*, etc) nor *Hansard* contain many references to demographic trends and elderly people which reflect the same degree of urgency as the demographic rhetoric of the early 1950s.

SEVEN

The restructuring of welfare services for elderly people

Introduction

The Seebohm Report recommended the establishment of:

> **... a new department to meet the social needs of individuals, families, and communities, which would incorporate the present functions of children's and welfare departments, together with elements from the education, health and housing departments, with important additional responsibilities designed to ensure an effective family service. (Seebohm Report, 1968, p 43)**

Most of these recommendations were incorporated into the 1970 Local Authority Social Services Act and the new social services departments came into operation in April 1971. These departments were headed by directors of social services whose backgrounds were in the personal social services and who normally possessed some form of social work qualification. Residential homes for elderly people, the home help service, meals and lunch club provision, laundry facilities, aids and adaptations and counselling services were all included in this new department.

A major reorganisation of the NHS was under consideration at the same time, with a focus on the need to reduce the inefficiencies associated with the tripartite structure established by the 1946 Act. (For general accounts of NHS reorganisation, see Brown, 1979 and Levitt and Wall, 1985.) Increasingly, the local authority health services had become seen as "a rag-bag of functions" (Brown, 1979, p 6) that needed to be integrated into the hospital and GP services. The end result of these deliberations was the 1973 Health Service Reorganisation Act, by which Brown has claimed that "basically, the local authority services were nationalised and brought under the same management as hospital services, while the administration of family practitioner services was aligned with the new authorities" (p 22). District nurses and health visitors were no longer to work in a local authority department; they were to be responsible to a district nursing officer who would be a member of a district management team of the health authority. It was the district nursing officer who would have primary responsibility for the allocation of district nursing and health visitor staff; this might or might not involve their location in GP practices. The post of medical officer of health was abolished. Each district management team instead included a community physician whose task was to assess needs and evaluate service provision within the community.

These major changes in the organisation of health provision and personal social services were obviously the product of complex macro and micro pressures that lie outside the immediate concerns of this research. The task of this chapter is to show the relationship between the narrow debate about the organisation of service provision for elderly people and the broad organisational changes that eventually took place. The obvious risk in attempting this is that one overemphasises concern about service delivery for elderly people as a factor in the impetus behind the changes. The intention, however, is to indicate the nature of this debate during the 1950s and 1960s and not to judge its overall importance relative to other factors. This is a crucial task because most of the existing accounts of these changes pay little if any attention to issues relating to older people.

The last two chapters have noted the growing interest of the Ministry of Health during the 1960s with issues of planning and coordination. Interest in planning was a feature of the period across a wide range of public services and not specific to the health and welfare services. The common response to these Ministry of Health planning initiatives is to criticise them as incompetent (see, for example, Meacher, 1970, pp 80-109). Ten-year plans and the subsequent rolling programmes failed to specify service objectives, were not based on an assessment of need, and contained no mechanism for imposing minimum standards upon all local authorities. Sumner and Smith showed that local authorities had little concept of how to engage in long-term planning. This was compounded by "lack of basic information and of the means to obtain it, doubts about what services to develop, and failures in the relationship between central and local government" (Sumner and Smith, 1969, p 359). The research by Moseley (1968) and Davies et al (1971) showed that the end product of this situation was enormous variation in service provision from one local authority to another which did not appear to bear any relationship to assessments of need.

In many ways, the situation in 1970 appeared the same as in 1960, when Ruck had lamented that "although there are many services for old age, there is no policy for old age" (Ruck, 1960, pp 120-31). Such a policy would need to contain decisions about the nature and objectives of specific services and the continuing debate about this was the subject of the previous two chapters. However, it would also need to contain decisions about who should administer and control the chosen services. Three main components of this debate can be separated:

- What kind of department should administer residential and domiciliary services for older people? Should it be the welfare department, the health department, or a new social services department?
- Who should be in charge of the development of such services at the local level? Chapter Five looked at this issue in relation to the residential home/hospital division; should a geriatrician, medical officer of health or a chief welfare officer control access to residential homes? Similar arguments existed in relation to domiciliary services as pointed out by Titmuss:

  > **In all this discussion at the present time of who is responsible for what, the family doctor is being cast for the role of co-ordinator, mobilizer, director, stage manager and leader of community care.... Others, however, are seeing the medical officer of health performing this role partly on the grounds that the family doctor is too busy and is trained as a clinician and medical diagnostician. Still others propose that the chief welfare officer and a family welfare service should assume some or most of these responsibilities. (Titmuss, 1968, p 100)**

- Who should be the key worker with elderly people and what skills should such a person possess? Should it be the health visitor, the district nurse or the social worker? Is their primary task to assess need, allocate services or provide counselling support?

This chapter will look at the various arguments advanced in response to such questions during the 1950s and 1960s. The emphasis is on the organisation of services for people who still live in their own homes, because organisational issues in relation to residential care have already been discussed in detail. A distinction will be made between the 'medical lobby' and the 'social work lobby' as offering competing definitions of how services should develop. This is not meant to imply that these lobbies were coherent entities or that professional associations were more influential upon thinking than other pressure groups.

Arguments for the medical control of welfare services for elderly people

Throughout the period 1948-71 the argument was made that there should be a combined health and welfare department under the control of the medical officer of health. Perhaps not surprisingly this view was advanced strongly by medical officers of health themselves. For example, in 1950, Irvine, Medical Officer of Health for Dewsbury, argued for such a combined department on the grounds that "the transference of old people from a home to a hostel, from a hostel to hospital, and vice versa can be most readily effected when the decisions lie with medical men who understand the medical basis of the case" (Irvine, 1950, p 74). He pointed out that Liverpool, Wigan, Preston, Reading and Kent had all made arrangements by which the health department was responsible for local authority services under the 1948 National Assistance Act.

Such views received support from the Guillebaud Committee on the cost of the NHS. This recommended "that all authorities who have not yet done so should review the working of their health and welfare services to see whether their efficiency might be improved, and the interests of patients better served, by combining their administration under one committee of the council, or under a joint sub-committee" (Guillebaud Report, 1956, p 200). The Report assumed that this would involve the assimilation of the welfare department into the health department rather than vice versa. The 1960 Royal Commission on Local Government in Greater London adopted a similar stance and claimed that:

> **... in view of the fact that so high a proportion of the work of the health department and all its branches in a county or county borough is concerned with the domiciliary care of old people, it is only logical and sensible that the health and welfare departments should be combined, with perhaps separate sub-committees looking after the residential homes and needs of the handicapped. (Herbert Report, 1960, pp 213-14)**

However, central government and its medical advisers were more concerned to emphasise the role of the family doctor as head of the domiciliary team. In the 1950s, the GP and medical officer of health were often seen as complementary, but it was the latter who was seen as having the central coordination and consultancy role in terms of domiciliary services (see, for example, Fry, 1957). However, by 1960 the Standing Medical Advisory

Committee of the Central Health Services Council was going much further than this. In relation to elderly people, the Committee argued that GPs were in contact with patients all their lives and were therefore in the best position to detect the earliest signs of decline. They were becoming increasingly involved with those who were just beginning to 'fail', medically or socially, so that they had the dual role of advising on preventive measures to maintain health and of treating established disease. Preventive work was seen as including advice on such matters as employment for disabled people, the development of leisure interests, the prevention of home accidents, and the means by which other services could be obtained (Central Health Services Council, 1961, p 12). Certain senior officials at the Ministry of Health were keen to push this concept even further. Russell-Smith, an Under Secretary, argued at the 1960 NOPWC annual conference that:

> **We have tried to build up the domiciliary personal services to serve as a kind of safety-net, and thus support old people in their own homes as long as possible. The domiciliary team comprises the home nurse, the health visitor, the home help, and the welfare officers for the handicapped under the National Health Service Act and the National Assistance Act. The team should be active under the leadership of the family doctor, who is in a position to call the various services into action when he thinks his patient has reached a stage at which the particular service is required. (Russell-Smith, 1960, p 46)**

It seems likely that Russell-Smith related the role of the GP to the needs of elderly people because she was speaking to an NOPWC audience. At the time, however, the Ministry of Health had a general concern with defining the overall field of work of family doctors because of their perceived lack of status in relation to hospital consultants.

This issue was explored in depth by the Gillie Report (1963) which was produced by a sub-committee of the Standing Medical Advisory Committee of the Central Health Services Council. A range of proposals were advanced by the report including an emphasis upon group practices, better post-qualification training and more opportunities to work in hospitals or clinics as part of normal professional life. However, the report also defined the role of family doctors as having three elements: the family doctors were the patient's first line of defence in times of illness; they were the essential intermediary in the transmission of specialised skills to the individual; and third, the family doctor was:

> **... the one member of the profession who can best mobilise and co-ordinate the health and welfare services in the interests of the individual in the community, and of the community in relation to the individual. (Gillie Report, 1963, p 9)**

This third role was seen as requiring teamwork between the doctors and the preventive services, especially in relation to the complex needs of elderly people. They also needed to monitor continuously the health of all their patients until full recovery was established. The Gillie Report argued that:

> **To achieve this the family doctor must have the help of the domiciliary team of workers which the preventive health service can supply. He needs the training and understanding to use the team as his ancillary staff in the home. (Gillie Report, 1963, p 38)**

However, the report was worried that the family doctor as 'the clinical leader of the domiciliary team' would remain a platitude unless field workers (for example, the nurse, midwife and health visitor) could be attached to individual practices. So long as this occurred, there would be no need to create a unified control for the two divisions of the health service concerned (that is, the general medical services and the local authority preventive health services). The Gillie Report did not specify the role of the medical officer of health in the process of service coordination.

Such arguments were not without their critics. Titmuss, for example, claimed "there is as yet little evidence that in his day-to-day medical work the family doctor is moving, or wishes to move, in this direction" (Titmuss, 1968, pp 100, 215). Indeed, Titmuss pointed out that consultation rates with elderly people had fallen since 1948 (p 96). One response to his criticism was to stress that the medical officer of health did still have a key role even if the family doctor was the head of the domiciliary team. The 1960 Royal Commission on Local Government in Greater London argued that the family doctor should be clinical head of the domiciliary team but that it was "the day-to-day work of the district nurse, health visitor and home help, the ancillary services such as laundry and chiropody, and the voluntary services such as meals on wheels that make it possible for so many old people to remain in their own homes" (Herbert Report, 1960, p 158). The GP could neither provide these services nor secure their efficiency. There must be an 'administrative head' to ensure that these services were available; and that those supplying the services worked together as a team. Many disagreed with the Gillie Report and believed that this could best be achieved by combining the GP and local authority health services. Brockington, for example, proposed a "community health authority" which could become "the friendly rival of the hospital" (Brockington, 1963, pp 1145-6).

However, the developing debate about family doctors and the domiciliary team did undermine the security and status of medical officers of health. It began to be asked whether an administrator of domiciliary services needed to be medically qualified especially when there was a shortage of doctors. This question was raised by Titmuss (1968, p 210) and perhaps more significantly by the 1967 Mallaby Report on the staffing of local government:

> **The legislation which governs the provision of health services requiring the employment of medical officers established patterns suited to the particular times. But the evolution of the National Health Service, and particularly the changes now coming about by reason of the increasing growth of specialisms in the hospital services, associated with the alterations in the pattern of general medical practice, make changes necessary in the present system of employing medical practitioners in local authority service. (Mallaby Report, 1967, p 39)**

In the short term, the Mallaby Report recommended that medical practitioners who transferred from clinical duties to administrative duties should receive training for their new responsibilities and that "the shortage of medical practitioners is such that they should not be charged with responsibility for services such as those provided under the National Assistance Act" (Mallaby Report, 1967, p 71). Medical officers of health were not in a strong position to oppose such recommendations. They had low status within the medical profession which was reflected in both their salary (p 39) and their composition. Warren and Cooper, in their 1966 study of 528 medical officers of health, found that they were an older group than consultants or GPs (see Table 13), that they had little opportunity to gain experience in other branches of the medical service and that they tended to remain a long time in their posts (Warren and Cooper, 1966, pp 3-12). Medical officers of health were in danger of being squeezed between the competing claims of family doctors and the emergent social work lobby.

Table 13: Distribution by age groups of medical officers of health, consultants and GPs

Age	Medical officers of health	Consultants	GPs
	%	%	%
Under 50 years	39	58	63
50-64 years	56	41	31
65 years and over	5	1	6

Source: Warren and Cooper (1966, p 7)

Table 14: Health visiting 1966-68: number of cases of certain types

	1966	1967	1968
Children born in calendar year	884,702	871,085	841,277
Children born during previous five years	2,735,672	2,772,830	2,663,581
Persons aged 65 or over	312,673	346.346	357,997
Mentally disordered persons	22,605	23,614	22,894
Persons excluding maternity cases discharged from hospital (other than mental hospitals)	39,891	43,753	46,160
Tuberculosis households	141,811	128,674	38,536

Source: DHSS (1969a, p 128)

So far the arguments have been about who should be the clinical and administrative leaders of the so-called domiciliary team. The eventual restructuring of services was, of course, based on assumptions about a distinction between medical services (GP, health visitor, district nurse and so on) and social services (social work, home helps and so on). One reason for this split was that no group within the old local authority health departments established their legitimacy as key workers in relation to elderly people. District nurses and home help organisers worked with elderly people on a regular basis, but they were never put forward as having a general preventive and liaison role outside the confines of their own particular service. This argument was made frequently for health visitors but they failed or were denied the opportunity to take on this role. Table 14 indicates the extent to which their work remained geared to children.

However, the health journals such as *The Lancet*, *British Medical Journal*, *The Medical Officer* and *Hospital and Social Services Journal* during the 1950s and 1960s had numerous references to the potential role of the health visitor in relation to elderly people. As early as July 1950, a leader in *The Medical Officer* was arguing that:

> **If health visitors can be adequately trained and be recruited in sufficient numbers we can think of no more suitable persons for the visitation of the aged, not only because they are best fitted to assist in the prevention of the disasters which at present unfortunately afflict too many in late life, but also because the employment of the one nurse in a district for all preventive health services is a sensible and economic way of securing adequate visitation without a multiplication of visitors. (*The Medical Officer*, 1950, Leader on 'The aged in hospital and at home', 15 July, p 26)**

In 1953, Wofinden similarly put heavy emphasis on the need to avoid multiple visiting. He claimed that it was theoretically possible for a household to be visited by any one of 35 field medico-social workers, and that he knew a number of families which had in fact been visited by at least seven or eight different workers within a space of six months. He concluded that the health visitor was the predominant medico-social worker in the home and that she should have the crucial coordination role in relation to services for the elderly sick (*The Medical Officer*, 1953, Letter from R.C. Wofinden on 'The elderly sick', 21 February, p 104). At a sessional meeting of the Royal Society of Health on 'The health visitor's contribution to the care of the aged', Akesler argued that the health visitor was the ideal person to marshal "all the various forms of statutory and voluntary aid for the people in her district" (*Hospital and Social Services Journal*, 12 September 1958, p 962)[1]. The health visitor could also apply pressure on 'the socially weak individuals and families' to ensure that they maintained high standards of cleanliness and obtained their welfare rights; and they could also put pressure on 'reluctant daughters and other relatives'. Williamson and his colleagues in their Scottish study of 'Old people at home' claimed that their research indicated a need for increased health visitor involvement. They could carry out initial medical assessments of all elderly people in their districts and refer to GPs where appropriate. They also argued:

> **There seems no reason why the health visitor could not carry out simple tests for mental deterioration or depression and gather corroborative evidence from relatives, neighbours, local shopkeepers, and others. She could put the old person in touch with appropriate social services and could advise about diet budgeting, and the avoidance of accidents in the home. (Williamson et al, 1964, p 1120)**

Rudd, on the other hand, stressed the role of health visitors as 'morale-builders' for families under strain from looking after elderly relatives (Rudd, 1962, p 395).

Why were health visitors not offered these various tasks in relation to elderly people on a more regular basis during the 1950s and 1960s? One reason was staff shortages. There was a general shortage of both nurses, and nurses trained as health visitors (Jameson Report, 1956). The consequent argument about priorities and boundaries was a major factor in the establishment of the 1956 Jameson Committee (Jameson Report, 1956) into the field of work, training and recruitment of health visitors. Employers, professional and educational organisations were asked about the range of duties on which health visitors should be employed. Among the range of duties suggested to these organisations by the Jameson Committee was the "care and after-care of acute and chronic illness" and "health and welfare of the aged and handicapped" (p 6). The response showed that "some medical opinion and some employing authorities favoured the limitation of work for the aged and handicapped to ascertainment and supervision of specific health problems" (p 7). One body representing English local health authorities had pointed out that inconsistency in the interpretation of the 1946 National Health Service Act had produced almost infinite variation in health visiting practice in different types of area. While expressing themselves as generally satisfied with present health visitors and the quality of their work, the Jameson Committee argued that a major decision was needed on whether they should concentrate primarily on the 'health' or on the 'social' aspects of the work. In relation to elderly people, the Jameson Report came down strongly in favour of the former:

> **We have said that Health Visitors can particularly help the doctor in the care of the aged sick. Their role with the failing and aged who need no medical attention is more problematical. Certainly failing strength and energy may lead to failure of health, in its turn often the beginning of a social problem. If the Health Visitor is brought in at an early stage, her encouragement and advice on diet, hygiene and general care could be invaluable, particularly to the elderly living alone. Some of the official services affording practical help to the aged are outside the ambit of the health services. A considerable amount of the domiciliary work with the aged is likely to be done by voluntary bodies, such as old people's welfare committees. Much of the Health Visitor's work will therefore consist of co-operation with welfare organisations and the welfare department of the local authority. She should have a recognised place in schemes of official or unofficial help – called in wherever there is a health problem with which she can assist or herself calling for the help of the appropriate organisation when, as may often be the case, she is first on the scene. (Jameson Report, 1956, p 113)**

In other words, the health visitor was skilled in the assessment of health problems. Other workers and other organisations were skilled in the assessment of social problems.

Despite these comments, the Jameson Report recommended an expansion of health visitor involvement with elderly people. Health visitors should visit all single people over 65 once a year and one quarter of all elderly married couples once a year. The proposals for all client groups meant an increase of visits from 12.5 million per year to 20.6 million, and of visits to the elderly from the existing figure which was in the range 900,000 to 1.4 million to 2.6 million visits per year. The Ministry of Health showed little interest in implementing these proposals, especially in so far as they affected elderly people. The 10-year plans for health and welfare services envisaged only a 40% increase in staff, and yet the 1956 report had called for a 66% increase in visits. As the National Labour Women's Advisory Committee pointed out, "in the 372-page Government Plan for Health and Welfare, exactly 82 words were devoted to the contribution to be made by health visitors to the elderly" (National Labour Women's Advisory Committee, 1965, p 15). The closing words of this brief section were that "in enabling the elderly to live at home, it is however, the home nurses and home helps who play the biggest part" (Ministry of Health, 1963a, p 17).

The preventive assessment of the medico-social needs of elderly people was thus given a low priority by central government. However, increasingly, those sympathetic to the emergent 'social work lobby' were arguing that 'social problem' assessment needed to be separated out from 'health problem' assessment. This required different skills and should be carried out by different workers. Jefferys, for example, argued for the appointment of "a social worker on the home front" (Jefferys, 1960, pp 2-9) who could assess the needs of elderly people and their relatives and how these could best be met by the range of existing social services. It was only the social worker (that is, from the welfare department) who had the necessary knowledge of the services, the technique of eliciting the patient's own feelings concerning his or her needs, or the time or interest to devote to the problem. These functions could not be taken over by the health visitor because "as long ... as a full nursing training is considered essential to health visiting, it is impracticable to suggest that health visitors should take over social work duties". Would central government be any more sympathetic towards the concept of the social worker as key worker with elderly people than it had been in relation to health visitors?

Arguments for the social work control of welfare services for elderly people

It was not obvious in 1948 that the newly created welfare departments would show much interest in the emergent 'profession' of social work. The new departments were expected to administer services in the same way as in the previous public assistance departments. However, the new arrangements had destroyed the old system of career development associated with the Poor Law Examinations Board. The 1948 'reforms' had not substituted an alternative system of career progression. This was made even more problematic by the fact that staff were split into smaller departments and units. Such anxieties were a major influence behind the setting up of the Institute of Social Welfare in 1955 by the Association of Directors of Welfare Services, the County Welfare Officers' Society and the Scottish Welfare Officers' Association. The objects of the Institute were to provide a professional staff association which would establish a system of training, education and qualification for its members so that the best possible standard of service was rendered by them to the public. The interesting question was: what kind of training, education and qualification would be appropriate for chief welfare officers and their colleagues?

The evidence (*Municipal Review Supplement*, January 1957, p 19) of the AMC in 1957 to the Younghusband Committee (Younghusband Report, 1959) on *Social workers in the local authority health and welfare services* listed the tasks of a district welfare officer. This list is quoted at length because it does bring out the extent to which much of their work was seen as essentially administrative during the 1950s. Such officers were seen as carrying out some or all of the following duties:

- receiving and investigating applications for admission to residential and temporary accommodation;
- periodical review of cases on the waiting list for residential accommodation, and ensuring that any necessary services are provided until accommodation is provided;
- investigating and taking appropriate action in connection with the temporary protection of the moveable property of persons admitted to hospital or residential accommodation;
- investigating cases where it is proposed to apply for the appointment of an officer of the council as receiver in respect of a mental patient under Section 5.1 of the 1908 Lunacy Act;
- making preliminary investigation of applications by handicapped persons, other than the blind and partially sighted, for services under the council's approved schemes;
- liaison with local OPWCs, old people's clubs and other statutory and voluntary organisations working for the welfare of old or disabled people;
- collection of contributions from residents in Part III accommodation;
- receiving and investigating applications for the disposal of the bodies and effects of certain deceased persons;
- other duties in connection with civil defence and the registration of births, deaths and marriages.

The existence of this attitude of mind has been confirmed by both Brown and Townsend. Brown stressed how the model of work in welfare departments with regard to the blind was very much that of the home teacher (Brown, 1972, p 252); the model of work with disabled people was that of administering practical aids, leisure facilities and occupational services (p 101). Townsend, in *The last refuge*, studied the role of welfare officers in the assessment of elderly people for a place in a residential home. Such officers had large caseloads and the emphasis was on the speedy turnover of interviews. This crucial decision about the remaining years of an elderly person's life "was taken after a superficial examination of the facts, without thorough inquiry into the alternatives, and without ensuring that individuals really did agree with the course of action proposed and were fully informed about its likely consequences" (Townsend, 1964, p 129). What information was collected did tend to reflect the administrative needs of the organisation rather than 'diagnostic' or 'therapeutic' objectives:

> **Care was taken to inquire into income, and the existence of a will and of a life insurance policy. The purpose of securing the name and address of next of kin was unashamedly stated sometimes by chief welfare officers to be 'for burial purposes' ... or 'to notify admission to hospital. (Townsend, 1964, p 128)**

And yet, by the late 1950s, this administrative definition of the work of the welfare worker was being challenged. It was argued that more emphasis should be placed upon the 'diagnostic' and 'therapeutic' elements and that this should be linked to broader assessments of whether care packages could be developed to enable more elderly people to remain in their own homes.

Most commentators claim the Younghusband Report was crucial in changing the climate of debate about the assessment skills required by welfare staff in their work with elderly people. Younghusband, herself, has explained the reason for its establishment by the Minister of Health in the following words:

> **The urgent case for training was argued by welfare and mental welfare workers who had had no chance to train since the vacuum left when the Poor Law Examinations Board ceased to exist in 1948. They thought that a national qualification would help recruitment and recognition that the social work function demanded both training and a high sense of responsibility, and that hard work, devotion to duty, and kindness to the mentally or physically handicapped and the old were insufficient without good training. (Younghusband, 1978b, p 218)**

The working party was established in 1955 to inquire into:

> **... the proper field of work and the recruitment and training of social workers at all levels in the local authorities' health and**

> **welfare service under the National Health Service and National Assistance Acts, and in particular whether there is a place for a general purpose social worker with an in-service training as a basic grade. (Younghusband Report, 1959, p 1)**

Brown has claimed that the subsequent report was the crucial development that brought professional social work into local authority welfare services (Brown, 1972, p 218). She feels it made clear that "if the various services which are being provided for the welfare of old people ... were to reach the people who needed them, at the right time and in an acceptable manner they had to be provided in a social work frame of reference" (p 47). And yet the Younghusband Report had very little to say about social work and elderly people which suggests that the development of interest in this issue had more complex origins than those put forward by Brown.

The Report defined the purpose of social work as being to help individuals or families with various problems, and to overcome them so that they might achieve a better personal, family or social adjustment. The task of the social worker was to assist individuals or families with a specific need, impairment or misfortune and that "the degree of skill needed in relation to the complexity of the situation should determine the worker required in any given case" (Younghusband Report, 1959, p 7). Three main categories of need were defined:

- People with straightforward or obvious needs who require material help, some simple service, or a periodic visit.
- People with more complex problems who require systematic help from trained social workers.
- People with problems of special difficulty requiring skilled help by professionally trained and experienced social workers. (Younghusband Report, 1959, p 7)

The first type of case should be dealt with by welfare assistants who would receive 'in-service' training. Much of the counselling for the second and third type of need should be carried out by general purpose social workers with a general training in social work equivalent to two years' full-time training. However, initial assessment and supervision would be carried out by professionally trained and experienced social workers (for example, almoners, psychiatric social workers) who should have a professional training in social work following a social science degree or other related qualification. These workers should also "undertake casework in problems of special difficulty" (Younghusband Report, 1959, p 8).

In other words, a new system of training was being proposed. There would be 'in-service' training for welfare assistants and the continuation of postgraduate diplomas for the social work 'elite'. However, a national system of two-year social work courses (Younghusband Report, 1959, p 246) was to be developed for non-graduates and this would be the relevant qualification for the bulk of health and welfare social work staff. Those officers in the health and welfare services without a social work qualification and over the age of 50 or with 15 or more years experience in a social work appointment would be recognised from the date of the new training scheme as "qualified by experience" (p 265). The resultant trained staff should be allocated work on the basis of "social and personal needs" (p 9) rather than by narrowly defined client groups. Specialisation should be by type of need not group and social workers needed to be willing to deal with a wide range of clients.

The Report argued that the new national system of social work training should be overseen by an independent representative body – a National Council of Social Work Training (Younghusband Report, 1959, p 247). To give impetus to these major training developments it was also proposed that "a national staff college" (p 272) should be created. Such a college could provide pioneer courses for selected officials to act as a nucleus of fieldwork supervisors in health and welfare departments for social work students. It could also offer a forum for discussion by senior administrators of social policy, social planning and social work method. These two bodies were established. The Council for Training in Social Work was initially set up in 1963 by the Health Visiting and Social Work (Training) Act. In 1961, the Nuffield Foundation and the Joseph Rowntree Memorial Fund provided the initial finance for the National Institute for Social Work Training to be a "focal point to which those concerned especially with the training of non-graduate social workers will look for guidance" (*Municipal Review Supplement*, September 1961, p 221). Non-graduate social work teaching did begin to develop in the early 1960s. The 1965 Annual Report of the Council for Training in Social Work indicated that the intake figures for all Certificate in Social Work courses in the UK was under 100 in 1962 but that the number was expected to rise to 400 in 1966 (Council for Training in Social Work, 1965). The National Institute was at the same time running a range of courses for those already employed as social workers in health and welfare departments (NISW, 1974).

Such developments suggest a growth in importance of local authority social work but so far little evidence has been provided that links this to concern about the welfare needs of elderly people. The Younghusband

Report, in fact, paid little attention to this group compared to other groups such as those with mental health problems, the sensory impaired and unmarried mothers. In the summary, it was asserted that "the proportion requiring the most skilled help is expected to be higher among the mentally ill and in certain family problems, than among the elderly or physically handicapped" (Younghusband Report, 1959, p 7). Welfare assistants were expected to do most of the work with elderly people. In the main report, brief mention was made of the importance of domiciliary services in the care of elderly people; the prime responsibility for their provision and coordination was seen as being with the voluntary organisations although the social worker could play an important liaison role (pp 132-7). Mention was made of the social work role in the assessment of applicants for residential homes; the Report denies this was a purely administrative task and indicates it requires "systematic help from a trained social worker" (p 160). However, there was no detailed consideration of the assessment task. The Report did not suggest that frail and sick elderly people would become the major component in the caseload of social workers in health and welfare departments.

However, only six years after the publication of the Younghusband Report, the Association of Directors of Welfare Services presented their evidence to the Seebohm Committee on the reorganisation of the personal social services, and they argued that elderly people "posed the biggest social problem for this country"[2]. Six pages of their evidence concerned the social work needs of elderly people and only two-and-a-half pages were devoted to 'handicapped persons'. With regard to elderly people, it was argued that "if the needs of the elderly are to be made known and dealt with at an early stage the most urgent requirement is for a rapidly expanding casework and advisory service such as is available to the various classes of handicapped persons"[3]. The Seebohm Report did not treat elderly people as 'the biggest social problem' and we have already suggested that service provision for this group was not a major area of debate among committee members. At the same time, the Report gave this area of work much more attention than the Younghusband Report. The Seebohm Report saw the social worker as the key assessor of the needs of elderly people for residential and domiciliary services (Seebohm Report, 1968, pp 90-9). Part of this function involved the full investigation of "the contribution which relatives, neighbours and the wider community can make and how the social service department can best enable such potential assistance to be realised" (Seebohm Report, 1968, p 96).

How did this shift of emphasis within the social work 'profession' come about? It is not possible to offer a complete answer but some of the influences can be identified. One of these influences was medical social work. Such workers were often appointed to geriatric units and their dominant task was achieving a speedy bed turnover for the consultants. This involved negotiating for residential care or domiciliary services; it also involved negotiating with relatives about the level of support that they might be willing to offer if the elderly person left hospital. Discussions about the use of casework with elderly people and their families seems to have developed earlier in medical social work as a result of these pressures than it did in local authority health and welfare departments. Jarvis referred to the almoner as a "buffer between the hospital and the patient's relatives" (Jarvis, 1950, p 324), while Sheridan spoke of how:

> **The almoner is the best qualified person on the hospital staff to evaluate the social position, including the amount of help available from relatives and friends. She can also advise staff of the practical position in the home and the degree to which domiciliary services can be supplemented in that particular district and household. (Sheridan, 1955, p 413)**

By the early 1960s, articles were appearing in *The Almoner* that stressed how such work should relate to the kind of casework principles associated with other fields of social work. Simmons and Van Emden spoke of how "like younger patients, they may need help in working through their fears and feelings generally, in order to free them for constructive action and at the same time to help them accept their disabilities" (Simmons and Van Emden, 1960, pp 325-32). The almoner had to tackle fear of dying, illness and ageing. Butrym (1963) attempted to apply the seven casework principles of Biestek (1961) to geriatric patients. Such an approach could sometimes deny the legitimacy of anger expressed by elderly clients. Butrym claimed "irrelevant sounding complaints about relatives or neighbours are often a similar reflection of insecurity and of a search for understanding and acceptance, and consequently the value of sharing these with the caseworker is not necessarily related to the degree of their authenticity" (Butrym, 1963, p 330).

Medical social work was exploring casework models of intervention with elderly people that focused upon the counselling of the patients and their relatives as well as the practical provision of domiciliary and residential services. However, the actual influence of such articles and debates upon the activities of welfare workers in welfare departments is difficult to assess.

Certainly, Sheridan did produce articles (1959) on the need for a more general application of casework techniques in welfare work with elderly people, and she was later appointed to a senior position at first the National Institute of Social Work Training and then the Welfare Division of the Ministry of Health.

Discussion about the needs of elderly people and their elderly relatives for counselling advice was also generated by voluntary organisations throughout the 1950s and 1960s, although it was never a dominating influence upon their overall thinking. Slack found there were 39 full-time and 9 part-time appointments in 20 OPWCs in London and that:

> **Whereas they were called variously, secretary, organiser, secretary/organiser, organising secretary, administrative assistant, welfare officer, welfare/organiser, social worker and counsellor, there was no notable difference, in the large number of cases, in their sphere of work. Secretaries or organising secretaries were also undertaking personal welfare work and welfare workers were undertaking administrative work. (Slack, 1960, p 75)**

Slack argued that this was inevitable so long as only one full-time official was appointed to most OPWCs. Many staff felt unhappy about the present situation, especially those appointed as welfare workers, but then submerged under administrative duties. Some of these workers were involved in developing contacts with other professionals involved in counselling elderly people. Slack indicated that since 1955 a group of geriatric almoners, OPWC secretaries and psychiatric social workers had met regularly at the Maudsley Hospital to discuss their work (Slack, 1960, p 85).

The need for counselling and casework skills was also raised in relation to visiting schemes. These were often criticised for being too unstructured (Shenfield, 1957, p 178). As one critic explained: "a friendly chat is not enough" (Baran, 1965, pp 17-18). The NOPWC discussed whether it had the resources in paid staff or trained volunteers to offer intensive support to very isolated and lonely elderly people. For example, the 1959 guidelines for visiting schemes stressed that one of their objectives was "to provide carefully selected and trained visitors for those with more difficult problems" (NOPWC, 1959, p 13). At the same time, the annual reports of the NOPWC indicated that better local administration was seen as a much higher priority than the establishment of a counselling or casework service (see, for example, the discussion in NOPWC, 1965, p 2).

The NCCOP also showed some interest in the development of social casework with elderly people. Their own staff concentrated upon advising elderly people and their relatives about placement in voluntary and private homes, but these workers found that "there are some problems met with by the elderly which can only be dealt with on the casework level". The secretariat believed:

> **... casework for old people is only at the beginning of an understanding of the job it has to do. Old people do have problems, attitudes and emotions, and experience physical, mental and spiritual needs which are to some extent peculiar to themselves, and social workers have not gone so far in understanding them as they have perhaps in other fields of casework.[4]**

The above is an extract from the proposed NCCOP evidence to the Younghusband Committee. The Governors refused to sanction it on the grounds that the Corporation had insufficient experience of the recruitment and training of social workers. Although this document was never made public, it still represented an important argument about the skills required by any key worker with elderly people. Such a worker was not involved in the simple administration of practical help. A more complex social assessment had to be made and this included the emotional problems associated with ageing and family relationships.

The proposed NCCOP evidence to Younghusband had argued that such a casework service should be a statutory duty. The campaign for extending the powers of the 1948 National Assistance Act was looked at in detail in Chapter Six. The lack of such powers in the 1950s may have encouraged the Younghusband Committee to ignore social work with elderly people. Nevertheless, staff in health and welfare departments were already in touch with large numbers of elderly people who wished to enter local authority residential care. It is possible that interest in social work with elderly people developed within local authorities because of this function. Brown, for example, has claimed:

> **... welfare became gradually conscious of the need for social work.... But as waiting lists for old people's homes increased, someone had to make the social diagnosis that decided who should be admitted and who asked to wait. Residential care did not operate on medical criteria of need but on the 'need for care and attention not otherwise available'. That criterion**

required an increasingly sophisticated assessment of the applicant's overall social situation. (Brown, 1972, p 252)

Sheridan offered a slightly different argument. The allocation of financial support, residential care places and domestic help should be attempted only after "an accurate social assessment of the individual's difficulties". However, this often did not occur and "attempts to work on a hit-and-miss basis are producing personality damage and economic waste" (Sheridan, 1959, p 289). *The last refuge* supported such criticisms with its descriptions of assessment for residential care as a narrow administrative task (Townsend, 1964, pp 128-9). The important point is that this view of welfare work with elderly people was beginning to be challenged by the late 1950s and early 1960s. The core of the argument was that casework was cost-effective. It enabled a full social assessment to take place of residential and domiciliary care needs and the relationship of these needs to personal and 'family' tensions. For instance, had the old person 'adjusted' to old age and did the female relative carry out the 'necessary' care functions? At the same time, the argument was developing for a family help service, as advocated by Townsend (1964, pp 202-7) that could 'support' elderly people and their relatives prior to any request for residential care.

So far two explanations have been offered for the development of such arguments between the publication of the Younghusband and Seebohm Reports. First, they were influenced by casework developments in medical social work and voluntary organisations. Second, they were a 'natural' product of the evolving activities of staff in welfare departments. Other possibilities exist. These are linked with the impact of the post-Younghusband training courses and the perceived self-interest of welfare departments. The Younghusband Report may have placed little stress on social work with elderly people, but this was not true of the consequent two-year certificate in social work courses or of the short courses run by the National Institute of Social Work Training. For example, Huws Jones claimed that in the two year courses:

The classroom teaching of the principles and practice of social work quite deliberately includes case material concerned, for instance, with elderly clients. The teaching, of course, is concerned with implications for casework in general but incidentally it conveys the significance of the needs of the elderly, the social and emotional effects of growing old, seeing that old

> **people are people first, but recognising that they are also old, and that this can make a difference. (Huws Jones, 1963, p 6)**

Such a message was being offered to students who were likely to be receptive. Most of them were seconded staff of health and welfare departments. This group are:

> **... likely to work in one way or another with old people and their families, with those who apply to enter communal homes, with those who struggle to live their independent lives, with the newly blind (80% of whom are old), with deaf and physically handicapped people and with people who are suffering from the mental frailty that comes in later life. (Huws Jones, 1963, p 5)**

The National Institute of Social Work Training was running shorter courses for senior management from the same departments; and these courses often contained discussion of social work with elderly people (Goldberg, 1966, pp 9, 34). The National Institute later became involved in a major research study into "how the use of trained and experienced social workers can contribute to the welfare of the old person and his or her family" (Goldberg, 1970, p 17). *Helping the aged* looked at the social needs of 300 clients who were over 70; half of them were allocated to trained social workers and the other half to untrained social welfare officers.

It is easy to exaggerate the importance of such training and research developments. They affected only some staff. Courses remained limited in how they addressed the social work task in relation to elderly people. *Introduction to a social worker* (National Institute of Social Work Training, 1964) which was produced by the National Institute in 1964 virtually ignored social work with elderly people. A 1967 Council for Training in Social Work discussion paper on *Human growth and behaviour* did have a section on 'Old age' but the author queried whether sufficient time was devoted in such courses to "the psychology of ageing" (Council for Training in Social Work, 1967; see especially Lloyd, pp 23-5).

Brown, however, was in no doubt about the overall impact of such training developments. She feels that they reinforced the growing interest in helping elderly people to delay having to enter residential care. The concept of 'community care', she believed, owed more to the development of social work, including group work and community work as well as individual casework, than it did to social medicine so that:

> **On a practical level, therefore, many welfare departments were finding a growing affinity with children's departments, for example, rather than with health. The introduction of more trained social workers to the departments, since the Younghusband Report and its resultant training schemes, tended to accentuate this feeling. Some authorities were even groping towards the formulation of a comprehensive welfare policy based on the broader concept of community care and involving a wide range of services. (Brown, 1972, p 51)**

This brings us back to the organisational politics of the period. If social workers were to become the key workers with elderly people because of their assessment and counselling skills, where should they be employed? In a combined health and welfare department? In general practice? In a welfare department? In a new social services department?

The case for the first alternative has already been considered. It tended to be made by medical officers of health who doubted the utility of social work. The second alternative was raised by authors such as Jefferys (1965, p 312)[5] but it does not seem to have been widely considered as feasible. Perhaps the most obvious answer was that they should remain in the existing welfare departments and be accountable to a chief welfare officer. The Younghusband Report accepted the existing diversity of arrangements but argued that all welfare staff should be under the direction of a senior officer trained and experienced in social work and administration (Younghusband Report, 1959, p 212). However, many chief and senior welfare officers were becoming persuaded of the need for a much larger grouping of services in a single department and their arguments tended to emphasise the importance of their work with elderly people. As early as 1959, Hansen had claimed that the key principle underlying the Younghusband Report was that all social work was about the process of helping people, and this suggested the need for "the formation in local areas of Departments of Social Work, whose function would be to provide a social work service to those people in need of help" (Hansen, 1959, pp 1042, 1050). In other words, the social work functions of health, welfare and children's departments would be combined. Four years later, he argued that extended training could have a profound impact upon service provision for elderly and handicapped people, and increasingly they would be seen in their community and family context:

> **Thus, the development of a comprehensive visiting service**

> **to the handicapped, including the aged, who cannot manage without support of some kind from the community care services may result in the recognition and constant reappraisal of primary aims. In turn, this may lead to consideration being given to the rationalisation of the welfare services, perhaps culminating in a family welfare service advocated by Donnison et al (1962, p 9) and Townsend (1964, pp 202-7; 1963, p 758) (Hansen, 1963, p 758)**

This chapter has already shown how such views were reflected in the evidence of the Association of Directors of Welfare Services to the Seebohm Committee. They not only emphasised the importance of service provision for elderly people but argued for "the creation of a single Social Services Department"[6]. This was supported by the evidence of the County Welfare Officers' Society which also noted that "many authorities have gone far beyond their statutory obligations in providing services notably for old people"[7]. The Institute of Social Welfare stressed the need for a new department which would concentrate "upon the provision of social work and welfare services, by whomsoever required, and looks beyond the interests of comparatively small classes or groups"[8].

The evidence of these organisations to the Seebohm Committee poses two questions. Why did senior welfare officers wish to see the establishment of a unified social services department? Why did they begin to give greater emphasis to social work with elderly people? One explanation is the large number of elderly people compared to more narrowly defined groups of 'the handicapped'. Hamson, the Deputy County Welfare Officer for Lindsey, was quite explicit about this. The development of casework with elderly people gave the chance for welfare departments to escape their 'ugly duckling of social work image'. The welfare department must "shed its drab plumage and join the other swans" (Hamson, 1965, p 751). The development of casework with elderly people, especially if the 1948 Act could be amended, offered the chance to achieve this. Such arguments helped to suggest that there was a distinctive role for welfare departments as opposed to health departments. They also offered a balance to the resource and staffing demands of children's departments, who could refer to their increased duties under the 1963 Children and Young Persons Act and their proposed new responsibilities for juvenile offenders in the White Paper on *The child, the family and the young offender* (Home Office, 1963). Hansen, again, summed up this strand of thought:

At this point, the suggestions in the Home Office White Paper that 1,000 extra social workers will be needed in the attack upon the problem of juvenile delinquency is most significant. The increasing number of social workers being trained for the local authority health and welfare services may not remain in those services if they continue to be planned and administered on out-dated concepts and principles. There may well be a 'drain' to other social work services offering a greater challenge – and better career prospects. (Hansen, 1962, p 666)

The new principles thus should revolve around prevention and 'community care' based on the assessment skills of social workers, and should be offered to a range of groups including elderly people.

Career prospects, however, may have suggested that this needed to occur in a unified social services department. Some may have seen this as the only way to avoid what Titmuss called "'balkanized' rivalry in the field of welfare" (Titmuss, 1968, p 80). There needed to be one large department built around the provision of personal social services and the 'skill' of social work. Others may have seen such a development not as a means to improve service delivery but as a prerequisite for the professional advancement of social work. Many commentators have, of course, seen the Seebohm Report as a reflection of professional self-interest (see, for example, Sinfield, 1970, pp 32-8). Most of these accounts, however, have emphasised how the call for reorganisation was led by the childcare side. This chapter has suggested similar sentiments were often expressed by senior welfare staff and that an important part of their argument concerned the growth of their work with elderly people. By the mid-1960s, welfare provision for elderly people had become less peripheral to the social work debate than it had been in the period of the Younghusband Report. There was growing acceptance of the social worker as the key worker with elderly people. However, these changes coincided with a reduced political interest in the hospital–residential care division. This had not yet been reawakened by concern about demographic trends and the rising number of over 75s. The growth of social work interest in elderly people was not very firmly based.

The Seebohm Report and the reorganisation of the personal social services

Hall (1976) and Cooper (1983) provide detailed accounts of the politics of both the Seebohm Report and the period from its publication in 1968 to the passing of the 1970 Local Authority Social Services Act. There is agreement that there was a long campaign to extend the work of children's departments into a family casework service that dealt with juvenile crime. These ideas were based upon a belief that the roots of such crime could be traced back to family malfunctioning. Such views dominated the 1964 Labour Party document *Crime: A challenge to us all* (Longford Report, 1964) which was the basis for the subsequent White Paper on the need to move from an emphasis on punishment to an emphasis upon treatment.

This strand of reasoning excluded any consideration of a reorganisation of health and welfare departments. However, Hall claims that "a number of prominent academics and practitioners within the social services, some closely connected with the Labour Party, became alarmed at the shape the proposals were taking" (Hall, 1976, p 22). An 'ad hoc' working group was formed and their main arguments were outlined by Titmuss at the Royal Society of Health Conference in April 1965.

> **It is fashionable at the present time to argue the case for Family Service Departments. As I understand it, the core of this new Department would be the Children's Department to which would be transferred certain other responsibilities at present carried in many areas by welfare departments. I must say, I am not happy about this proposal, and for the following reasons. In the first place, it is too family-centred and child-centred.... We have to remember that a larger number of needs arising in the community are not essentially 'family needs'; mentally ill migrants, elderly widows and widowers, the isolates and childless, unmarried mothers and other categories of people who, in an increasingly mobile society might well hesitate before turning to a 'Family Department'.... Secondly, I suggest that the conception of a Family Service Department is not broad enough. Important welfare responsibilities both residential and domiciliary might remain well outside the province of a Family Service Department (FSD).... Thirdly, I am doubtful whether a FSD would effectively bring together within one administrative structure all social workers in the employ of a single local authority. (Hall, 1976, p 22; an extended version of this speech can be found in Titmuss, 1968, pp 83-90)**

By late May 1965, the group had produced a memorandum pointing out that previous committees which considered aspects of the social work services had been precluded by their terms of reference from a comprehensive survey of these services. Since 1948 there had been a great expansion of services in which social workers were required but this had occurred in an 'ad hoc' way. This created serious problems of overlap between services and departments, which was "confusing for the people being helped, uneconomic for the community and frustrating for the social worker" (see Appendix Two of Hall, 1976, pp 142-3 for a copy of 'The ad hoc group's memorandum on the need for an enquiry into the integration of social work services at the local level'). Clients failed to obtain services to which they were entitled. Preventive work was being obstructed. Resources could not be effectively planned. Scarce staffing resources could not be allocated in the most appropriate way. These difficulties were occurring at a time when the common basis of social work was "affirmed by recent developments in the training of social workers and by the coming together of social workers from different fields of work in the Standing Conference of Social Workers". The 'ad hoc' group, therefore, proposed:

> **That an enquiry should be undertaken forthwith into the departmental structure and organisation of social work services at the local level and their relation to other relevant services in the community. The enquiry should be concerned with all the work of local authority children's and welfare departments of health, education and housing; it must also take account of probation and aftercare and social work in hospitals, in the social security services and in relevant voluntary bodies.**

Hall suggests that leading members of the 'ad hoc' group (Titmuss, Huws Jones and Morris) were able to persuade certain members of the Labour government of the need for an enquiry (Hall, 1976, p 25). The Seebohm Committee was appointed in December 1965 "to review the organisation and responsibilities of the local authority personal social services in England and Wales, and to consider what changes are desirable to secure an effective family service" (Seebohm Report, 1968, p 11).

The Seebohm Committee appeared to be faced with a bewildering array of organisational possibilities. The final report listed the following seven possibilities:

- the existing structure but with a more formalised and effective machinery for coordination;

- two social services departments, one responsible for social work services for children and families with children, and the other for old people and handicapped adults;
- personal social services divided between an enlarged children's department and a combined health and welfare department;
- a social casework department acting on an agency basis for other departments;
- personal social services absorbed into enlarged health, or health and education departments;
- taking the personal social services away from local government;
- a social services department. (Seebohm Report, 1968, pp 38-43)

Evidence to the committee has been well summarised by Hall (1976, pp 42-58)[9]. It underlined the extent of conflict between medical and social work interests. The medical lobby argued that health and welfare department services should remain under medical control and some felt that this control should be extended to the work of children's departments. The British Medical Association, for example, called for the establishment of "the all-purpose social welfare service" which would "come within the ambit of the Health Department, which could then be renamed the Health and Social Services Department"[10]. The Association of County Medical Officers of Health argued for no major change; existing services should be developed to the full, which offered the prospects of better provision than any form of major reorganisation[11]. The Society of Medical Officers of Health called for combined health and welfare departments and stated that the medical officer of health should be responsible in clearly defined terms for the coordination of all health and social services[12]. Such views were opposed by what could be called the welfare side of the social work lobby, that is, the Association of Directors of Welfare Services, the County Welfare Officers' Society and the Institute of Social Welfare. All of these organisations called for a unified social services department. They were broadly supported by the rest of the 'social work lobby' although some of the childcare organisations did claim that a reorganisation of children's services should occur before the addition of social work from the other departments[13].

What evidence and suggestions were offered by central government, the local authority associations and the main voluntary organisations? The Home Office claimed that the best solution was the creation of a social work department but there was a danger of a dilution of childcare standards as resources were spread too thin. The scope of the new department had to be 'kept within bounds' and for this reason school attendance enforcement, child guidance, social work with unmarried mothers and mental health social work should remain with the existing departments, and accommodation for the elderly and the home help service should be among the last to be considered for a place in the new department[14]. Hall believed that "the strategy behind the proposal appears to have been to retain the predominance of child care in any new department by excluding the major competing services and thereby preserve the standard of that service" (Hall, 1976, p 44). The Ministry of Health was more circumspect. Detailed consideration was given to the amalgamation of the health, welfare and children's departments and also to the creation of a new social welfare department. However, the disadvantages of both these potential solutions were outlined at length and no final recommendation about reorganisation was offered. The main disadvantage of a social welfare department was seen as being the weakening of the health department. The closest possible relationship between health and welfare services was essential, but "this relationship would be hampered by the reorganisation of responsibilities on this basis"[15].

The AMC listed a series of service reorganisation models but refused to specify which it preferred. The AMC felt 'radical reorganisation' was essential because the present system had been "rendered obsolete by the development of new skills and an expansion of personal social services"[16] but that at the same time there should be as much discretion as possible to enable local authorities to develop their services in a way which was best suited to their own local circumstances and needs. The CCA were much clearer about the necessary direction for change. Most of the personal social services should be combined within one department "leaving the health and education departments to concentrate on what can best be described as their specialist functions"[17]. The voluntary organisations found it very difficult to address the overall issue of reorganisation and few made detailed proposals. The NOPWC, the NCCOP, the WVS and the Red Cross all decided to avoid engaging in the overall debate and restricted their evidence to stressing that voluntary organisations would continue to have a crucial preventive role irrespective of the future pattern of local authority services.

How could the Seebohm Committee cope with such a plethora of advice? What led them to support the creation of social services departments and so undermine local authority health departments and the status of medical officers of health? This chapter has shown how the debate about these issues preceded the intervention of the 'ad hoc' group and the setting up of the Committee. The membership of the Committee seemed almost certain to produce the eventual main recommendation on reorganisation, namely the need to establish unified social services departments. Sinfield took a jaundiced view of the Committee membership:

> **The committee itself consisted essentially of the various vested interests particularly from the National Institute of Social Work Training, the staff college of the social work profession. By the end it could be said to be represented by its chairman, its principal, one of its lecturers and perhaps too its president's wife – four out of ten. (Sinfield, 1970, p 41)**

Several members of the Seebohm Committee had already indicated their desire for some form of unified social services department. Both Huws Jones and Morris had been members of Titmuss' 'ad hoc' group which had not specified the details of reorganisation but had been quite clear about the overall arguments for change as being based upon the definable skill of social work. Huws Jones had been a member of the Younghusband Committee, was a strong believer in the need to avoid narrow social work specialisms, and by 1963 was calling for "an integrated local authority family welfare department", one component of which would be a comprehensive service "to help old people themselves and the families of handicapped and old people" (*Hospital and Social Service Journal*, 31 May 1963, p 627; see Report of Proceedings of the 64th Annual Conference of the Association of Hospital and Welfare Administrators). Mike Simson was secretary of the NCCOP and the proposed evidence of this organisation to Younghusband had called for a statutory casework service for elderly people but one integrated into "a family service including old people automatically and incidentally in its work"[18]. Huws Jones and Morris had both contributed to the *Socialist Commentary* pamphlet on *Our old people: Next steps in social policy.* This considered coordination of services, and argued:

> **It is, in fact, impossible to contemplate a social service for old people built up in isolation from other social services. Some administrative reorganisation will have to bring all the local services and the workers in them closer together. (Morris et al, 1966, p xvii)**

However, the authors did not feel that this made a case for a combined health and welfare department; such a department might become "unwieldy, generating sub-departments and committees that will still leave the very real problems of co-ordination unsolved".

These known positions of Committee members raise important questions about the logic of their selection by the central departments. Did the Ministry of Health obtain the report it wanted despite the denial of an overall position in its official evidence? Medical interests were not reflected strongly in the composition of the committee. The only doctor (Professor Morris) was, in any case, a member of the 'ad hoc' group and unsympathetic to the concept of combined health and welfare departments. Both Hall and Cooper indicate that the main decisions were taken early in the life of the Committee and were little influenced by the evidence. Hall has indicated that draft chapter headings, which bore a remarkable similarity to those of the final report, had been circulated by September 1966 (Hall, 1976, p 61). Members of the Committee have told Cooper that the written evidence was considered for the most part to be partial, and defensive of traditional loyalties to client groups and areas of skill (Cooper, 1983, p 170). Perhaps the most crucial decision taken by the committee members was their definition of 'the family' which they defined as 'everybody' so that the restrictions of the terms of reference could be sidestepped. Members explained this decision to Cooper on the grounds that "any restrictive definition would have left out some group and a service for families with children would have drained off staff and financial resources from other less popular groups, and especially from the growing elderly population which needed an expansion of services" (Cooper, 1983, p 120). The way was thus left open for the recommendation of a unified social services department.

Finally, the main direction of thinking of Committee members was supported strongly by social work developments in Scotland. The Kilbrandon Committee was established in May 1961 to look at certain aspects of the juvenile justice system in Scotland. The Committee's report proposed the creation of a social education department to combine education and childcare functions. However, mention was also made of how:

> **In discussions before us, reference was made by some of the witnesses to the possibility in the long term of an even wider measure of reorganisation of services so as to provide a comprehensive 'family service', catering for the needs of adults of all ages, as well as those of children in the family. Such a**

> **concept may have validity if it implies the need for better co-ordination of existing services, and we would expect that our own proposals, if adopted, would go a considerable way to improve the channels of communication necessary for concerted action relating to those, young or old, within a particular family unit, and irrespective of the initial source of referral. (Kilbrandon Report, 1964)**

Cooper gives an idea of the complex coalition of politicians, academics, civil servants and social workers that developed in support of the establishment of broadly defined social work departments in Scotland that would cater for all age groups (Cooper, 1983, pp 33-53). An Advisory Group (including Richard Titmuss) was appointed by the Scottish Office to advise on the feasibility of such a proposal. The 1966 White Paper on *Social work and the community* concluded that "in order to provide better services and to develop them economically it seems necessary that the local authority services designed to provide community care and support, whether for children, the handicapped, the mentally and physically ill or the aged, should be brought within a single organisation" (Scottish Education Department, Scottish Home and Health Department, 1966). The Seebohm Committee were considerably helped by developments taking place in other parts of Britain.

The reactions to the Seebohm Report were as varied as one might expect. Donnison called it "a great state paper" (Donnison, 1968, p 3). Townsend felt the report was constructive but "lacking in analysis, drive and vision" (Townsend, 1970, p 7). Authors in the medical journals tended to be less complimentary. Gordon in *The Lancet* spoke of "Seebohm sophistry" (Gordon, 1969, pp 299-300) which had enabled the Committee to demonstrate the need to keep health and social services together yet demand their separation. This conflict of opinion was no doubt a factor in the protracted debate about whether to implement the main recommendations of the Seebohm Report. Hall (1976, pp 81-110) suggests that for a long period their implementation appeared unlikely. Crossman, Secretary of State for Social Services, was not convinced of the virtues of social work. The government was preoccupied with NHS reorganisation. There was conflict over whether the Home Office or the new DHSS should control the proposed social services departments.

The micropolitics of how and why this opposition was overcome are not outlined in this book. It is more relevant to stress that the Seebohm Report reflected the growing belief that it was possible to distinguish between services that were social and those that were medical. Certainly, the 1970 Local Authority Social Services Bill received all party support. Crossman claimed that the aim of the bill was "to forestall family breakdown and avoid wherever possible moving people to old people's homes, to remove the danger of institutionalising the life of children and to move them into children's homes, foster homes or hospitals" (*Hansard*, House of Commons, vol 796, 26 February 1970, col 1408). Lord Balniel, replying for the opposition, argued that the Local Authority Social Services Bill and the proposed NHS reorganisation were based upon the following logic:

> **It is a demarcation based, to use his phrase, on primary skill. It is a demarcation so that on one side there should be services which are primarily medical in content and, on the other side, the services which are primarily social in content. I do not think one can try to separate services along the lines of one suggestion, considered and rejected by the Seebohm Committee, some being for children and some being for the elderly. It is the primary skill which is the only conceivable, logical line of demarcation in this field. (*Hansard*, House of Commons, vol 796, 26 February 1970, col 1424)**

Social services departments came into operation on 1 April 1971.

The reorganisation of the voluntary sector

An important theme throughout this book has been the changing role of voluntary organisations in relation to welfare provision for elderly people. The voluntary sector had not expressed clear views about how the personal social services should be reorganised but this did not mean that they would not be heavily affected by the eventual restructuring.

The Seebohm Report had some strong opinions about the future role of volunteers and voluntary organisations. It questioned the extent to which voluntary organisations should provide services as direct agents of the local authority. This could "present problems to the local authority, which may be led to neglect its own responsibilities and to the voluntary organisation which may be prevented from developing its critical and pioneer role" (Seebohm Report, 1968, p 182). The need was for new radical voluntary bodies with a youthful membership rather than the kind of organisation that attempted to act as "vehicles for upper and middle class philanthropy appropriate to the social structure ofVictorian Britain" (p 153). The proposed social services departments would not reduce the need for volunteers. Many of these would still be organised through voluntary organisations but others could use the social services department as their focal point. Volunteers could "complement the teams of professional workers" (p 153). This discussion took place in the chapter on 'The community' and the overall message was that a preventive policy of community care required increased involvement from neighbours and volunteers in supporting those 'at risk'.

The Seebohm Report noted that the role and preparation of voluntary workers were being considered by a committee, set up by the National Council of Social Service (NCSS) and the National Institute of Social Work Training, under the chairmanship of Dame Geraldine Aves (Aves Report, 1969). The Foreword (Farrer-Brown and Seebohm, 1969) to the Aves Report claimed that it had been financed from a desire to clarify how volunteers should fit into the total structure of the social services and how they should relate to professional staff. The Aves Report followed Seebohm in noting that:

> **Although we are left with some services where the independent role of the voluntary organisation remains unimpaired, the main feature of the current scene is the ever increasing responsibility of statutory bodies for meeting individual needs and their growing awareness of their own need for voluntary reinforcements. A partnership of some kind inevitably develops. (Aves Report, 1969, pp 22-3)**

The Aves Report also supported the rhetoric of 'community care'. Volunteers were the means by which the community itself could participate in meeting the needs of its members. Such volunteers could give the 'special gift' (Aves Report, 1969, p 90) of time and so they had more freedom to continue caring relationships than pressurised paid staff. However, volunteers still needed to be organised, managed and trained if their contribution was to be maximised. These tasks could be carried out by both voluntary and statutory bodies but extra finance would be required. At the local level, joint committees for the training of voluntary workers should be established, composed of representatives from both the statutory and voluntary sector. Local authorities needed to be more willing to pay the administrative costs of voluntary organisations. At the national level, a volunteer foundation "should be established, to be concerned not only with training, but with many aspects of voluntary work; and to provide a focus for the local co-ordinating bodies" (Aves Report, 1969, p 167). Such a foundation would need to be of 'independent status' although some central government funding would be required. The Aves Report specifically stresses that no existing body could perform such a function and that "the National Council of Social Service is not sufficiently identified with studies, training, or professional groups" (p 192). In September 1973, the Volunteer Centre was established as a charity with finance from both government and voluntary trusts.

It would be easy to exaggerate the influence and importance of comments about the voluntary sector in the Seebohm and Aves Reports and yet they do seem to express common themes and anxieties. Voluntary organisations needed to place less emphasis upon direct service provision. Coordination of volunteers and voluntary organisations was weak and this failure was out of keeping with the planning ethos of the period; local authorities should perhaps be given a more central coordination role for the voluntary sector. Voluntary organisations needed to adjust to social policy trends by stressing their potential role in 'community care'. Many of these themes were summed up by Morris in the conclusion to her 1969 study of *Voluntary work in the welfare state*:

> **The expansion of welfare services by central and local government should mean not only the overall provision will be increased but that some tasks which are now being carried out by unpaid labour will be transferred to the salaried staff of statutory authorities. This should be welcomed by the voluntary bodies and by all 'good neighbours' since it should set them free to concentrate on tasks for which they are specially suited, instead of having to fill gaps which could be better filled by paid workers. There will always be such tasks since it is inconceivable that the State could ever meet all social needs without voluntary assistance – indeed the very concept of community care which is central to present social policy involves the active participation of ordinary members of the community. (Morris, 1969, p 213)**

Morris warned voluntary bodies that they had to coordinate and stop bickering over sectional interests as in the past. The extent of such conflict within the voluntary sector with regard to welfare provision for elderly people has been seen in earlier chapters. Morris suggested (1969, p 219) and the Aves report implied (1969, p 192) that the NCSS had failed to overcome this problem by providing the necessary coordination through which influence could be exerted upon the Ministry of Health at an early stage in the planning process. These difficulties were perhaps highlighted by the arrival in the mid-1960s of voluntary pressure groups such as Shelter which took a campaigning stand on social issues. The NCSS was particularly vulnerable to such criticism. Lapping, in an article in *New Society* in 1966, attacked the NCSS for three main reasons. It failed to coordinate the voluntary sector and stop unnecessary overlap. It had a 'too cosy' relationship with senior civil servants, and it failed to pressurise the government on behalf of minorities in marked contrast to newer voluntary groups such as the Child Poverty Action Group, the Campaign Against Racial Discrimination and the Disablement Income Group. It was failing to develop good relationships with the statutory sector and especially social work. As a result the organisation was "much less than the sum of its parts" (Lapping, 1966, p 760). She concluded:

> **Statutory bodies are, quite rightly, taking on more functions. If voluntary organisations do not want to become increasingly irrelevant they must not compete with them, but outflank them with plans for so far uncovered areas of need. And they must put public pressure on the government to do things it has been shirking, or has never thought of. (Lapping, 1966, p 761)**

What were the implications of this analysis for the main voluntary organisations associated with welfare provision for elderly people?

The WVS had strong central and local government funding. The organisation continued to provide meals services and to maintain its own residential homes. The WVS had remained an organisation that wanted to deal direct with government rather than through any other voluntary organisation. It remains available as a national organisation in a time of national emergency. The BRCS did decide to reduce some elements of its service provision (especially meals services[19]) but it also changed little as a result of the 1970s restructuring. Overall, these two organisations seem to have experienced a slow reduction of their overall influence upon policy development and implementation.

The NCCOP and the NOPWC were to be much more obviously influenced by the late 1960s debate about the role of the voluntary sector in social policy provision. Two main possibilities were discussed during the late 1960s. Should the NOPWC 'break away' from the NCSS and become a completely independent body? Should the NOPWC and NCCOP amalgamate because of their overlapping functions? Tension between the NCSS and the NOPWC had always existed. In November 1940, the NCSS Executive Committee had agreed to provide the new old people's organisation with office and clerical assistance but also stressed that the organisation "should, as soon as possible, be given an independent existence"[20]. However, by 1944, this position was revised and it was agreed that "the Committee would become an autonomous group associated with the Council and would take responsibility for work in its own field"[21]. The NCSS would provide premises, the secretariat, certain basic services and a major proportion of the general expenses.

The annual reports of NOPWC through the 1950s and 1960s (1963, pp 35-6; 1964, pp 34-6) often hinted that this arrangement did not always work satisfactorily, especially over the issue of finance. NOPWC received some finance direct and it also received a grant from the NCSS. NOPWC felt that this second grant was too low and failed to reflect how many donations to NCSS were from individuals keen to see an expansion of voluntary work with elderly people. The establishment of Help the Aged in the mid-1960s probably increased the sensitivity of NOPWC to the whole issue because they now had a rival asking for donations even if the focus of the second organisation was more upon work abroad[22]. By 1966, Lapping was able to indicate that there were "rumblings of rebellion" (Lapping, 1966, p 760) from NOPWC over finance and shared premises, and she expected a breakaway group to be formed by 1970 when the lease on the NCSS' present home was up. During 1968, NOPWC tried to negotiate more money from NCSS but these negotiations failed. By November 1968, the following statement was being discussed by NOPWC as part of a grant application to the NCCOP:

> **For some time the Council has been aware that, to provide a fully effective service, more money is needed than is available at present; and extended discussions with NCSS have shown conclusively that substantially increased financial resources cannot be expected while the Council remains an associated group of that body. NCSS must, naturally, pay regard to the position of all its associated groups. It takes the view that it would be detrimental to its work as a whole to single out one group for specially favourable financial treatment. This view is understood but it inevitably means that continued association on these terms must preclude the Council from making effective**

> **use of the fund raising potential of its work for old people, a potential which, it feels must be greater than that of any of the other associated groups.**[23]

Money was needed to establish a larger headquarters staff that could impose a more coordinated response from local OPWCs to social policy developments. Independence would also create a clearer image to the outside world so that the Council could "reinforce its status as the national focal point of voluntary effort in the service of the elderly". On 10 July 1969, the NCSS Executive Committee agreed that NOPWC should become an independent body from 1 April 1970[23]. The Annual Report of NOPWC for 1969-70 reviewed the reasons for these changes. The Foreword from the chairwoman stressed the need for restructuring in the voluntary sector to reflect new thinking about statutory services from central government. Greater emphasis needed to be given to improving communication with local committees. Voluntary potential needed to be mobilised by "a strong independent body" so that it could respond to "current and impending legislation under which statutory bodies will increasingly wish to co-operate with the voluntary sector" (NOPWC, 1970, pp 2-3).

However, it had not always been clear in the period 1968-69 that the eventual 'solution' would be a new organisation that was completely separate from the NCCOP. Possible overlap between the two organisations had often been discussed. For example, a joint working party was set up in 1957 "to discuss the question of the spheres of work of the two organisations in more detail"[24]. In 1964, the NCCOP considered a change of name because "the better the Corporation becomes known the more confusion there seems to be in the minds of many people between it and the National Old People's Welfare Council"[25]. The NCCOP began to discuss the conflict between the NCSS and NOPWC in early Summer 1968 and at first the discussion was about whether the NCCOP would be willing to help finance the establishment of an independent NOPWC[26]. However, by May 1969, the Secretary of NCCOP was informing his governors that the DHSS were "firmly behind the proposal for NOPWC and NCCOP to get together more closely and seem to have been exhorting NOPWC to leave NCSS and join NCCOP"[27]. The agenda had changed. Should the NCCOP and NOPWC amalgamate in some form? The Secretary of NCCOP warned his governors that "if the Corporation are asked to take over NOPWC it might find that its own work was swamped by the routine work of NOPWC"[27], such as the coordination of all the local OPWCs. The DHSS continued to press for a merger and "to have some doubts about the immediate future of NOPWC"[28]. The NCCOP resisted this but did agree that their secretary should be seconded to NOPWC to help with their establishment as an independent organisation. In July 1970, the governors confirmed their commitment to the maintenance of NCCOP and NOPWC as separate organisations[29]. In December 1970, David Hobman was appointed as Director of NOPWC and in January 1971 the name of NOPWC was changed to Age Concern. The main focus of Age Concern was to be the creation of national publicity about the needs and aspirations of elderly people rather than the service delivery by local committees.

Elderly people and the personal social services after 1971

Hope Murray, in her review of the development of services for elderly people provided by social services departments in the latter half of 1972, took a largely optimistic view of the future, since:

> **It was evident that many directors and senior staff were seized with the importance of encouraging new ideas of seeking more ways of preserving independence among the elderly and of considering alternative forms of care. There was concern about the quality of life in many residential homes and some early effort to obtain the views of elderly people about their needs and the services which they felt to be required. Others saw services for the elderly as part of wider social services to the community and considered that past concentration on residential services was changing in favour of a variety of methods of community care. A few were already engaged in reviewing the needs of elderly people in care to see whether some might live more independently, given appropriate housing and domiciliary support. (Hope Murray, 1977, p 15)**

Many commentators would feel such 'hopes' were never realised. Most local authorities failed to reduce their reliance upon residential care and to develop community care services. Qualified social workers proved reluctant to work with elderly clients.

Bosanquet complained in 1978 that "we are spending far more on keeping residents in homes than we are on the elderly in the community in face of evidence that the great majority even of the severely handicapped housebound live in the community" (Bosanquet, 1978, p 120). He pointed out that this was unlikely to change according to the 1976 priorities document from the DHSS (1976). By this time, the dynamics of the overall situation were changing on a dramatic scale. There was growing concern about future demographic trends combined with the development of pressures upon local government to control their spending. It was the interaction of these two trends that initially persuaded the authors of the need for this research.

Notes

[1] The proceedings of the conference are summarised in an article on 'The health visitor and the aged'.

[2] Family Service Committee Papers (FSCP) 104. Evidence from The Association of Directors of Welfare Services, p 7.

[3] Ibid; p 12.

[4] NCCOP Archives: Governor's Minutes – Book 4. Report on 'Evidence to Working Party on Social Workers' for 59th Meeting, 31 July 1956.

[5] She argued that GPs should work in "home based health units" with health visitors and social workers.

[6] FSCP 104, p 9.

[7] FSCP 241. Evidence from the County Welfare Officers' Society.

[8] FSCP 51. Written Evidence from the Institute of Social Welfare, p 4.

[9] The evidence is summarised in FSCP 364(i) and FSCP 364(ii).

[10] FSCP 148.

[11] FSCP 241.

[12] FSCP 161.

[13] FSCP 95, p 10. Evidence of the Association of Children's Officers.

[14] FSCP 35.

[15] FSCP 116.

[16] FSCP 221. See also *Municipal Review Supplement,* November 1966, pp 293-8, for a copy of the AMC evidence.

[17] FSCP 207. See also *CCA Gazette,* July 1966, pp 166-70, for a copy of the CCA evidence.

[18] NCCOP Archives: Governor's Minutes – Book 4. Report on 'Evidence to Working Party on Social Workers' for 59th Meeting, 31 July 1956.

[19] The exact date of the decision by the BRCS to reduce meals service as a priority is not known because the relevant files have been destroyed. BRCS staff suggest it was in the mid-1970s.

[20] Age Concern Archive: Box File 29, *NOPWC independence from NCSS, 1968-1969.* See Extract from OPWC Minutes, 22 November 1940.

[21] Ibid; see extract from NOPWC Minutes, 23 February 1944.

[22] Help the Aged were not welcomed by NOPWC who were very suspicious of the 'newcomer'. See Age Concern Archives: Box File 26, *Voluntary and Christian Service.*

[23] Age Concern Archives: Box File 29, *NOPWC independence from NCSS, 1968-69.* See draft statement appended to letter from Sir Harold Fieldhouse, 27 October 1968.

[24] NCCOP Archives: Governor's Minutes – Book 5. See Minutes of 66th Meeting, 19 November 1957.

[25] Ibid. Governor's Minutes – Book 10. See Minutes of 96th Meeting, 12 May 1964.

[26] Ibid; Governor's Minutes – Book 12. See Minutes of 112th Meeting, 7 June 1968 and 113th Meeting, 30 July 1968.

[27] Ibid; see report of Secretary to 116th Meeting, 6 May 1969.

[28] Ibid; see report of Secretary to 118th Meeting, 24 November 1969.

[29] Ibid; see minutes of 121st Meeting, 21 July 1970.

EIGHT

Community care and older people: reflections on the past, present and future

Introduction

In various talks and lectures to managers and practitioners from social services, health and housing, the authors have often run what they like to call a community care quiz. It usually comprises the following questions:

- When did it become mandatory for social services authorities to provide a home help service?
- What change was brought in by the 1948 National Assistance Act 1962 (Amendment) Act?
- "The importance of enabling older people to go on living in their own home where they most wish to be ... is now generally recognised". What was the date of the government publication from which this quotation is drawn?
- When did government start to include equity tied up in one's house in assessing the client contribution to residential care fees?
- When did government introduce charges for domiciliary services such as home care?

Thorough readers of this book should be in a position to answer all these questions!

Our starting point in this chapter has to be to emphasise once again the relevance of such 'knowledge' to an understanding of present community care debates. In saying this, we make no claim to have offered a factual objective history of the past. This book is partial in what it has covered and the sources it has drawn upon, and the information collected has been shaped into a 'story' through the influence of our theoretical assumptions. Nevertheless, we believe that our study helps to undermine both 'the Golden Age' myths of the left and 'the Disaster Years' myths of the right about the early development of community care policy and practice in this country. This book concludes by considering a number of the present day issues in terms of what we have concluded about how they were or were not addressed in the past.

The health and social care interface

One of the clearest messages which emerges from our study of the development of welfare services for elderly people is that politicians and policy makers have struggled to define 'what is health' and 'what is welfare' right back into the Poor Law period. Initially the distinction was between being ill and hence not to blame for being destitute and being a welfare case and hence deserving of the label of 'pauper'. Older people challenged this distinction because their problem was often seen to be frailty through ageing which meant that they could no longer support themselves in the workplace. How to respond to the elderly infirm was an ongoing issue during the Second World War (see Chapters Two and Three).

The 1948 National Assistance Act attempted to resolve the dilemma through the creation of a category of those in need of 'care and attention' only to find out, as we saw in Chapter Five, that this had not resolved the issue of 'the partly sick and partly well' in terms of whether they should be in a local authority residential home or a patient in NHS long-term care. Ministry of Health *Circular 14/57* (1957a) attempted to resolve this problem by offering 'a working guide' to enable local authorities and health authorities to resolve how best to respond to borderline cases. In reality, the Circular was riddled with interpretative problems and hence a major source of conflict at the local level.

Nearly 40 years later, we see an almost identical story emerging. The 1990 National Health Service and Community Care Act places the responsibility on local authorities to fund nursing home care for elderly people on low incomes, causing Henwood to argue:

> **Despite the claim that the responsibilities of the NHS are unchanged, nursing home care is apparently now viewed as social care, not health. Is this contradictory, or are we to accept that there is a real distinction between those needing nursing home care for reasons of ill health and those needing it for other reasons? Surely this is playing *Alice in Wonderland* games with words and semantics? (Henwood, 1992, p 28)**

As we have argued elsewhere, such a situation was bound to encourage health authorities to run down their remaining nursing homes and continuing care bed provision (Means and Smith, 1998). It was also inevitable that local authorities would feel tempted to reject some people referred to them from acute hospitals by claiming that their needs remained those of healthcare and not social care.

By the mid-1990s there was extensive conflict over how to interpret the health and social care interface as redefined by the 1990 Act with health authorities using the Act to justify a major reduction in the provision of NHS continuing care (Wistow, 1995). The then Conservative government responded to this situation by setting out *NHS responsibilities for meeting continuing health care needs* (DoH, 1995). In terms very similar to *Circular 14/57* (Ministry of Health, 1957a), it argued that after a multidisciplinary assessment and consideration of local eligibility criteria, the consultant (or GP in some community hospitals) together with the disciplinary team would decide whether:

- the patient needs continuing inpatient care arranged and funded by the NHS because:
  – either he or she needs ongoing and regular specialist clinical supervision (in the majority of cases this might be weekly or more frequent) on account of:
  the complexity, nature and intensity of his or her medical, nursing or other clinical needs;
  the need for frequent not easily predictable interventions;
  – or because after acute treatment or inpatient palliative care in hospital or hospice his or her prognosis is such that he or she is likely to die in the very near future and discharge from NHS care would be inappropriate;
- the patient needs a period of rehabilitation or recovery arranged and funded by the NHS to prepare for discharge arrangements breaking down;
- the patient can be appropriately discharged from NHS inpatient care with:
  – either a place in a nursing home or residential care home arranged and funded by social services or by the patient and his or her family;
  – or a package of social and healthcare support to allow the patient to return to his or her own home or to alternatively arranged accommodation. (DoH, 1995, p 9)

Again, a government had responded to a dispute over how to define the boundaries between health and welfare with working guidance for local agencies which is itself open to differing interpretations by health and local authorities.

Our historical perspective on the health and social care interface underlines that the latest guidance is unlikely to resolve where the boundary lies and that there is a tendency for each redefinition to include ever more frail and sick old people within the term 'care and attention' under the 1948 National Assistance Act. This has meant that more and more older people can be means tested on their ability to contribute to the cost of meeting their health and welfare needs in later life.

Lead agency? Lead profession?

The main emphasis of the White Paper on community care (DoH, 1989) and the subsequent 1990 Act was on social services as the lead agency in community care for older people. There was far less clarity over who should be the lead profession, although social workers along with home care organisers and occupational therapists were seen as central to the development of care management.

There have been signs that the Labour government is not fully convinced by these arrangements and that they have little faith in the ability of social services authorities to meet community care objectives, partly because of the continued lack of integration between social services and the health service in terms of both hospital provision (Wistow, 1995) and primary healthcare (Thistlethwaite, 1996). There is frustration at what Frank Dobson, Secretary of State for Health has called the Berlin Wall (Dinsdale, 1998, p 7) between health and social care. One possibility is that the government will allocate much more responsibility for community care within what the 1997 White Paper on the NHS calls the "modern and dependable NHS" (DoH, 1997) with its emphasis on the replacement of GP fundholding with primary care groups and primary care trusts. The purchase of community care services might become the responsibility of health authorities and/or primary care groups/trusts over time on the grounds that total purchasing strategies need to place the provision of health and welfare service for older people within a single budget. The previous chapter illustrated the long history of debate about lead agencies and lead professions with regard to welfare services for older people. The GP and what we would now call the primary healthcare team have long been seen as one option even though the creation of social services departments in the early 1970s, as a result of the Seebohm Report

(1968), seemed to shift the debate decisively in favour of social services.

The rationale for the creation of social services departments was that they would be responsive to local communities. Welfare services for elderly people were included in the new departments because they were seen as primarily social rather than medical in content, and hence needed to be part of the same department as children's services. As Chapter Seven outlined, a common and expanding need for social casework and trained social workers were seen as ensuring a growing common agenda.

However, Chapter One stressed that qualified social workers proved themselves extremely reluctant to work with older people in these new social services departments, and their managers felt such work could be safely left to unqualified staff. One irony is that the community care reforms could be argued as opening up opportunities for greater involvement of qualified social workers with older people rather than squeezing them out, as has been argued (Dominelli and Hoogvelt, 1996).

However, community care is still seen as about organising and rationing 'practical' help while childcare services are seen as much more about responding to the emotional needs of families. Hallett (1991) among others, has argued that community care and childcare are becoming increasingly separate activities in social services in terms of legislation, philosophy and organisational structure. As such, the argument for the retention of social services as the lead agency in community care may be being undermined on the grounds that they now have much more in common with primary healthcare.

Cinderella groups, folk devils and family care

The late 1980s and the 1990s has seen an extensive debate about the future affordability of the welfare state. A key element of this has been predicted demographic changes in terms of a rise in the overall numbers of elderly people and the ageing of the elderly population (Evandrou, 1997). Both Conservative and Labour governments have been concerned about the social security, health and welfare expenditure implications of such trends. Of particular relevance to us is the debate about how to shift the costs of continuing care away from the state without undermining the housing inheritance of the next generation, as the equity tied up in the homes of former owner-occupiers is used to pay for their residential and nursing home care. A wide range of proposals now addresses how this could best be tackled (Barclay Report, 1996; Richards et al, 1996). The former Conservative government favoured a long-term insurance scheme approach (Chancellor of the Exchequer et al, 1996) while the 1997 Labour government established a Royal Commission to review the whole area.

We have seen throughout this book that older people have often been a cinderella group in terms of their lack of priority for resources from health and welfare agencies. This has been demonstrated by both the shocking conditions in PAIs (Chapters Three and Four) and the low priority given to the development of domiciliary options (Chapter Six). Nevertheless, demographic fears have still meant that governments worry periodically about the public expenditure 'burdens' placed upon the rest of society by older people. Will such burdens undermine the welfare state, a key focus of both the Phillips (1954) and Guillebaud Reports (1956) in the 1950s (see Chapter Five)?

As a result, older people have sometimes been used to spark off what Cohen would call "a moral panic", which occurs when "a condition, episode, person or group of persons" become seen as "a threat to societal values and interests" (Cohen, 1973, p 9). Cohen was primarily concerned with the youth culture of the 1960s and how society amplified or exaggerated existing deviant behaviour (that is, violence between mods and rockers) in order to address societal concerns about the changing role of young people in society. Elderly people seem to have performed a similar 'moral panic' role in terms of being presented as undermining the affordability of welfare provision.

Cohen also argues that those at the centre of moral panics are often presented as "folk devils". This seems not to happen to older people as such but rather to their families who are seen as likely to abandon older people to the state, if given the opportunity to do so, because of the slackening of the moral fibre and the lack of filial piety in modern society (see Chapter Six). Such terminology may seem old fashioned in the late 1990s but the same concerns still exist. We have seen that one explanation for the slow development of domiciliary services was a fear that this would provoke the abandonment of older people, and legislative support for their development materialised only after studies such as that by Townsend and Wedderburn (1965) proved that such services enabled families to carry on caring. As such, the emphasis of the 1989 White Paper on community care that "carers need help and support if they are to continue to carry out their role" (DoH, 1989, p 4) represents an important continuity with past debates. The key role in supporting older people should come from the family, and any breakdown in a willingness to offer that support is seen by governments as representing a major threat to society.

A focus on institutional care

One of the key messages of this book is that debates about welfare services and older people have tended to be dominated by issues relating to institutional care. In the 1930s, the policy focus was on the PAI and how to reform it. In the 1950s and the early 1960s, it was on the interface between local authorities' residential homes and long-stay nursing care available from the NHS. It is depressing to realise that little has changed. By the late 1980s, the emphasis was on how to control expenditure on independent sector residential and nursing home care while in the mid-1990s the focus switched to how to fund continuing care. Far less attention has been given to the provision of complex care packages to people in their own homes, let alone to the need to develop more preventative services before older people meet a major crisis and hence become eligible for care management (Means and Smith, 1998, ch 9; Wistow and Lewis, 1996; Harding, 1997). Yet the vast bulk of older people with support needs continue to live in their own homes and not in some form of institutional provision.

Key misconceptions

As already indicated on a number of occasions, present debates about the impact of the community care reforms and their implications for future policy developments are often based on false and superficial pictures of the past. Some of these false pictures have already been identified in this chapter, but others include:

Older people were seen as 'best off' in residential care in the 1950s and 1960s

We have shown that this was very much not the case, one example being how Ministry of Health annual reports nearly always stressed that older people should stay in their own homes for as long as possible. Governments want older people to live in their own homes and to be looked after by their families. What has changed is a recognition that informal carers are more likely to carry on caring if they receive support services. However, it is important to note that the ideology of family care is 'toned down' in periods of national emergency, such as a world war when extensive use may need to be made of female labour in the formal parts of the economy (see Chapters Two and Three).

Local authorities had the power to provide a full range of domiciliary services from 1948 onwards

Chapters Four and Six illustrate how far from the truth this is. For example, the general preventative power of local authorities to promote the welfare of older people and the turning of home care into a mandatory responsibility rather than a permissive power did not occur until 1 April 1971. In the ensuing years, the death of Maria Colwell ensured that policy priority would be given to childcare within the newly created social services departments, while the mid-1970s oil crisis saw the end of a welfare consensus in the UK about the need for incremental growth (Means, 1995). Local authorities have had less time to develop the full range of community care services than is often assumed.

The mixed economy of social care developed in the 1980s

This book demonstrates the historical reliance on the voluntary sector as a major provider of welfare services for older people. In the 1950s , the Red Cross, the W(R)VS, local OPWCs (now Age Concern) and others played the dominant role in the provision of most domiciliary services.

Chapter Three illustrated the role of these agencies in the development of many of these services in the latter part of the Second World War and Chapter Four showed how they were keen to restrict the legal power of local authorities to provide services directly. It was the failure of voluntary agencies to develop domiciliary services such as meals on wheels on a national scale which resulted in "the wind of discontent" (Slack, 1960) from local authorities as they began to argue forcibly for wider legal powers to provide domiciliary services.

However, important differences between the mixed economy of the 1950s and 1960s and the present time need to be noted. It was not until the mid-1980s that the private sector as well as the voluntary sector emerged as a major service provider (Means and Smith, 1998, ch 3), and this took the form of a major expansion of residential and nursing home care for older people rather than of domiciliary services (Wistow, 1996). And it was not until the 1990 reforms that the concept of developing a quasi-market (Le Grand and Bartlett, 1993) controlled through contracts and the purchaser–provider split began to emerge (Means and Smith, 1998, ch 5). Community care in the UK has had a strong reliance on the independent sector as a provider of services since the Second World War, but the nature of the mixed economy has undergone significant changes.

Rationing was introduced by recent Conservative governments

This history of the development of welfare services for elderly people underlines Cranston's (1976) point that few social rights can be universal rights because they are expensive and have to be rationed even in times of a commitment to increased public expenditure. A theme running throughout this book is the ever changing nature of eligibility criteria for institutional care, as we moved from the issue of who was entitled for consideration for evacuation hostels (Chapters Two and Three) through to the need to assess who should have priority for local authority residential care in the late 1960s (Chapter Five).

In saying this, it does need to be recognised that the initial conception of local authority residential homes was of places where older people might choose to enter if they felt that they could no longer manage in their own homes. However, this philosophy was soon abandoned as a result of the very slow pace of construction of new homes after the Second World War because of the shortage of building materials. It also needs to be remembered that rationing can take many forms. To offer nearly all elderly applicants home care for just two hours per week irrespective of their need for this service is a form of rationing which if many of those applicants need much more intensive help than is on offer. However, it is less explicit that modern systems of rationing which deny services to a high percentage of applicants in order to release resources to those assessed as in greatest need. Finally, to acknowledge the inevitability of some rationing is not to deny the need to campaign for more resources to underpin community care provision for older people.

Charging was introduced by recent Conservative governments

Once again, this is a major misconception. In terms of local authority residential care, the principle of means testing was embedded in the 1948 National Assistance Act and this included an assessment of housing equity where the applicant was an owner-occupier (see Mackintosh et al, 1990, ch 5). Chapters Four and Six tracked the complex history of charging for domiciliary services but with a clear overall theme that charging for such services was seen as the norm for most clients.

This does raise the issue of why charging and means testing have proved to be such controversial issues in recent years (Chetwynd et al, 1996; Baldwin and Lunt, 1996). With regard to domiciliary services, it seems likely that many local authorities stopped charging for most services because the income generated from low income clients did not justify the costs of fee collection. By the early 1990s many local authorities, and most organisations of service users and disabled people, saw free services as a principle to be protected.

The big issue in charging for residential care is home equity. It has emerged in recent years as a contentious topic for two main reasons. First, the number of elderly owner-occupiers seeking local authority residential care prior to the 1980s would have been minuscule. However, by the late 1990s, owner-occupation had become the dominant tenure of later life (Means, 1997), and the inheritance of home equity had become a major source of wealth for the next generation (Hamnett, 1995). Second, continuing care has shifted from being a free service provided by the NHS to a service provided by the independent sector for a fee and public subsidy is provided following a means tested assessment by local authorities.

Absent voices and new discourses

This chapter has stressed the enormous insights to be gained about community care policy and practice in the late 1990s from a detailed consideration of earlier developments and debates. However, in doing this, it is crucial to be sensitive to what voices are absent from these earlier debates and when new discourses emerge. This is a slightly more complex task than might at first appear. The fact that an issue has not been addressed in Chapters Two to Seven may indicate that it was absent from policy and practice discussions, or that the researchers failed to highlight their existence because such debates were seen as marginal to their main concerns. As explained in Chapter One, the fieldwork for the book was carried out in the early 1980s and so the material collected was shaped by the concerns of over 15 years ago. The absent voices which most strike us as we re-read our original work are as follows:

- ***Empowerment*** – if empowerment is what Clarke and Stewart (1992) have called a theme for the 1990s, it was certainly not a theme for the 1940s, 1950s and 1960s. Not only does the word not appear but there is little if any reference to involving older people in service planning or in shaping the services they are to receive. Older people are conceptualised in nearly all policy documents as passive and dependent.

- ***Black and minority ethnic elders*** – not only did the research fail to uncover any reference to the community care needs of black and minority ethnic elders but we failed to comment upon this at all in the 1985 edition. Indeed, it was not really until the mid-1980s that a race and community care literature began to emerge in the UK (see, for example, Barker, 1984). Although this is now extensive (Ahmad and Atkin, 1996; Blakemore and Boneham, 1994, chs 7 and 8), it has not necessarily meant that black and minority ethnic elders now receive a more appropriate response from social services (Askham et al, 1995). Although this 'absence' may be partially explained by the very low numbers of such elderly people in the 25 years after the Second World War, it still does not explain why so little thought was being given to future trends.

- ***Dementia*** – earlier chapters have made frequent reference to categorisations of older people which use terms such as 'senile confused', 'senile infirmity' and , elderly mentally infirm' as groups needing accommodation in either residential or nursing care. The Aid for the Elderly in Government Institutions (AEGIS) campaign of the late 1960s was driven by the mistreatment of elderly people in long stay psychiatric hospitals, while *Taken for a ride* by Michael Meacher (1972) was an attack upon the growth of specialist homes for the 'confused elderly'. Therefore, at one level it could be argued that the care of older people with dementia is not an absent discourse in this book. However, not only has terminology undergone striking change, but there is also the complete failure of the 1985 book to get to grips with dementia as a major challenge facing the future provision of health and welfare services for older people. Indeed, there remains a lack of detailed thinking about older people with dementia in much of the present day general literature on community care.

- ***Elder abuse*** – in a similar vein, the 1985 book chronicled the repeated abuse of older people in both residential care and hospital care. Such violence was understood in terms of the overall political economy perspective of the book. However, in the mid-1980s elder abuse had not emerged as a policy and practice issue in its own right (Bennett et al, 1997), and so some of the true significance of this long history of abuse was not appreciated. Certainly, in modern writings on elder abuse the emphasis is as much on the abusive behaviour of family members as on that by professionals (Kingston and Penhale, 1995). There is also a tendency (including in some of our work) to see abuse by paid staff as likely to increase within a mixed economy, where it is very hard to regulate and supervise the quality of care provided by small voluntary and private sector agencies (Means and Langan, 1996). Chapters Two to Six illustrate how local authority residential homes and NHS hospitals have often been the site of violence towards older people. Abuse is not restricted to the independent sector.

- ***Housing*** – earlier chapters have briefly considered sheltered housing in the traditional way that assumes that housing and older people issues are synonymous with sheltered housing. Yet the first page of Chapter Six presents the classic quotation from Townsend (1963, p 38) in terms of the strong attachment of many older people to their terraced houses despite their often poor physical condition and lack of basic amenities. However, the housing and community care implications of this were not pursued in the policy debates of the period and not drawn out by us in the 1985 book. Ironically, one of us became the co-author just five years later of a report called *Housing: The essential element in community care* (Harrison and Means, 1990) which looked at the potential community care contribution of home improvement agencies which advise elderly and disabled people on how they might improve and/or adapt their property. However, even today, there is not a complete acceptance that the availability of affordable accessible housing in good condition is crucial to the achievement of community care objectives for older people (Means and Smith, 1998, ch 7; Watson, 1997).

- ***The 1970s and 1980s*** – the timeframe of the detailed fieldwork for this study ended on 1 April 1971. The whole period from the establishment of social services departments through to the implementation of the main elements of the 1990 Act reforms in April 1993 is, therefore, not covered in either the 1985 or this edition of the book. So many of the myths perpetuated about community care prior to the 1990 changes draw upon assumptions about what did or did not happen in the period 1971-93. We are therefore delighted to be presently engaged in a research project funded by the ESRC (Grant Reference Number R 000 23 1648) which is examining this period in terms of how four contrasting local authorities (Devon, Hammersmith and Fulham, Oxfordshire and Stockport) were or were not developing community care services for older people.

Future prospects

Perhaps the most important message of this book is the ageism which has been so embedded in the history of welfare services for elderly people. They have been a low priority for resources, the services offered have often been of a low standard, they have been patronised by policy makers and sometimes abused by practitioners.

What are the prospects of this changing? It is possible to argue that future cohorts of older people will be far more assertive about their rights and far more demanding of policy makers and practitioners. As Evandrou has said of the soon to retire 'baby boom' generation:

> **The baby boomers are better educated than previous generations and have become sophisticated consumers. The notion of retirement is taken for granted and there are clear expectations associated with it. Most see it as a period of leisure in return for a lifetime of work and expect to have a period of active and relatively healthy old age.... The new millennium elders who were nurtured on megabytes, microfibre and media imaging are likely to be more discerning consumers both of leisure activities and of health and welfare services. (Evandrou, 1997, p 174)**

But Evandrou also acknowledges that differences among these future cohorts of older people will be enormous with the poorest in real danger of being residualised and excluded.

This could mean that the better-off will finally escape dependence upon 'Cinderella' health and welfare services even if they have to make a much larger personal contribution to access these services than ever envisaged by Beveridge. But this could still mean 'poorer' older people remaining dependent not only upon second-class 'free' services but services which risk imposing a 21st century equivalent to the stigma of pauperism.

The 1997 Labour government is, in 1998, reviewing both the funding of continuing care and the role of social services as the lead agency in community care. We believe that these reviews need to answer the following questions:

- To what extent should community care services be funded through public expenditure?

- Who should be the lead agency in the strategic planning of community care services?
- What balance of mechanisms should be used to deliver services?
- To what extent should the "better off" be expected to pay for social care?
- How can the chosen system be made to be 'user'-driven and non-stigmatising for all older people and not just for the more wealthy?

We also believe that answers to these questions require a detailed consideration of the past history of health and welfare provision for older people.

Bibliography

Abel-Smith, B. (1964) *The hospitals, 1800-1948*, London: Heinemann.

Abel-Smith, B. and Townsend, P. (1965) *The poor and the poorest,* London: Bell.

Addison, P. (1975) *The road to 1945: British politics and the Second World War,* London: Jonathan Cape.

Agate, J. (1970) 'The old: hospital and community care', in P. Townsend et al (eds) *Social services: A critical analysis of the Seebohm proposals*, London: Fabian Society, p 116.

Ahmad, W. and Atkin, K. (eds) (1996) *'Race' and community care,* Buckingham: Open University Press.

Amulree, Lord (1951a) *Adding life to years,* London: NCSS.

Amulree, Lord (1951b) 'Half-way houses', *Social Service Quarterly*, vol 25, no 1, p 8.

Amulree, Lord (1953) 'Modern hospital treatment and the pensioner', *The Lancet*, 17 September, p 574.

Amulree, Lord and Sturdee, E. (1946) 'Care of the chronic sick and the aged', *British Medical Journal,* 20 April, p 617.

Amulree, Lord, Arnold, P. and Polak, A. (1952) 'Length of stay in hospital of the aged sick', *The Lancet,* 26 July, p 191.

Anderson Report (1947) *The care and treatment of the elderly and infirm,* London: BMA.

Andrews, C. and Wilson, T. (1953) 'Organisation of a geriatric service in a rural area', *The Lancet*, 18 April, pp 785-9.

Askham, J., Henshaw, L. and Tarpey, M. (1995) *Social and health services for elderly people from black and minority ethnic communities,* London: HMSO.

Assistance Board (1946) *Report of the Assistance Board for the year ended 31st December 1945*, Cmd 6883, London: HMSO.

Aves, G. (1964) 'The relationship between homes and other forms of care', in K. Slack (ed) *Some aspects of residential care of the elderly*, London: NCSS, p 12.

Aves Report (1969) *The voluntary worker in the social services,* London: Allen and Unwin.

Baldwin, S. and Lunt, N. (1996) *Charging ahead: The development of local authority charging policies for community care*, Bristol: The Policy Press.

Baran, S. (1965) 'A friendly chat is not enough', *New Society,* 25 February, pp 17-18.

Barclay Report (1982) *Social workers: Their role and tasks,* London: Bedford Square Press.

Barclay Report (1996) *Meeting the costs of continuing care: Report and recommendations*, York: Joseph Rowntree Foundation.

Barker, J. (1984) *Black and Asian older people in Britain*, Mitcham: Age Concern Research Unit.

Barton, R. (1959) *Institutional neurosis,* London: John Wright and Sons.

Beauman, K. (1977) *Green sleeves: The story of WVS/WRVS,* London: Seeley and Co.

Beglin, M. (1965) 'Residential accommodation', in J. Farndale (ed) *Trends in social welfare,* Oxford: Pergamon.

Bennett, G., Kingston, P. and Penhale, B. (1997) *Dimensions of elder abuse: Perspectives for practitioners*, Basingstoke: Macmillan.

Beveridge Report (1942a) *Social insurance and allied services*, Cmd 6404, London: HMSO.

Beveridge Report (1942b) *Social insurance and allied services: Memoranda from organisations,* Cmd 6405, London: HMSO.

Beveridge, W. (1948) *Voluntary action,* London: Allen and Unwin.

Beveridge, W. and Wells, A. (eds) (1949) 'Women's Voluntary Services', in *The evidence for voluntary action,* London: Allen and Unwin.

Biestek, F. (1961) *The casework relationship,* London: Allen and Unwin.

Black, J. et al (1983) *Social work in context: A comparative study of three social services teams,* London and New York: Tavistock.

Blakemore, K. and Boneham, M. (1994) *Age, race and ethnicity: A comparative approach*, Buckingham: Open University Press, chs 7 and 8.

Bligh, E. (1951) 'Welfare of the aged', *Journal of the Royal Sanitary Institute*, vol LXX1, no 1, p 46.

BMA (British Medical Association) (1948) *The right patient in the right bed*, First Supplement to the Report of the Committee on the Care and Treatment of the Elderly and Infirm.

Board of Trade (1940) *Statistical abstract for the United Kingdom for each of the fifteen years 1924 to 1939*, Cmd 6232, London: HMSO.

Bond, M. (1982) *Women's work in a woman's world*, Working Paper No 25, Bristol: SAUS, University of Bristol.

Bosanquet, N. (1978) *A future for old age*, London: Temple Smith/New Society.

Boucher, C. (1958) 'The aged and infirm', *The Journal of the Institute of Home Help Organisers*, vol 7, December, p 8.

Boucher Report (1957) *Survey of services available to the chronic sick and elderly 1954-55*, Reports on Public Health and Medical Subjects No 98, London: HMSO.

Bransby, E. and Osborne, B. (1953) 'A social and food survey of the elderly living alone or as married couples', *British Journal of Nutrition*, vol 7, p 164.

BRCS (British Red Cross Society, (1946) *Report of the British Red Cross Society for the year 1945*.

BRCS (1947) *Report of the British Red Cross Society for the year 1946*.

BRCS (1948) *Report of the British Red Cross Society for the year 1947*.

BRCS (1955) *Report of the British Red Cross Society for the year ended 1955*.

BRCS (1962) *Report of the British Red Cross Society for the year ended 1962*.

Brewer, C. and Lait, J. (1980) *Can social work survive?*, London: Temple Smith.

Brittain, V. (1953) *Lady into woman*, London: Andrew Dakers.

Brockington, R. (1963) 'A community health authority', *Hospital and Social Service Journal*, 20 September, pp 1145-6.

Brooke, E. (1950) 'The aged in hospital and at home: the need for cooperation between the authorities concerned', in *Welfare Problems of Old People*, Fifth National Conference of NOPWC, London: NCSS.

Brown, M. (1965) 'A welfare service not a welfare department', *Social Services Quarterly*, vol 37, no 3, p 92.

Brown, M. (1972) 'The development of local authority welfare services from 1948-1965 under Part III of the National Assistance Act, 1948', PhD thesis, University of Manchester.

Brown, R. (1979) *Reorganising the National Health Service*, Oxford: Blackwell.

Bruce, M. (1961) *The coming of the welfare state*, London: Batsford.

Burr, N. (1949) *The home help service*, London: Henry Morris.

Butler, A., Oldham, C. and Wright, R. (1979) *Sheltered housing for the elderly: A critical review*, Department of Social Policy and Administration Research Monograph, University of Leeds.

Butrym, Z. (1963) 'Introduction to a discussion on casework with geriatric patients', *The Almoner*, vol 15, no 11, pp 325-32.

Calder, A. and Sheridan, D. (1984) (eds) *Speak for yourself: A mass-observation anthology, 1937-49*, London: Jonathan Cape.

Campbell, J. and Oliver, M. (1996) *Disability politics: Understanding our past, changing our future*, London: Routledge.

Cambray, P. and Briggs, G. (1949) *British Red Cross and St John: The official record of the humanitarian services of the war organisation of the British Red Cross Society and Order of St John of Jerusalem*, BRCS.

Central Health Services Council (1961) *Report of the Central Health Services Council for the year ended December 31st 1960*, London: HMSO.

Chalke, H. and Benjamin, B. (1953) 'The aged in their own homes', *The Lancet*, 21 March, p 589.

Challis, D. and Davies, B. (1980) 'A new approach to community care for the elderly', *British Journal of Social Work*, vol 10, no 1, pp 1-18.

Chancellor of the Exchequer et al (1996) *A new partnership in old age*, Cm 3563, London: HMSO.

Chetwynd, M., Ritchie, L., Reith, L. and Howard, M. (1996) *The cost of care: The impact of charging policy on the lives of disabled people*, Bristol: The Policy Press.

Christie, K. (1964) 'Welfare authorities and the aged', *The British Hospital and Social Service Journal*, 14 February, p 213.

Clarke, J. (1948 edn) 'The Assistance Board', in W. Robson (ed) *Social security*, London: Allen and Unwin.

Clarke, M. and Stewart, J. (1992) 'Empowerment: a theme for the 1990s', *Local Government Studies*, vol 18, no 2, pp 18-26.

City of Birmingham (1940) *Public Assistance Committee: Handbook and diary*, Birmingham: City of Birmingham.

Cohen, S. (1973) *Folk devils and moral panics: The creation of mods and rockers*, St Albans: Paladin.

Cooper, J. (1983) *The creation of the British personal social services 1962-74*, London: Heinemann.

Cosin, L. (1947) 'Organising a geriatric department', *British Medical Journal*, 27 December, p 1046.

Council for Training in Social Work (1965) *Second Report 1965: Social work training – numbers, standards and social needs*, London: CTSW.

Council for Training in Social Work (1967) *Human growth and behaviour as a subject of study for social workers*, CTSW Discussion Paper No 2.

Cranston, M. (1976) 'Human rights: Real and supposed', in N. Timms and D. Watson *Talking about welfare*, London: Routledge, pp 133-44.

Crowther, M. (1981) *The workhouse system 1834-1929*, London: Batsford.

Curtis Report (1946) *Report of the Care of Children Committee*, Cmd 6422, London: HMSO.

Davies, B. (1968) *Social needs and resources in local services*, London: Michael Joseph.

Davies, B., Barton, A., McMillan, I. and Williamson, V. (1971) *Variations in services for the aged*, Occasional Paper in Social Administration, No 40, London: Bell.

Davies, M. (1979) 'Swapping the old around', *Community Care*, 18 October, p 16-17.

Deacon, A. (1981) 'Thank you, God, for the means-test man', *New Society*, 25 June, pp 519-20.

Dearlove, J. (1973) *The politics of policy in local government*, London: Cambridge University Press.

DHSS (Department of Health and Social Security) (1969a) *Annual report of the DHSS for the year 1968*, Cmnd 4100, London: HMSO.

DHSS (1969b) *Circular 10/69*, 'Local authority health and welfare services: programme of capital projects', 25 June.

DHSS (1969c) *Circular 19/69*, 'Census of residential accommodation', 12 December.

DHSS (1971a) *Circular 53/71*, 'Help in the home: Section 13 of the Health Services and Public Health Act', 28 October.

DHSS (1971b) *Annual Report 1970*, Cmnd 4714, London: HMSO.

DHSS (1972) *Annual Report 1971*, Cmnd 5019, London: HMSO.

DHSS (1975) *The census of residential accommodation 1970: 1 – Residential accommodation for the elderly and for the younger physically handicapped*, London: HMSO.

DHSS (1976) *Priorities for health and personal social services in England*, London: HMSO.

DHSS (Department of Health and Social Security) (1978a) *A happier old age: A discussion document on elderly people in our society*, London: HMSO.

DHSS (1978b) *Social service teams: The practitioner's view*, London: HMSO.

DHSS (1981) *Growing older*, Cmnd 8173, London: HMSO.

DHSS (1983) *Elderly people in the community: Their service needs*, London: HMSO.

DHSS (1989) *Caring for people: Community care in the next decade and beyond*, Cm 849, London: HMSO.

DHSS (1995) *NHS responsibilities for meeting continuous health care needs*, London: DoH.

Digby, A. (1978) *Pauper palaces*, London: Routledge and Kegan Paul.

Digby, A. (1989) *British welfare policy: Workhouse to workforce*, London: Faber and Faber.

Dinsdale, P. (1998) 'Pilot lights new way forward', *Guardian Society*, 4 February, p 7.

DoH (Department of Health) (1989) *Caring for people: Community care in the next decade and beyond*, Cm 849, London: HMSO.

DoH (1995) *NHS responsibilities for meeting continuous health care needs*, London: DoH.

DoH (1997) *The new NHS – Modern, dependable*, Cm 3807, London: The Stationery Office.

Dominelli, L. and Hoogvelt, A. (1996) 'Globalisation and the technocratisation of social work', *Critical Social Policy*, vol 16, no 2, pp 45-62.

Donnison, D., Jay, P. and Stewart, M. (1962) *The Ingleby Report: Three critical essays*, Fabian Research Series No 231.

Donnison, D. (1968) 'Seehohm: The Report and its implications', *Social Work (UK)*, vol 25, no 4, p 3.

Douglas, W. (1950) 'Plans and achievements since the passing of the National Assistance Act by local authorities and voluntary organisations', *The interests of the aged*, Fourth National Conference of the NOPWC, London: NCSS.

Doyal, L. with Pennell, I. (1979) *The political economy of health*, London: Pluto Press.

Dunn, G. (no date) *The story of the National Federation*, Blackburn: NFOAPA.

Easton, H., Clark, R. and Harper, W. (1945) *The hospital services of the Yorkshire area*, London: HMSO.

Eckstein, H. (1959) *The English health service*, London: Oxford University Press.

Engels, F. (1969 edn) *The condition of the working class in England*, London: Panther.

Euson, H., Clark, R. and Harper, W. (1945) *The hospital services of the Yorkshire area*, London: HMSO.

Evandrou, M. (ed) (1997) *Baby boomers: Ageing in the 21st century*, London: Age Concern (England).

Exley, C. (ed) (1932) *The guide to poor relief*, Liverpool: Meek, Thomas & Co.

Exton-Smith, A. (1952) 'Investigation of the aged sick in their homes', *British Medical Journal*, 26 July, pp 182-6.

Farrer-Brown, L. (1980 edn) 'Foreword', in B.S. Rowntree, *Old people: Report of a survey committee on the problems of ageing and the care of old people*, New York: Arnos Press.

Farrer-Brown, L. and Seebohon, F. (1969) 'Foreword' in Aves Report, *The voluntary worker in the social services*, London: Allen and Unwin.

Finer, S. (1955) 'Voluntary social services in the changing welfare state', *Social Service Quarterly*, June/August, p 8.

Ford, P. (1939) *Incomes, means tests and personal responsibility*, London: King and Son.

Fraser, D. (1973) *The evolution of the British welfare state*, London: Macmillan.

FRS (Friends Relief Service) (1945) *Hostels for old people*, Friends Book Centre.

Fry, J. (1957) 'Care of the elderly in general practice: A socio-medical reassessment', *British Medical Journal*, 21 September, pp 666-70.

Garland, R. (1948) 'End of the Poor Laws - and a new era dawns in British social welfare', *Social Welfare*, vol 11, no 2, p 36.

Geffen, D. and Warren, M. (1954) 'The care of the aged', *The Medical Officer*, 18 June, p 289.

George, V. (1973) *Social security and society*, London: Routledge and Kegan Paul.

Gibbs, G. (1961) 'Foreward', in A. Harris, *Meals on wheels for old people*, NCCOP.

Gilbert, B. (1970) *British social policy 1919-39*, London: Batsford.

Gillie Report (1963) *The field of work of the family doctor*, Report of the Sub-Committee of the Standing Medical Advisory Committee of the Central Health Services Council, London: HMSO.

Gilmour, R. (ed) (1951) *British Red Cross Society: Welfare services manual*, No 12, London: Cassell and Company.

GLC (Greater London Council) Records Office (1940) *London County Council Civil Defence and General Purposes Committee Papers,* No 11, December, Report by Chief Officer, Rest Home Services, 26 November.

Godlove, C. and Mann, A. (1980) 'Thirty years of the welfare state: current issues in British social policy for the aged', *Aged Care and Services Review*, vol 2, no 1, p 3.

Goffman, E. (1968 edn) *Asylums: Essays on the social situation of mental patients and other inmates*, Harmondsworth: Penguin.

Goldberg, E. (1966) *Welfare in the community: Talks on social work to welfare officers*, London: NCSS.

Goldberg, E. (1970) *Helping the aged: A field experiment in social work*, London: Allen and Unwin.

Goldberg, E. and Connelly, N. (1982) *The effectiveness of social care for elderly people*, London: Heinemann, pp 92-5.

Goodin, R. and Gibson, D. (1997) 'Rights, young and old', *Oxford Journal of Legal Studies*, vol 17, no 2, pp 190-203.

Gordon, I. (1969) 'Seebohm sophistry and Green-Paper gallimaufry', *The Lancet,* 8 February, pp 299-300.

Gough, I. (1979) *The political economy of the welfare state*, London: Macmillan.

Graham, W. (1954) 'The aged sick: admission to hospital or care at home?', *The Lancet*, 6 February, p 304.

Graves, C. (1948) *Women in green: The story of the WVS in wartime*, London: Heinemann.

Gray, A. and Topping, A. (1945) *The hospital services of London and the surrounding area*, London: HMSO.

Gray, J. M. (1977) 'Why wardens should come out of the shelter', *Community Care*, 23 March, pp 20-1.

Griffith, J. (1966) *Central departments and local authorities*, London: Allen and Unwin.

Guillebaud Report (1956) *Report of the Committee of Enquiry into the cost of the National Health Service*, Cmd 9663, London: HMSO.

Gyford, J. and James, M. (1982) 'The development of party politics in the local authority associations', *Local Government Studies*, vol 8, no 2, p 23.

Haber, C. (1983) *Beyond sixty-five: The dilemma of old age in America's past*, Cambridge: Cambridge University Press.

Hadley, R. and Clough, R. (1996) *Care in chaos: Frustration and challenge in community care*, London: Cassell.

Hall, P., Land, H., Parker, R. and Webb, A. (1975) *Change, choice and conflict in social policy*, London: Heinemann.

Hall, P. (1976) *Reforming the welfare: The politics of change in the personal social services*, London: Heinemann.

Hallett, C. (1991) 'The Children Act 1989 and community care: comparisons and contrasts', *Policy and Politics*, vol 19, no 4, pp 283-92.

Ham, C. and Smith, R. (eds) (1978) *Policies for the elderly*, Working Paper No 4, Bristol: SAUS, University of Bristol.

Ham, C. (1981) *Policymaking in the National Health Service*, London: Macmillan.

Hamnett, C. (1995) 'Housing, equity release and inheritance', in I. Allen and E. Perkins (eds) *The future of family care for older people*, London: HMSO, pp 163-80.

Hamson, J. (1965) 'Casework for the aged' *Hospital and Social Service Journal*, 23 April, p 751.

Hansen, J. (1959) 'Administrative principles and the Younghusband Report', *Hospital and Social Service Journal*, 9 October, pp 1042 and 1050.

Hansen, J. (1962) 'Challenge in the welfare services', *Municipal Review*, November, p 666.

Hansen, J. (1963) 'Welfare services for the old and handicapped in a new society', *Hospital and Social Service Journal*, 28 June, p 758.

Harding, T. (1997) *A life worth living: The independence and inclusion of older people*, London: Help the Aged.

Harris, A. (1961) *Meals on wheels for old people*, NCCOP.

Harris, A. (1968) *Social welfare for the elderly: vol 1, Comparison of areas and summary*, Government Social Survey, London: HMSO.

Harris, J. (1977) *William Beveridge: A biography*, Oxford: Clarendon Press.

Harris, J. (1981) 'Some aspects of social policy in Britain during the Second World War', in W. Mommsen (ed) *The emergence of the welfare state in Britain and Germany*, London: Croom Helm, pp 247-62.

Harrison, L. and Means, R. (1990) *Housing: The essential element in community care*, Oxford: SHAC, London and Anchor Housing Trust.

Harrison, T. (1976) *Living through the Blitz*, London: Collins.

Heb, J. (1981) 'The social policy of the Attlee Government', in W. Mommsen (ed) *The emergence of the welfare state in Britain and Germany*, London: Croom Helm, pp 296-314.

Heclo, H. (1974) *Modern social politics in Britain and Sweden: From relief to income maintenance*, New Haven and London: Yale University Press.

Henwood, M. (1992) 'Twilight Zone', *Health Service Journal*, 5 November, p 28.

Hepworth, N. (1976 edn) *The finance of local government*, London: Allen and Unwin.

Herbert Report (1960) *Royal Commission on local government in greater London 1957-60,* Cmnd 1164, London: HMSO.

Heywood, J. (1959) *Children in care: The development of the service for the deprived child*, London: Routledge and Kegan Paul.

Higham, T. (1953) 'Health and welfare organisation: The results of a national survey', *Hospital and Social Service Journal*, 20 February, pp 201-3.

Hill, M. (1961) *An approach to old age and its problems*, Edinburgh and London: Oliver and Boyd.

Home Office (1943) *Civil Defence Circular 87/1943*, 'Future of the Women's Voluntary Service', London: HMSO.

Home Office (1947) *Civil Defence Circular 8/1947*, 'Future of the Women's Voluntary Service', London: HMSO.

Home Office (1963) *The child, the family and the young offender*, Cmnd 2742, London: HMSO.

Honigsbaum, F. (1979) *The division in British medicine: A history of the separation of general practice from hospital care, 1911-68*, London: Kegan Paul.

Hope Murray, E. (1977) 'Development of services for the elderly provided by social services departments in England in 1972', *Social Work Service*, December, p 15.

Horder, Lord (1941) 'The modern troglodyte', *The Lancet*, 19 April, pp 499-502.

Howell, T. (1946) 'Social medicine in old age', *British Medical Journal*, 16 March, p 399.

Howell, T. (1948) 'Care of the aged sick', *Problems and progress in old people's welfare*, Third National Conference of NOPWC, London: NCSS.

Hubback, E. (1947) *The population of Britain*, West Drayton: Penguin.

Hughes, H. (1951) 'The care of the aged who are chronically sick', *Journal of the Royal Sanitary Institute*, vol LXX1, no 1, p 38.

Hunt, A. (1970) *The home help service in England and Wales*, Government Social Survey, London: HMSO.

Huws Jones, R. (1952) 'Old people's welfare - successes and failures', *Social Service Quarterly*, vol 26, no 1, pp 19-22.

Huws Jones, R. (1963) *Discussion of the need for more adequate teaching of gerontology in the training of social workers*, International Society of Gerontology Conference, Copenhagen, mimeo.

Irvine, E. (1950) 'The place of the health department in the care of the aged', *The Medical Officer*, 12 August, p 74.

Isaacs, B. and Thompson, J. (1960) 'Holiday admissions to a geriatric unit', *The Lancet*, 30 April, pp 969-71.

Isaacs, S., Brown, C. and Thorless, J. (1941) *The Cambridge evacuation study*, London: Methuen.

Jameson Report (1956) *An inquiry into health visiting*, London: HMSO.

Jarvis, E. (1950) 'Some thoughts on the work of a geriatric almoner', *The Almoner*, vol 3, no 9, p 324.

Jefferys, M. (1960) 'Some aspects of social work in local authority health and welfare departments', *Case Conference*, vol 7, no 1, pp 2-9.

Jefferys, M. (1965) *An anatomy of welfare*, London: Michael Joseph.

Jones, K. (1972) *A history of the mental health services*, London: Routledge and Kegan Paul.

Jordan, F. (1967) 'Welfare services statistics 1965-66', *County Councils Gazette*, July, p 179.

Judge, K. and Matthews, J. (1980) *Charging for social care*, London: Allen and Unwin.

Kay, D., Beamish, P. and Roth, M. (1962) 'Some medical and social characteristics of elderly people under state care', in P. Halmos (ed) *Sociology and medicine: Studies within the framework of the British health service*, Sociological Review Monograph No 5, University of Keele, pp 173-93.

Kay, D., Roth, M. and Hall, M. (1966) 'Special provision problems of the aged and the organisation of hospital services', *British Medical Journal*, 22 October, p 968.

Keeling, D. (1961) *The crowded stairs*, London: NCSS.

Kelsall, R. (1967) *Population*, London: Longman.

Kemp, M. (1973) 'An update on the workhouse', *Built Environment*, vol 2, no 9, p 496.

Kilbrandon Report (1964) *Children and young persons in Scotland*, Cmnd 2306, Edinburgh: HMSO.

Kingston, P. and Penhale, B. (1995) *Family violence and the caring professions*, Basingstoke: Macmillan.

Lapping, A. (1966) 'Too grand a council', *New Society*, 17 November, p 760.

Le Grand, J. and Bartlett, W. (eds) (1993) *Quasi-markets and social policy*, Basingstoke: Macmillan.

Levitt, R. and Wall, A. (1985) *The reorganised National Health Service*, 3rd edn, London: Croom Helm.

Lindsay, A. (1962) *Socialised medicine in England and Wales: The National Health Service 1948-61*, Chapel Hill: University of North Carolina Press.

Longford Report (1964) *Crime: A challenge to us all*, Labour Party Standing Group.

Lord Mayor's National Air Raid Distress Fund (1954) *The final survey of the work of the Fund to 13 January 1954.*

Lowther, C. and Williamson, J. (1966) 'Old people and their relatives', *The Lancet,* 31 December, p 1460.

Macdonald, D. (1950) 'Whither the geriatric almoner', *The Almoner,* vol 2, no 10, pp 227-9.

Macintyre, S. (1977) 'Old age as a social problem', in R. Dingwall et al (eds) *Health care and health knowledge,* London: Croom Helm.

Mackintosh, S., Means, R. and Leather, P. (1990) *Housing in later life,* Bristol: SAUS Publications.

Macnicol, J. (1981) *Social policy in Britain during and after the Second World War,* Paper given at the 5th Lelio Basso International Week of Studies, Turnin, December.

Maddison, A. (1954) 'Mental sickness provision', *Hospital and Social Service Journal,* 26 September, p 983.

Mallaby Report (1967) *Committee on the staffing of local government,* London: HMSO.

Markham/Hancock Report (1945) *Report on post-war organisation of private domestic employment,* Ministry of Labour and National Service, Cmd 6650, London: HMSO.

Marsh, D. (1965 edn) *The changing social structure of England and Wales, 1871-1961,* London: Routledge and Kegan Paul.

Marshall, H. (1948) 'Public assistance', in W. Robson (ed) *Social security,* London: Allen and Unwin, pp 38-60.

Matthews, O. (no date) *Housing the infirm* [self-published and originally distributed through WH Smith and Son].

McEwan, P. and Laverty, S. (1949) *The chronic sick and elderly in hospital,* Bradford (B) Hospital Management Committee.

McKeown, T. and Lowe, C. (1950) 'Care of the chronic sick', *British Medical Journal,* 11 February, p 323.

Meacher, M. (1970) 'The old: the future of community care', in P. Townsend et al (eds) *Social service: A critical analysis of the Seebohm proposals,* London: Fabian Society.

Meacher, M. (1972) *Taken for a ride*, London: Longman.

Means, R. (1995) 'Elderly people and the personal social services', in D. Gladstone (ed) *British Social Welfare*, London: UCL Press, pp 195-217.

Means, R. (1997) 'Time for partnership?: Reflections of a "jobbing" researcher', in R. Sykes (ed) *Putting older people in the picture?*, Oxford: Anchor Trust.

Means, R. (1997) 'Housing options in 2020: a suitable home for all?' in M. Evandrou (ed) *The baby boomers: Ageing in the 21st century*, London: Age Concern , pp 142-64.

Means, R. and Langan, J. (1996) 'Charging and quasi-markets in community care: implications for elderly people with dementia', *Social Policy and Administration*, vol 30, no 3, pp 244-62.

Means, R. and Smith, R. (1985) *The development of welfare services for elderly people,* London: Croom Helm.

Means, R. and Smith, R. (1998) *Community care: Policy and practice*, 2nd edn, Basingstoke: Macmillan.

Ministry of Health (1940a) *Circular 2061, Evacuation of civil population – special scheme* , 21 June.

Ministry of Health (1940b) *Circular 2000*, 'Public assistance', 19 April.

Ministry of Health (1940c) *Circular 2251*, 'Hostels' , 27 December.

Ministry of Health (1942a) *Summary report by the Ministry of Health for the period 1st April 1941 to 31st March 1942*, Cmd 6394, London: HMSO.

Ministry of Health (1942b) *Current trends of population in Great Britain*, Cmd 6358, London: HMSO.

Ministry of Health (1944) *Circular 179/44*,'Domestic help' , 14 December.

Ministry of Health (1946a) *Circular 195/46*, 'Government evacuation scheme and homeless service. Aged persons who are without suitable accommodation to which to return' , 28 October.

Ministry of Health (1946b) *Circular 110/46*, '"Home helps" and "domestic help"', 6 June.

Ministry of Health (1947a) *Circular 49/47*, 'The care of the aged in public assisitance homes and institutions', 6 June.

Ministry of Health (1947b) *Circular 118/47*, 'National Health Service Act: health services to be provided by local health authorities under Part III of the Act'.

Ministry of Health (1947c) *Report of the Ministry of Health for the year ended 31st March 1946 (including the Report of the Chief Medical Officer on the state of the public health for the year ended 31st December 1945)*, Cmd 7119, London: HMSO.

Ministry of Health (1947d) *Summary of the provisions of the National Assistance Bill*, Cmd 7348, London: HMSO.

Ministry of Health (1947e) *Circular 172/47*, 'National Assistance Bill – future of public assistance institutions', 11 December.

Ministry of Health (1948a) *Circular 85/48*, 'Closing-down of the government evacuation scheme'.

Ministry of Health (1948b) *Report of the Ministry of Health for the year ended 31st March 1947 (including the Report of the Chief Medical Officer on the state of the public health for the year ended 31st December 1946)*, Cmd 7441, London: HMSO.

Ministry of Health (1948c) *Circular 87/48*, 'National Assistance Act 1948'.

Ministry of Health (1949a) *Circular 50/49*, National Assistance Act 1948: Training of matrons and assistant matrons of old people's homes, 16 May.

Ministry of Health (1949b) *Circular 51/49*, 'Contributions to old people's welfare organisations', 20 May.

Ministry of Health (1950a) *Circular 11/50*, 'Welfare of old people', 23 January.

Ministry of Health (1950b) *Report of the Ministry of Health for the year ended 31st March 1949*, Cmd 7910, London: HMSO.

Ministry of Health (1950c) *Circular HMS 50/25*, 'Care of the aged mentally infirm cases'.

Ministry of Health (1950d) *Circular 25/50*, National Assistance Act 1948: Training course for workers and matrons of old people's homes, 3 March.

Ministry of Health (1952) *Report of the Ministry of Health covering the period 1st April 1950 to 31st December 1951*, Cmd 8655, London: HMSO.

Ministry of Health (1953) *Report of the Ministry of Health for the year ended 31st December 1952*, Cmd 8933, London: HMSO.

Ministry of Health (1954a) *Circular 26/54*, 1: National Health Service - Local health services; 2: National Assistance Act, 1948 - Part III: Local authority services, 18 November.

Ministry of Health (1954b) *Report of the Ministry of Health for the year ended 31st December 1953*, Cmnd 8329, London: HMSO.

Ministry of Health (1955a) *Report of the Ministry of Health for the year ended 31st December 1954*, Cmnd 9566, London: HMSO.

Ministry of Health (1955b) *Circular 3/55*, 'Residential accommodation for old people: homes for the more infirm', 25 February.

Ministry of Health (1956) *Circular 3/56*, 'Restriction of local government expenditure', 17 February.

Ministry of Health (1957a) *Circular 14/57*, 'Local authority services for the chronic sick and infirm', 7 October.

Ministry of Health (1957b) *HM(57)86*, 'Geriatric services and the care of the chronic sick', 7 October.

Ministry of Health (1958) *Report of the Ministry of Health for the year ended 31st December 1957*, Cmnd 495, London; HMSO.

Ministry of Health (1959a) *Circular 25/59*, National Health Service Act, 1946: National Assistance Act 1948 - Local health and welfare services: Building programmes for the financial years 1960/61 and 1961/62, 15 September.

Ministry of Health (1959b) *Report of the Ministry of Health for the year ended 31st December 1958*, Cmnd 806, London: HMSO.

Ministry of Health (1959c) *Circular 9/59*, 'Mental health service: residential accommodation for the mentally disordered', 4 May.

Ministry of Health (1959d) *Circular 11/59*, 'National Health Service Act 1946', Section 28, Chiropody Services, 21 April.

Ministry of Health (1960) *Report of the Ministry of Health for the year ended 31st December 1959*, Cmnd 1086, London: HMSO.

Ministry of Health (1961) *Report of the Ministry of Health for the year ended 31st December 1960*, Cmnd 1418, London; HMSO.

Ministry of Health (1962a) *Local authority building note no 2: Residential accommodation for elderly people.*

Ministry of Health (1962b) *Report of the Ministry of Health for the year ended 31st December 1961,* Cmnd 1754, London: HMSO.

Ministry of Health (1962c) *A hospital plan for England and Wales*, Cmnd 1604, London: HMSO.

Ministry of Health (1962d) *Circular 7/62*,'Development of local authority health and welfare services: cooperation with voluntary organisations', 12 April.

Ministry of Health (1962e) *Circular 12/62*,'National Assistance Act 1948 (Amendment) Act 1962', 3 July.

Ministry of Health (1962f) *Circular 18/62*, 'Development of health and welfare services: cooperation with voluntary organisations', August.

Ministry of Health (1963a) *Health and welfare:The development of community care,* Cmnd 1973, London; HMSO.

Ministry of Health (1963b) *Circular 91/63*, Development of local authority health and welfare services, 11 October.

Ministry of Health (1963c) *Circular 25/65*, 'The home help service', 10 December.

Ministry of Health (1964a) *Health and welfare:The development of community care – revision to 1973-74 of plans for the health and welfare services of the local authorities in England and Wales*, Cmnd 3022, London: HMSO.

Ministry of Health (1964b) *Circular 18/64*,'Voluntary effort in the health and welfare services', 20 November.

Ministry of Health (1965a) *Circular 18/65*, 'The care of the elderly in hospitals and residential homes', 20 September.

Ministry of Health (1965b) *Circular 14/65*, Development of local authority and welfare services, 30 July.

Ministry of Health (1965c) *Circular 25/65.*

Ministry of Health (1966) *Annual Report of the Ministry of Health for the year 1965,* Cmnd 3039, London: HMSO.

Ministry of Health (1967) *Circular 10/67*, 'Local authority health and welfare services: development plans and programme of capital projects', 22 May.

Ministry of Health (1968a) *Annual Report for the year 1967*, Cmnd 3702, London: HMSO.

Ministry of Health (1968b) *Circular 19/68*, 'Local authority health and welfare services: development plans and programme of capital projects, 13 May.

Ministry of Health and Ministry of Home Security (1940) *Recommendations of Lord Horder's Committee regarding the conditions in air-raid shelters with special reference to health; and a brief statement of action taken by the government thereon*, Cmd 6234, London: HMSO.

Ministry of Housing and Local Government (1958) *Flatlets for old people,* London: HMSO.

Ministry of Housing and Local Government (1962) *Some aspects of designing for old people*, London: HMSO.

Ministry of Housing and Local Government (1969) *Circular 82/69*, 'Housing standards and costs: accommodation specially designed for old people', 24 October.

Ministry of Local Government and Planning (1950) Housing Manual Sub-Committee of the Central Housing Advisory Committee, *Housing for special purposes: Supplement to the Housing Manual 1949*, London: HMSO.

Ministry of Reconstruction (1944) *Social insurance,* part one, Cmd 6550, London: HMSO.

Minns, R. (1980) *Bombers and mash: The Domestic Front, 1939-45*, London: Virago.

Morgan, W. (1944) *The future institutional service*, National Association of Administrators of Local Government Establishments.

Moroney, R. (1976) *The family and the state: Considerations for social policy*, London: Longman.

Morris, C. (1940) 'Public health during the first three months of war', *Social Work (London)*, January, pp 186-96.

Morris, J. et al (1966) *Our old people: Next steps in social policy*, reprinted from *Socialist Commentary*, January, p ix and xvii.

Morris, M. (1969) *Voluntary work in the welfare state,* London: Routledge and Kegan Paul.

Moseley, L. (1968) 'Variations in socio-medical services for the aged', *Social and Economic Administration*, vol 2, no 3, pp 169-83.

Moss, J. (1947) 'The year's development in work for old people', in *Working together for old people's welfare: Report of the Second National Conference on 'The care of old people'*, 14-15 November, NOPWC, mimeo.

Muir Gray, J. (1981) *Section 47, The compulsory removal of old people from their homes*, MD Thesis, University of Glasgow.

Myrdal, A. and Klein, V. (1956) *Women's two roles: Home and work,* London: Routledge and Kegan Paul.

National Institute of Social Work Training (1964) *Introduction to a social worker,* London: Allen and Unwin.

NISW (National Institute for Social Work) (1974) *An introductory account 1961-1974*, London: NISW.

National Labour Women's Advisory Committee (1964) *National survey into care of the elderly*, Interim Report, Labour Party.

National Labour Women's Advisory Committee (1965) *Labour Women's national survey into care of the elderly: Second interim and final report*, Labour Party.

NCCOP (National Corporation for the Care of Old People) (1948) *First Annual Report for the year ending 30 September 1948.*

NCCOP (1950) *Third Annual Report for the year ended 30th September 1950.*

NCCOP (1951) *Fourth Annual Report for the year ended 30th September 1951.*

NCCOP (1953) *Sixth Annual Report for the year ended 30th September 1953.*

NCCOP (1960) *Thirteenth Annual Report for the year ended 30th September 1960*, Appendix.

NCCOP (1962) *Fifteenth Annual Report for the year ended 30th September 1962.*

NCCOP (1969) *Twenty-second annual report for the year ended 30th September 1969.*

NCSS (National Council of Social Service) (1954) *Over seventy: Report of an investigation into the social and economic circumstances of one hundred people of over seventy years of age,* London: NCSS.

Nepean-Gubbins, L. (1958) 'The contribution of the home help organiser to the welfare of the aged', *Royal Society of Health Journal*, vol 78, no 6.

Nepean-Gubbins, L. (1972) 'The home help service: past, present and future', *Community Health*, vol 4, no 2, pp 77-82.

NISW (National Institute for Social Work) (1974) *An introductory account 1961-74*, London: NISW.

Nixon, B. (1980) *Raiders overhead*, London: Scolar/Gullivar.

NOPWC (National Old People's Welfare Committee) (1952) *Progress Report, October 1950- March 1952*, London: NCSS.

NOPWC (1950) *Annual Report for the year ending 31st March 1950.*

NOPWC (1950) *Third Annual Report for the year ended 30th September 1950.*

NOPWC (1951) *Fourth Annual Report for the year ended 30th September 1951.*

NOPWC (1952) *Progress report, October 1950-March 1952,* London: NCSS

NOPWC (1953) *Progress report for the year ending 31st March 1953.*

NOPWC (1954) *Progress report for the year ending 31st March 1954.*

NOPWC (1955) *Progress report for the year ending 31st March 1955.*

NOPWC (1957) *Progress report for the year ending 31st March 1957.*

NOPWC (1959) *Annual report for the year ending 31st March 1959.*

NOPWC (1960) *Annual Report for the year ending 31st March 1960.*

NOPWC (1961a edn) *Age is opportunity*, London: NCSS.

NOPWC (1961b) *Annual Report for the year ending 31st March 1961.*

NOPWC (1962) *OPWCs: Why they are needed; how they are started; what they do*, London: NCSS, March.

NOPWC (1962) *Fifteenth Annual Report for the year ended 30th September 1962.*

NOPWC (1963) *Annual Report for the year ending 31st March 1963.*

NOPWC (1964) *Annual Report for the year ending 31st March 1964.*

NOPWC (1965) *Annual Report for the year ending 31st March 1965.*

NOPWC (1970) *Annual Report 1969-70.*

Norman, A. (1980) *Rights and risk: A discussion document on civil liberty in old age*, London: NCCOP.

Norman, A. (1982) *Mental illness in old age: Meeting the challenge*, London: Centre for Policy on Ageing.

Nuffield Provincial Hospitals Trust (1946) *The hospital surveys: The Domesday Book of the hospital services*, Oxford: Oxford University Press.

Oliver, B. (1966) *The British Red Cross in action*, Basingstoke: Macmillan.

Oliver, M. (1990) *The politics of disablement*, London: Faber and Faber.

Packman, J. (1975) *The child's generation*, Oxford: Blackwell.

Parker, J. (1965) *Local health and welfare services*, London: Allen and Unwin.

Parker, J. (1968) 'The trained home help in the domiciliary services', *The Medical Officer*, 16 February, pp 85-7.

Parker, R. (1983) 'The gestation of reform: the Children Act 1948', in P. Bean and S. MacPherson (eds) *Approaches to welfare*, London: Routledge and Kegan Paul, pp 196-217.

Parker, R. (1988) 'An historical background', in L. Sinclair (ed) *Residential care: The research reviewed*, London: HMSO.

Pater, J. (1981) *The making of the National Health Service*, London: King Edward's Hospital Fund.

Phillips Report (1954) *Report of the Committee on the economic and financial problems of the provision for old age*, Cmd 9332, London: HMSO.

Phillipson, C. (1977) *The emergence of retirement*, Working Paper in Sociology, No 14, University of Durham.

Phillipson, C. (1982) *Capitalism and the construction of old age*, Basingstoke: Macmillan.

Rackstraw, M. (1944) 'An old people's hostel', originally published by *Social Work (London)*, January; reprinted by OPWC.

Reading, Lady (1948) 'Foreword', in C. Graves (1948) *Women in green: The story of the WVS in wartime*, London: Heinemann.

Reeve, R. (1953) 'Care of the elderly sick and infirm', *Hospital and Social Service Journal*, 29 May, p 394.

Richards, E., Wilsdon, T. and Lyons, S. (1996) *Paying for long-term care*, London: Institute for Public Policy Research.

Richey, M. (1951) *The home help service*, National Association of Home Help Organisers.

Riley, D. (1981) 'The free mothers: pronatalism and working women in industry at the end of the last war in Britain', *History Workshop Journal*, Spring, p 60.

Robb, B. (1967) *Sans everything: A case to answer*, London: Nelson.

Roberts, F. (1949) 'The cost of the National Health Service', *British Medical Journal*, 19 February, pp 293-7.

Roberts, N. (1970) *Our future selves*, London: Allen and Unwin.

Robson, W. (1948) 'Introduction: present principles', in W. Robson (ed) *Social security*, London: Allen and Unwin.

Rooff, M. (1957) *Voluntary societies and social policy*, London: Routledge and Kegan Paul.

Rowntree, B.S. (1980 edn) *Old people: Report of a survey committee on the problems of ageing and the care of old people*, New York: Arno Press (originally published in 1947 by Oxford University Press for the Nuffield Foundation).

Royal Commission on the Law relating to mental illness and mental deficiency (1957) Cmnd 169, London: HMSO.

Royal Commission on Population (1949) Cmd 7695, London: HMSO.

Ruck, S. (1960) 'A policy for old age', *Political Quarterly*, vol 31, no 2, pp 120-31.

Ruck, S. (1963) *London government and the welfare services*, London: Routledge and Kegan Paul.

Rudd, T. (1958) 'Basic problems in the social welfare of the elderly', *The Almoner*, vol 10, no 10, pp 348-9.

Rudd, T. (1962) 'The home care of old people', *The Medical Officer*, 29 June, p 395.

Russell-Smith, E. (1960) 'Residential care for the physically and mentally infirm', *Ageing: Its changes and its promise*, Tenth National Conference of NOPWC, London: NCSS.

Ryan, T. (1966) 'The workhouse legacy', *The Medical Officer*, 11 November, pp 270-1.

Sainsbury, S. (1964) 'Home services for the aged', *New Society*, 2 April, pp 11-12.

Samson, E. (1944) *Old age in the new world*, London: Pilot Press.

Sanderson, W. (1949) 'Employment for old people - its scope and possibilities', *The interests of the aged*, Fourth National Conference of the NOPWC, London: NCSS.

Scottish Education Department, Scottish Home and Health Department (1966) *Social work and the community*, Cmnd 3065, Edinburgh: HMSO.

Seebohm Report (1968) *Report of the Committee on local authority and allied personal social services*, Cmnd 3703, London: HMSO.

Seldon, A. (1981) *Churchill's Indian summer: The Conservative Government, 1951-55*, London: Hodder and Stoughton.

Shanas, E., Townsend, P., Wedderburn, D., Friis, H., Milhoj, P. and Stehouwer, J. (1968) *Old people in three industrial societies*, London: Routledge and Kegan Paul.

Sheldon, J. (1948) *The social medicine of old age*, London: Oxford University Press.

Sheldon, J. (1950) 'The role of the aged in modern society', *British Medical Journal*, 11 February, p 319.

Sheldon, J. (1955) 'The social philosophy of old age', in *Old Age in the Modern World*, Report of the Third Congress of the International Association of Gerontology, Edinburgh and London: Livingstone.

Sheldon, J. (1960) 'Problems of an ageing population', *British Medical Journal*, 23 April, p 1225.

Shenfield, B. (1957) *Social policies for old age: A review of social provision for old age in Great Britain*, London: Routledge and Kegan Paul.

Sheridan, A. (1955) 'A sense of responsibility', *The Almoner*, vol 7, no 11, p 413.

Sheridan, A. (1959) 'The need for diagnosis in the problem of old age', *Hospital and Social Service Journal*, 20 March, pp 289-90.

Simmons, E. and Van Emden, D. (1960) 'Casework and the older patient', *The Almoner*, vol 15, no 11, pp 325-32.

Sinfield, A. (1970) 'Which way for social work?', in P. Townsend et al (eds) *The fifth social service: Nine Fabian essays*, London: Fabian Society.

Sissons, M. and French, P. (eds)(1963) *Age of austerity, 1945-51*, London: Hodder and Stoughton.

Slack, K. (1960) *Councils, committees and concern for the old*, Occasional Paper on Social Administration, No 2, Welwyn: Codicote Press.

Slack, K. (1961) *Councils, committees and concern for the old*, Occasional Paper on Social Administration, No 2, Welwyn: Codicote Press.

Slack, K. (1970) *Old people and London government*, Occasional Paper on Social Administration, no 36, London: Bell.

Speed, M. (1967) 'The future development of welfare services for the aged', Report of a conference on 'Prospects for the Elderly', Devon County Council, mimeo.

Stacey, M. and Price, M. (1981) *Women, power and politics*, London: Tavistock.

Staley, A. (1948) *Hostels for old people: The contribution of the Quaker Relief Organisations, 1940-46*, Thesis submitted for Diploma in Social Studies, London University, mimeo.

Stevenson, O. (1973) *Claimant or client?*, London: Allen and Unwin.

Sub-Committee of the Geriatric Almoners' Group (1951) 'Medical social work for the aged in the United Kingdom', *The Almoner*, vol 4, no 6, pp 252-4.

Summer, G. and Smith, R. (1969) *Planning local authority services for the elderly*, London: Allen and Unwin.

Thistlethwaite, P. (ed) (1996) *Finding common cause*, London: Association of County Councils.

Thompson, A. (1949) 'Problems of ageing and chronic sickness (1)', *British Medical Journal,* 30 July, p 250.

Thomson, D. (1983) 'Workhouse to nursing home: residential care of elderly people in England since 1840', *Ageing and Society*, vol 3, part 2, pp 47-69.

Titmuss, R. (1955) 'Age and society: some fundamental assumptions', in *Old Age in the Modern World*, Report of the Third Congress of the International Association of Gerontology, Edinburgh and London: Livingstone.

Titmuss, R. (1961) *Essays on 'the welfare state'*, London: Unwin University Books.

Titmuss, R. (1963 edn) *Essays on 'the welfare state'*, London: Unwin University Books.

Titmuss, R. (1968) *Commitment to welfare*, London: Allen and Unwin.

Titmuss, R. (1976 edn) *Problems of social policy*, London: HMSO.

Townsend, P. (1962) *The last refuge,* London: Routledge and Kegan Paul.

Townsend, P. (1963 edn) *The family life of old people*, Harmondsworth: Pelican.

Townsend, P. (1964 edn) *The last refuge: A survey of residential institutions and homes for the aged in England and Wales*, London: Routledge and Kegan Paul.

Townsend, P. (1970) 'The objectives of the new local social service', in P. Townsend et al (eds) *The fifth social service*, London: Fabian Society.

Townsend, P. (1981) 'The structural dependency of the elderly: the creation of social policy in the twentieth century', *Ageing and Society*, vol 1, part 1, pp 5-28.

Townsend, P. and Wedderburn, D. (1965) *The aged in the welfare state,* London: Bell.

Tunstall, J. (1963) 'Selling services to old people', *New Society*, 8 July, pp 17-18.

Vaughan-Morgan, J., Maude, A. and Thompson, K. (1952) *The care of old people*, London: Conservative Political Centre.

Wade, B., Sawyer, L. and Bell, J. (1983) *Dependency with dignity: Different care provision for the elderly*, London: Bedford Square Press.

Walker, A. (1981) 'Towards a political economy of old age', *Ageing and Society*, vol 1, no 1, pp 73-94.

Walker, S. (1974) 'Meals-on-wheels', *Health and Social Service Journal*, 25 May.

Warren, M. (1946) 'Care of the chronic aged sick', *The Lancet*, 8 June, p 843.

Warren, M. (1951) 'The elderly in the community', *Social Service Quarterly*, vol 24, no 3, pp 102-6, 120.

Warren, M. and Cooper, J. (1966) 'Medical officer of health: the job, the man and the career', *The Medical Officer*, 15 July, pp 3-12.

Watson, L. (1997) *High hopes: Making housing and community care work*, York: Joseph Rowntree Foundation.

Wheeler, R. (1982) 'Staying put: a new development in policy?', *Ageing and Society*, vol 2, part 3, pp 299-330.

Wilkinson, S.F. (1947) 'The place of home helps in the National Health Service', pp 3-6 from proceedings of the 'Conference on Some Aspects of the Home Helps Scheme', Caxton Hall, London, 11-12 November 1947 [a copy of the proceedings can be found in WRVS Archives: *Miscellaneous Memoranda*].

Williams Report (1967) *Caring for people: Staffing residential homes,* London: Allen and Unwin.

Williamson, J. et al (1964) 'Old people at home', *The Lancet,* 23 May, p 1120.

Willinck, Sir H. (1961) 'Foreword', in M. Hill, *An approach to old age and its problems*, Edinburgh and London: Oliver and Boyd.

Wilson, E. (1980) *Only halfway to paradise: Women in postwar Britain 1945-68*, London: Tavistock.

Wilson, E. (1982) 'Women, the "community" and the "family"', in A. Walker (ed) *Community care: The family, the state and social policy*, Oxford: Blackwell.

Wistow, G. (1995) 'Aspirations and realities: community care at the crossroads', *Health and social care in the community*, vol 3, no 4, pp 227–40.

Wistow, G. (1996) 'The changing scene in Britain', in T. Harding, B. Meredith and G. Wistow (eds) *Options for long term care*, London: HMSO.

Wistow, G. and Lewis, H. (1996) *Preventive services for older people: Current approaches and future opportunities*, Oxford: Anchor Trust.

Women's Group on Public Welfare (1943) *Our towns: A close-up*, London: Oxford University Press.

Woodroffe, C. and Townsend, P. (1961) *Nursing homes in England and Wales: A study of public responsibility*, London: NCCOP.

Wright, C. and Roberts, L. (1958) 'The place of the home-help service in the care of the aged', *The Lancet*, 1 February, pp 235-6.

Wright, E. (1964) 'Helping the aged at home: a course for home helps', *The Medical Officer,* 3 January, pp 7-8.

WRVS (1978) *Stella Reading: Some recollections by her friends*, London: WRVS.

Younghusband Report (1959) *Report of the Working Party on social workers in the local authority health and welfare services,* London: HMSO.

Younghusband, E. (1978a) *Social work in Britain 1950-75: A follow-up study*, vol 2, London: Allen and Unwin

Younghusband, E. (1978b) *Social work in Britain: 1950-75*, vol 1, London: Allen and Unwin.

Appendix

List of those interviewed

Dame Geraldine Aves, OBE
Lord Amulree, KBE
Marjorie Burke, OBE
Elizabeth Carnegy-Arbuthnott, OBE
Sir Harold Fieldhouse, KBE
Jack Hanson, OBE
Kathleen Halpin, CBE
Elspeth Hope Murray, OBE
David Hobman, CBE
Robin Huw Jones, CBE
Hugh Mellor
Laura Nepean-Gubbins
Professor Roy Parker
John Peter, CB
Dorothea Ramsey
Dame Enid Russell-Smith
Mike Simpson, OBE
Alice Sheridan
Maurice Speed
Professor Peter Townsend
S.F. Wilkinson, CB

Correspondence was exchanged with

Kathleen Slack
William K. Sessions
Professor Roger Wilson

Index

A

B

C

D

M

N

O

S

T